"This book puts the weight of analytical frameworks and evidence behind the all too common tragedies of avoidable death, unnecessary illness, and health injustices that beset so many girls and women and also boys and men. It pushes the frontiers of our thinking about the barriers to justice and also provides compelling contemporary material which can—and should—be marshalled to support a right-to-health approach to gender and health."

Paul Hunt
UN Special Rapporteur on the Right to the Highest Attainable Standard of Health (2002–2008)

"This volume is a unique source of knowledge, inspiration and practical recommendations that go beyond the scope of many previous publications on gender and health. It brings together the evidence base, reflects on and synthesizes key messages, and crosses the needed extra mile to tie research to policy. An extraordinary mix of experiences and backgrounds have shaped it to be truly special. A must read for the many constituencies that are troubled by gender injustices and are seeking to reform the muted and often ill-conceived policy actions that attempt to deal with them."

Hoda Rashad
Research Professor and Director, Social Research Center, American University in Cairo

"One cannot act on the social determinants of health globally without considering the position of women. This book lays out most impressively how the structures of society impact on women's health. It brings together an impressive group of authors and presents the definitive view of gender inequity and what to do about it."

Michael Marmot
Chair, WHO Commission on Social Determinants of Health

Gender Equity in Health

Routledge Studies in Health and Social Welfare

Ipas Resource Center

Gender Equity in Health

The Shifting Frontiers of Evidence and Action

Edited by Gita Sen and Piroska Östlin

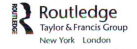

Routledge
Taylor & Francis Group
New York   London

First published 2010
by Routledge
270 Madison Ave, New York, NY 10016

Simultaneously published in the UK
by Routledge
2 Park Square, Milton Park, Abingdon, Oxon OX14 4RN

Routledge is an imprint of the Taylor & Francis Group, an informa business

Typeset in Sabon by IBT Global.
Printed and bound in the United States of America on acid-free paper by IBT Global.

Library of Congress Cataloging in Publication Data

Gender equity in health : the shifting frontiers of evidence and action / edited by Gita Sen and Piroska Östlin.
   p. ; cm. — (Routledge studies in health and social welfare ; 5)
Includes bibliographical references and index.
1. Social medicine. 2. Equality—Health aspects. 3. Sex discrimination.
4. Women—Medical care. I. Sen, Gita. II. Östlin, Piroska, 1958– III. Series:
Routledge studies in health and social welfare ; 5.
[DNLM: 1. Health Status Disparities. 2. Sex Factors. 3. Socioeconomic Factors. 4. Women's Health. WA 300.1 G325 2009]
   RA418.5.S63G46 2009
   362.1—dc22

ISBN10: 0-415-80190-7 (hbk)
ISBN10: 0-203-86690-8 (ebk)

ISBN13: 978-0-415-80190-4 (hbk)
ISBN13: 978-0-203-86690-0 (ebk)

"For my mother, Lakshmi, whose concern, confidence and courage have so inspired and protected me."

Gita

"Édesanyámnak, Borikának, sok hálával és köszönettel a szívből áradó őszinte szeretetéért és gondoskodásáért."

Piroska

Contents

Tables

Figures

Boxes

Preface

This volume brings together the work of leading researchers working on the question of gender equity in international health. It traces its origins to a research synthesis project undertaken in 2006 and 2007 by the Women and Gender Equity Knowledge Network (WGEKN) of the World Health Organization's Commission on Social Determinants of Health (CSDH). The WGEKN was set up to draw together the evidence base on health disparities and inequity due to gender, on the specific problems women face in meeting the highest attainable standards of health, and on the policies and actions that can address them. The editors of this volume were coordinators of the WGEKN.

The 18 Members and 29 Corresponding Members of the WGEKN represent policy, civil society, and academic expertise from a variety of disciplines, such as medicine, biology, sociology, epidemiology, anthropology, economics, and political science. The work was therefore able to draw on knowledge bases from a variety of research traditions and to identify intersectoral actions for health based on experiences from different fields.

The key research questions were the following:

How do essential structural dimensions of gender inequality affect women's health and what should be the priority actions to protect women's human rights and to expand women's opportunities and capabilities?

How do gendered norms in health manifest in households and communities and how can these norms, values, and practices be challenged through multilevel strategies?

How do different health conditions of women and men reflect a combination of biological sex differences and gendered social determinants? What are the relative roles of biological sex differences and social bias in our understanding of women's and men's differential exposure and vulnerability?

What are the root causes and consequences of the gendered politics of health care systems for women's health, and how we can minimize gender bias in health systems?

What mechanisms and policies need to be developed to ensure that gender imbalances in both the content and processes of health research are avoided and corrected?

How can we overcome the organizational rigidities and lacunae that seriously hinder the implementation of gender-equal policies both within and outside the health sector? What is required for building effective leadership, creating well-designed organizational mandates, structures, incentives, and accountability mechanisms that would ensure gender equitable laws, policies, and programs?

To answer these questions, the WGEKN commissioned a number of review papers, which provide useful in-depth analysis especially of frontier areas and difficult policy questions. In addition, civil society organizations and the members and corresponding members of the WGEKN provided information including cases that were more difficult to access.

The proposed volume goes beyond the scope of many previous publications on gender and health by detailing and recommending policy approaches and agendas that incorporate but go beyond commonly acknowledged issues relating to women's health and gender equity in health. It uses a newly developed conceptual framework for the role of gender as a social determinant of health (Chapter 1, Figure 1.1), and the chapters of this volume highlight aspects of the different components and pathways in that framework. Convincing arguments and evidence are provided of the importance of intersecting social hierarchies (e.g., gender, class, and ethnicity) for understanding health inequities and their implications for health policy. The volume brings together evidence from both lower- and higher-income countries.

Throughout the volume there is a robust evidence base on the association between gender inequality and health. Where the evidence base is most tentative is in demonstrating the health effects of some of the policies and interventions among different segments of women and men. Although many of the interventions presented in the chapters have been evaluated, there are some that are still awaiting systematic assessment. Nonetheless, these actions were assessed by the Knowledge Network members as important and innovative, and with great potential for making a difference on the ground and holding promise for the future.

The editors and authors of this volume would like to express their gratitude for the collective patience and expertise generously offered by Knowledge Network Members, Corresponding Members and the anonymous reviewers. The core members of the network were Rebecca Cook, Claudia Garcia Moreno, Adrienne Germain, Veloshnee Govender, Caren Grown, Afua Hesse, Helen Keleher, Yunguo Liu, Piroska Östlin, Rosalind Petchesky, Silvina Ramos, Sundari Ravindran, Alex Scott-Samuel, Gita Sen, Hilary Standing, Debora Tajer, Sally Theobald, and Huda Zurayk. We are also indebted to the CSDH Commissioners, especially Hoda Rashad, Monique Begin, Mirai Chatterjee, Ndioro Ndiaye, and Denny Vågerö, for their guidance and support. We are grateful for the generous financial support provided by the Swedish Ministry for Foreign Affairs through the World Health Organization, the Swedish National Institute of Public

Health (SNIPH), and the Open Society Institute. The editors thank also their institutions, the Indian Institute of Management Bangalore and the Karolinska Institutet in Sweden, for giving a home to the organizational hubs of the Knowledge Network.

We greatly appreciate the support provided by Charlotta Zacharias, Benjamin Holtzman and Terence James Johnson as we put this volume together.

Acknowledgments

The chapters in this volume are based on the detailed background papers commissioned by the WGEKN of the WHO's Independent CSDH. Short versions of all the papers, except Chapter 5 by Batthyany and Corrêa, were published in Gita Sen and Piroska Östlin (eds.), 2008, "Gender Inequity in Health: Why It Exists and How We Can Change It, Special Supplement," *Global Public Health* 3 (2): Supplement 1. The chapters here are substantially longer versions based on the original background papers. Permission to use the material in the GPH Special Supplement has been granted by its publishers, Taylor and Francis.

1   Gender as a Social Determinant of Health

Evidence, Policies, and Innovations[1]

Gita Sen and Piroska Östlin

Gender relations of power constitute the root causes of gender inequality and are among the most influential of the social determinants of health. They operate across many dimensions of life affecting how people live, work, and relate to each other. They determine whether people's needs are acknowledged, whether they have voice or a modicum of control over their lives and health, whether they can realize their rights. Addressing the problem of gender inequality requires actions both outside and within the health sector because gender power relations operate across such a wide spectrum of human life and in such interrelated ways. Taking such actions is good for the health of all people—girls and boys, women and men. In particular, intersectoral action to address gender inequality is critical to the realization of the Millennium Development Goals (MDGs) as has been shown by the report of Taskforce 3 on Gender Equality of the UN Millennium Project (Grown et al., 2005a, 2005b). Each one of the MDGs[2] requires that strong efforts be made towards gender equality if the goal is to be achieved. Some of these efforts need to be within the health sector but many are outside. The health sector may take leadership but it must also act in collaboration with other sectors if these goals are to be achieved.

Some might argue that gender inequalities in health are a natural consequence of biological difference and therefore difficult to change. We show that gender inequality and inequity in health are socially governed and therefore actionable. We draw on a growing body of research and program evidence that even in health (where the physical body has a central place), biology is not destiny. Sex and society, nature and nurture, chromosomes and environments interact in fascinating ways to determine, among other things, who is well or ill, who is treated or not, who is exposed or vulnerable to ill-health and how, whose behavior is risk-prone or risk-averse, and whose health needs are acknowledged or dismissed. The interactions between nature and nurture are probably more complex in the case of gender equity in health than in almost any other aspect of social hierarchy.

However, it can be difficult to understand how gender power relations work to reproduce health inequity without also understanding how gender intersects with economic inequality, racial or ethnic hierarchy, caste domination, differences based on sexual orientation, or a number of other social markers. Not all of these will be relevant in all communities or societies, barring economic inequality or class differences that are pervasive everywhere. However, only focusing on economic inequalities among households can seriously distort our understanding of how inequality works and who actually bears much of its burdens. Health gradients can be significantly different for men and women; medical poverty may not trap women and men to the same extent or in the same way. The picture becomes more complex when stratifiers[3] such as race or caste are added to the analysis. These findings challenge how many of those concerned about the social determinants of health understand the workings of social inequality. It calls for finer nuance in research and analysis, and greater sensitivity in policies and actions to the interactions among multiple sources of power and hierarchy.

They also challenge how one interprets human rights principles. The right to health is affirmed in the Universal Declaration of Human Rights (United Nations, 1948) and is part of the WHO's core principles. Yet the egregious violation of women's human rights through violence was only globally recognized at the World Conference on Human Rights in Vienna in 1993. This volume is grounded in the affirmation of equal and universal rights to health for all people, irrespective of economic class, gender, race, ethnicity, caste, sexual orientation, disability, age, or location, and it stresses the Commission on Social Determinants of Health (CSDH) belief that "The function of a just society is to do more than simply open the way for individuals to make use of their opportunities, it is to organize in such a way that, where people are deprived of opportunity to lead meaningful lives, deprived of freedoms or empowerment, such effects can be detected and changed" (CSDH, 2007, p. 3).

Gender analysis itself has been challenged more recently by work deriving from social movements for sexual rights, in particular the lesbian/gay/bisexual/transgender (LGBT) movement. These movements have challenged feminist movements to be more inclusive and to recognize sexual and gender orientation as an important source of discrimination, bias, violence, and challenges to health. The challenge is not only to policy but to the very concept of gender itself. Biological sex has never only consisted of the simple binaries—women and men. The presence of transgender people has been rendered socially invisible in some societies; in others their presence is socially recognized but they are relegated to the margins of society through discrimination and violence. But the challenge to heterosexual norms by the LGBT movement goes beyond biology to the social and ideational realms where sexuality and gender are defined, negotiated, and expressed. If the feminist movement has challenged masculinist norms, the LGBT movement challenges heterosexual norms that are also sources of discrimination and bias.[4] For the purposes of this chapter and the work of the CSDH, the effects of sexuality-based discrimination on the health of people are vitally important (Parker and Aggleton, 2007; Currah et al., 2006; Misra and Chandiramani, 2005; Butler, 2005; Fausto-Sterling, 2000).

While the conceptual frontiers are shifting, norms and policies have been slower to change. Even for the, by now, well-accepted notion of gender inequality between women and men, it is often the case that public speeches and stated commitments are not followed by action. Gender equality remains in a limbo where everyone agrees publicly about the need to act but resources are not allocated and follow-up action is weak or nonexistent. A recent example is from HIV policy where major agencies have agreed about its critical links to violence against women but action has been weak (Fried, 2007). Policy sensitivity to what has to be done *organizationally* is crucial to understanding whether and why policies to address women's health needs or gender inequity in health can misbehave or evaporate. The heart of the problem is that gender discrimination, bias, and inequality permeate the organizational structures of governments and international organizations, and the mechanisms through which strategies and policies are designed and implemented. People within these structures are themselves often deeply invested in the gender status quo. Focusing on how organizational changes happen has to be central to policy changes that hope to alter gender power relations (Ashcraft and Mumby, 2004). This requires attention to beliefs and values, incentive and disincentive structures, clear mechanisms to ensure action, strong organizational placement of gender equality champions within the system, and opening of spaces to civil society actors who are often the ones who can tell when the emperor has no clothes! The devil is often in the details of governance structures and organizational processes.

FRAMEWORK FOR THE ROLE OF GENDER AS A SOCIAL DETERMINANT OF HEALTH

The conceptual framework elaborated by the report of the Women and Gender Equity Knowledge Network (WGEKN) and the chapters in this volume proposes several pathways to explain how different factors interact, at the individual and collective levels, to generate inequalities that influence the health status of women and men in a given population. The pathways from the gendered structural determinants (see explanation following) to the intermediary factors that determine inequitable health outcomes are multiple, and can be complex. The intermediary factors are broadly four-fold: (a) discriminatory values, norms, practices, and behaviors, in relation to health within households and communities; (b) differential exposures and vulnerabilities to disease, disability, and injuries; (c) biases in health systems; and (d) biased health research. These intermediary factors result in biased and inequitable health outcomes, which, in turn, can have serious economic and social consequences for girls and boys, women and men, their families and communities, and their countries. Feedback effects, from outcomes and consequences to the structural determinants or to intermediary factors, can also be important. Figure 1.1 summarizes these relationships.

GENDERED STRUCTURAL DETERMINANTS OF HEALTH

Gender systems have a variety of different features, not all of which are the same across different societies. Women have less land, wealth, and property in almost all societies; yet they have higher burdens of work in the economy of 'care'—ensuring the survival, reproduction, and security of people, including young and old. Girls, in some contexts, are fed less, educated less, and more physically restricted; and women are typically employed and segregated in lower-paid, less secure, and 'informal,' occupations. Gender hierarchy governs how people live, and what they believe, and claim to

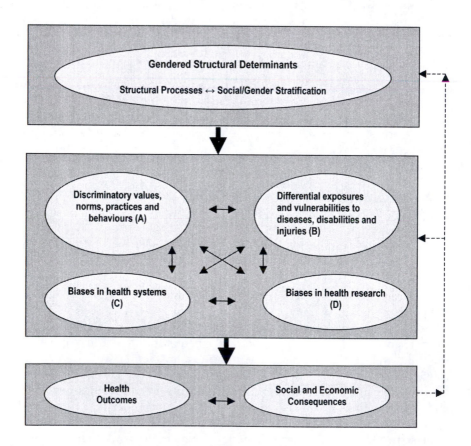

Figure 1.1   Framework for the role of gender as a social determinant of health.

know about, what it means to be a girl or a boy, a woman or a man. Girls and women are often viewed as less capable or able, and in some regions are seen as repositories of male or family honor and the self-respect of communities (Fazio, 2004). Restrictions on their physical mobility, sexuality, and reproductive capacity are perceived to be natural; and, in many instances, accepted codes of social conduct and legal systems condone, and even reward, violence against them (Garcia-Moreno et al., 2006).

Women are thus seen as objects rather than subjects (or agents) in their own homes and communities, and this is reflected in norms of behavior, codes of conduct, and laws that perpetuate their status as lower beings and second-class citizens. Even in places where extreme gender inequality may not exist, women often have less access to political power, and lower participation in political institutions, from the local municipal council or village to the national parliament and the international arena. While this is true for women as a whole vis-à-vis men, there can be significant differences among women themselves based on age or lifecycle status, as well as on the basis of economic class, race, caste, and ethnicity.

Intersecting Inequalities

Examination of the intersections among different social hierarchies—intersectionality—has begun in recent years to yield new insights about the social determinants of health (Iyer et al., 2007; Crenshaw, 1991; Iyer, 2007; Krieger et al., 1993; Ravindran, 1991; Breen, 2002; Schulz and Mullings, 2006; Geronimus and Thompson, 2004; Geronimus, 1996). Unfortunately, this has not yet permeated the health equity field generally. For many who work on or advocate health equity, the sources of inequity are primarily viewed as linked to gender-blind concepts of economic class differentials.

Recent work holds promise for the development of simple techniques for answering such questions (Iyer, 2007; Iyer et al., 2008; Sen et al., 2008). The chapter by Iyer, Sen, and Östlin in this volume (Chapter 3) reviews recent literature on intersectionality, and suggests that intersecting stratification processes can significantly alter the impact of any one dimension of inequality taken by itself. Important inferences for policy flow from this. For instance, the challenge of improving access to health care at a time of rising health care costs may best be met by a combination of universal systems (of provisioning or health insurance) across households coupled with forms of targeting or other mechanisms to ensure that they actually reach women and girls within households. Insufficient attention to intersectionality in much of the health literature has significant human costs, because those affected most negatively tend to be those who are poorest and most oppressed by gender and other forms of social inequality.

The other side of the coin of women's subordinate position is that men typically have greater wealth, better jobs, more education, greater political clout, and fewer restrictions on behavior. Moreover, men in many parts of the world exercise power over women, making decisions on their behalf, regulating and constraining their access to resources and personal agency, and sanctioning and policing their behavior through socially condoned violence or the threat of violence. Again, not all men exercise power over all women; gender power relations are intersected by age and lifecycle, as well as the other social stratifiers, such as economic class, race, or caste. The impact of gender power for physical and mental health—of girls, women, and transgender /intersex people, and also of boys and men—can be profound.

Education Deficits

Despite recent advances, a gender gap in literacy and education persists in many parts of the world as documented by Herz and Sperling (2004), and by the reports of Taskforce 3 on Education and Gender Equality of the UN Millennium Project (Grown et al., 2005a, 2005b; Birdsall et al., 2005). Significant numbers of women reach adulthood with no education, especially in South Asia where the literacy rate for women (equal to and over 15 years of age) in 2004 was as low as 48%, only two-thirds the rate for men (HDR, 2006). The children of women who have never received an education are 50% more likely to suffer from malnutrition or to die before the age of five (UNFPA, 2002). An in-depth review of the results of 44 scientific studies found that patients with low literacy had poorer health outcomes, including knowledge, intermediate disease markers, measures of morbidity, general health status, and use of health resources. Patients with low literacy were generally 1.5 to 3 times more likely to experience a given poor health outcome (Dewalt et al., 2004). Children and especially girls with low levels of schooling assume the work burdens of adults prematurely and are deprived of the opportunity for learning in an institutional setting outside the family. In many countries millions of girls 'disappear' into early traditional marriages, hazardous labor, or even combat roles (UNICEF, 2006).

Barriers to the education of girls include negative perceptions about women that devalue their capabilities, strong beliefs about the division of labor that places inequitable burdens on females, gender-biased beliefs about the value of educating girls, and curricula that are seen as inappropriate for girls (Abane, 2004). Such beliefs are exacerbated by structural barriers such as school fees or school-going costs; distance from schools; perceived or actual lack of safety for girls going to school; absence of female teachers; lack of gender sensitivity in schools, including absence of decent toilet facilities for adolescent girls; and inflexibility of classroom programs. These barriers work especially for postprimary education.

Demographic Changes and Women's Burdens

Changes in the demand for and supply of education have been fuelled in part by the demographic transition in birthrates and death rates. The pace and pattern of demographic change is different in different regions of the world. Some countries have seen falls in death rates without corresponding declines in birthrates. The resulting increase in the absolute and relative numbers of young people in these countries has gone hand in hand with the ageing of populations in other, usually high- or middle-income countries (UNFPA, 2003). In regions seriously affected by the HIV/AIDS pandemic, the age pyramid appears hollowed out in the middle ages due to the high infection rates among women and men in the reproductive ages. In regions with endemic son-preference, the availability of ultrasound technologies has significantly altered the sex-ratio in the population as a whole and particularly the child sex-ratio against girls and women (UNFPA, 2006).

These processes have important implications not only for the kind of demands placed on health services, but specifically on girls and women as the first-line providers of all forms of care, including health care within and outside the home. A large young population typically means an increase in women's work in maternity and caring for children. In most countries, this work is unsupported and usually unpaid. When children fall ill, it is women who have to juggle the multiple responsibilities of double and triple burdens of work. When mothers work for an income (as most poor mothers do), girls are recruited to care for siblings at the expense of their own education (Herz and Sperling, 2004). When parents die due to HIV, it is often grandparents or children (often girls) who are left to care for young children and households (Monash and Buerma, 2004). Highly biased population sex-ratios result in larger spousal age-difference and phenomena such as kidnapping of brides, or wife-sharing among brothers, all of which impact negatively on women's power within the home. (Hudson and den Boer, 2004)

The ageing of populations also increases women's care work burdens in supporting the elderly who usually also require more health care (WHO, 2003b). Ageing also hits women in another way, especially in countries that are experiencing greater longevity for women. Although there is evidence that widowers are less able to care for themselves and manage their lives than widows (Fry, 2001), the absolute numbers of widows tends to be greater. This is when the cumulative effect of women's lower economic position and dependency throughout their lives is felt. Widows tend to be poorer, and their rates of impoverishment and destitution higher than widowers and many other subsets of the population. In poor and middle-income countries where it is acceptable for older men to marry much younger women, and remarriage for widows is frowned on, there are many more widows than widowers. Here widows may be at greater risk of poor health if they live alone (having outlived their older spouse and, for one reason or another, not living with one of their children). For example, in Lebanon this is especially challenging for mothers of adult children who moved during the civil war to find work; 15% of elderly women live alone, compared to 1% of elderly men (Sibai et al., 2004). A study in Egypt and Tunisia found that older women, regardless of their residential status, appeared to experience more morbidity and disability than older men, and report using medication and visiting providers more often than men (Yount and Agree, 2005; Yount et al., 2004).

The extent to which the needs of young populations, as well as older populations, have to be met through the unpaid 'care' work of women, is exacerbated by crumbling health services and vanishing paid health staff. Women become the shock absorbers in the system, expected to act as such in both normal economic and health times, and during the bumps caused by health crises and emergencies. This is especially true for women who bear multiple and intersecting burdens of poverty and, for example, race, ethnicity or caste. Geronimus (1992) proposed the "weathering hypothesis" as a plausible explanation for racial differences in maternal age patterns for births and birth outcomes in the US. The "weathering hypothesis" suggests that the health of African-American women may begin to deteriorate in early adulthood as a physical consequence of cumulative socioeconomic disadvantage. As a consequence, teenage might be a healthier time for them to become pregnant and bear children than early adulthood. The weathering hypothesis has also been tested and found valid for US-born Mexican-American women with clear correlates in extraordinarily high levels of neonatal mortality and pregnancy-related hypertension in early adulthood (Wildsmith, 2002). This work implies an urgent need to reduce the socioeconomic stressors that women with multiple, intersecting oppressions face (Geronimus and Thompson, 2004; Geronimus et al., 2006).

Globalization

During the last four decades, the effect of demographic transitions and of increased education have been crosscut by technological and other changes that have brought local, national, and regional economies ever closer. Countries and their economic systems have become more strongly intertwined through large flows of money, goods, and people, through global assembly lines and commodity chains, greater information and knowledge, and stronger cross-national impacts of policies and actions (Labonté et al., 2007). Fuelled by the revolution in information technology and its penetration to the core of economic and production systems, this globalization, which has been driven by the rising dominance of highly volatile finance capital, has also given birth to social movements (environment, women, racism, and indigenous people) that are more global in scope. It has also been associated with (even if not always causally) increased militarization and warfare, and a rise in wars over energy and mineral resources, leading to a rising number of internal refugees, displaced persons, and trafficking in women and children.

Three implications of globalization are of particular significance for our focus on gender relations. The *first* is how it has transformed the composition of workforces, and the resulting impacts on women's health. Feminization of workforces has gone hand in hand with increased casualization, and continuing unequal burdens for unpaid work in the household, with serious implications for women's occupational health and the consequences of insufficient rest and leisure (Joekes, 1995; Standing, 1997; Messing and Östlin, 2006).

A *second* gendered consequence of globalization is through its narrowing of national policy space resulting in reducing funds for health and education with negative impacts on girls' and women's access (Stiglitz and Charlton, 2005; Herz and Sperling, 2004). In the 1990s, these policies springing from the so-called Washington Consensus were modified. Commitment to Poverty Reduction Strategies (PRS) or equivalent National Development Strategies (NDS) by countries were made the basis of foreign lending. Direct program lending for health increased in a number of cases, but has often been associated with pressures for privatization and increases in user fees. The modified approach has had mixed results in terms of actually being able to reverse negative trends in health systems.[5] Such policies have also been carried out in related spheres such as pension reforms with significant increases in inequality. Several Latin American countries have fully or partially privatized their public pensions since the 1980s. For instance, in 1995, Mexico privatized its public pension system, including a shift from a defined benefit to a defined contribution system based on privately administered individual accounts (Dion, 2006). Another study shows that the new privately managed pension system in Chile has increased gender inequalities (deMesa and Montecinos, 1999). Women are worse off than they were under the previous pay-as-you-go system of social security, in which the calculation of benefits for men and women did not differ and women could obtain pensions with fewer requirements than men. Currently, benefits are calculated according to individuals' contributions and levels of risk. Such factors as women's longer life expectancy, earlier retirement age, lower rates of formal labor-force participation, lower salaries, and other disadvantages in the labor market directly affect their accumulation of funds in individual retirement accounts, leading to lower pensions especially for poorer women.

A *third* aspect of globalization of importance for health is the rise in violence linked to the changing political economy of nation-states in the international order. The chapter by Petchesky and Laurie, in this volume (Chapter 4), applies the political theory of Agamben on 'states of exception' as a way of understanding current gender dynamics in reproductive health, militarization, and camps for refugees and internally displaced persons. It argues that a human rights approach to gender and health equity is essential in such sites of exclusion. Importantly, gendered violence does not only affect girls and women, but includes violence against boys and men, as well as transgender and intersex persons, and all those who do not meet heterosexual norms.

Deepening the Human Rights Agenda

Some of the negative consequences of globalization contrast with the deepening, during recent decades, of the normative framework of human rights. This deepening has been important in altering values, beliefs, and knowledge about gender systems and their implications for health and human rights. The social upheavals set off by the civil rights and women's movements of the 1960s and the intensified focus on a broad human rights agenda at the United Nations conferences of the 1990s[6] have challenged the narrower understanding of human rights that had prevailed until those times (Laurie and Petchesky, 2008). Hitherto unrecognized dimensions of inequality and inequity—gender, sexual orientation, ethnicity, race, caste, and disability—began to be debated. All of these new elements drew their inspiration from the Universal Declaration of Human Rights (UDHR) and referred to its various clauses and principles. But they also provided new interpretations to these same clauses, grounded in the realities of the lives of people who were subject to discrimination and inequality, or who were vulnerable for other reasons such as age.

The explicit recognition of 'lived' realities—for example, of rape as a violation of women's human rights (United Nations, 1993), or racism as a violation of the human rights of specific racial or ethnic groups (United Nations, 2001)—was critical to their being acknowledged as needing legal and policy remedies. One important precursor at the global level was the adoption of the Convention on the Elimination of All Forms of Discrimination against Women (CEDAW) in 1979. CEDAW provided a broad framework for women's rights that has been used in a number of countries to advance action at the national level. It also has an accountability mechanism built in whereby member states of the United Nations have to report on a regular basis on actions taken towards its implementation.

A further important way in which the human rights framework has been deepened is through interpreting the right to health to include reproductive and sexual health and reproductive rights (United Nations, 1994) and sexual rights (United Nations, 1995). In 2007, a distinguished group of international human rights experts launched the Yogyakarta Principles on the application of international human rights law to sexual orientation and gender identity.[7] Human rights violations targeted toward persons because of their actual or perceived sexual orientation or gender identity include extrajudicial killings, torture and ill-treatment, sexual assault and rape, invasions of privacy, arbitrary detention, denial of employment and education opportunities, and serious discrimination in relation to the enjoyment of other human rights. The Yogyakarta Principles affirm 29 key rights, many of which have implications for health, and affirm the primary obligation of states to guarantee these rights. Of particular note are Principles 17 (the right to the highest attainable standard of health) and 18 (the right to protection from medical abuses).

Transforming the Gendered Structural Determinants of Health

Deepening the recognition of human rights is, however, only half the needed action. The other half is to turn such norms into reality through mechanisms for implementation and accountability. This requires creation of organizational mechanisms, funding for implementation, and accountability structures that create incentives for appropriate action. The critique of structural adjustment programs and neoliberal economic reforms has clarified the need to ensure that resources for and attention to access, affordability, and availability of health services are not damaged during periods of economic reforms, and that women's entitlements, rights, health, and gender equality are protected and promoted, because of the close connections between women's rights to health and their economic situation. In a just world, responsibilities for domestic work and caring for people would be equally shared by women and men. Until then, providing women with the support that will minimize the health-damaging consequences of their double burdens, and especially their unpaid responsibilities for daily household needs such as gathering fuel, fetching water and fodder, cooking, washing, and cleaning, requires sustained public policy attention. In addition to these tasks women need support for their work of caring for the young, old, and the ailing within families.

Task Force 3 on Education and Gender Equality of the UN Millennium Project identified a set of strategic priorities in this regard (Grown et al., 2005a, 2005b). Of special importance for health are the specifications of efficient sources of energy, better transport systems, and clean water and sanitation as priorities. The substitution of biomass by cleaner and more efficient fuels will reduce both the time women spend and the problem of kitchen pollutants. Ensuring clean water and sanitation has well-known health implications for children and girls and women. However, the planning and implementation of such infrastructure can be most effective if girls and women are themselves involved.

To improve hygiene behavior requires an understanding of women's tasks, the choices they have, and the local constraints they experience— such as time constraints, poverty, and lack of support from the health and social authorities. Expecting women to change their behavior is unrealistic unless there are serious attempts to improve accessibility and reliability of water supplies, and the safe disposal of sewage and waste water (Watts, 2004; Zwane and Kremer, 2007). "A study of community water and sanitation projects in 88 communities in 15 countries finds strong evidence that projects designed and run with the full participation of women are more sustainable and effective than those that ignore women" (Gross et al., 2001). This finding corroborates an earlier World Bank study that found that women's participation was strongly associated with water and sanitation project effectiveness (Fong et al., 1996; United Nations, 2005). For example, "The Blue Nile Health Project" in Sudan with the objective to control water-associated diseases was perceived as very successful, thanks to the particular emphasis in the program on gender-related aspects that defined women's role and participation (Rahman et al., 1996).

Women's ability to play such a role depends at least partly on their educational capabilities. An earlier review of the links between education and economic well-being found that education enhances labor market productivity and income growth for all, and educating women also has beneficial effects on social well-being. For instance, it increases women's productivity in the home, which in turn can increase family health, child survival, and investment in children. It has been estimated that countries can expect per capita annual growth in GDP of between one to three percentage points higher with more gender-equal education levels, while each year of schooling lost means a 10–20% reduction in girls' future incomes (Herz and Sperling, 2004).

However, primary education is insufficient to provide women with the knowledge and skills to improve and sustain their own health or economic independence. A study analyzing the impact of female education on the use of maternal and child health services by women in Thailand during pregnancy found that secondary education was the most consistent predictor of health service use for three services—tetanus toxoid inoculations, prenatal care, and assistance by formal providers during delivery (Raghupathy, 1996). Higher levels of education can also give girls and women more ability to challenge gender norms provided their 'fallback' position in terms of control over economic assets or incomes also improves. Resistance and opposition to violence and genital mutilation is higher among women with at least some secondary education (Global Campaign for Education, 2005). Based on the report of the UN Millennium Project's Task Force 3 on Education and Gender Equality, it has been argued by Grown, Rao-Gupta, and Pande (2005b) that secondary education for girls also influences later age at marriage, improved ability by women to manage their fertility, smaller and more sustainable families, improved material care for children, including nourishment and success at school, and reduced vulnerability to HIV/AIDS.

What needs to be done to break the barriers to education for girls? Many of the actions may be the same for both primary and postprimary education.

> These include making schooling more affordable by reducing costs and offering targeted scholarships, building secondary schools close to girls' homes, and making schools girl-friendly. Additionally, the content, quality, and relevance of education must be improved through curriculum reform, teacher training, and other actions. Education must serve as the vehicle for transforming attitudes, beliefs, and entrenched social norms that perpetuate discrimination and inequality (Grown et al., 2005b).

Bangladesh's Female Secondary School Assistance Program began in 1994 with the aim of increasing the secondary school enrolment and retention rates of rural girls. Over the years, it has provided full scholarships covering tuition and all other costs, increased the numbers of female teachers, educated communities and parents about the value of girls' education, improved school infrastructure, and added occupational skills to the curricula. By 2002, the expanding program was supporting 5,000 schools in the 118 poorest rural districts with around a million girls getting scholarships, and almost 40% of the teachers being female. The enrolment and attendance rates for girls improved sharply and surpassed that for boys. Furthermore, the proportions of married girls among ages 13–19 dropped significantly (Herz and Sperling, 2004).

Cultural norms about teen pregnancy vary widely. But even where there may be little stigma attached to it, as in many parts of sub-Saharan Africa, pregnancy and motherhood can make it very difficult for a girl to continue schooling. Systematic actions to break these barriers are therefore required. Botswana's Diphalana Initiative shows how an integrated approach across social sectors—health, education, and social welfare—can address the needs of pregnant schoolgirls. Unlike many other areas where pregnancy for a schoolgirl can lead to her dropping out because it is too difficult for her to combine multiple roles and because of legal restrictions, this initiative explicitly has worked to tackle such barriers (United Nations, 2005).

INTERMEDIARY FACTORS—DISCRIMINATORY VALUES, NORMS, PRACTICES, AND BEHAVIORS

Gendered norms in health manifest in households and communities on the basis of values and attitudes about the relative worth, or importance, of girls versus boys and men versus women; about who has responsibility for different household/community needs and roles; about masculinity and femininity; who has the right to make different decisions; who ensures that household/community order is maintained and deviance is appropriately sanctioned or punished; and who has final authority in relation to the inner world of the family/community and its outer relations with society (Quisumbing and Maluccio, 1999). Norms around masculinity not only affect the health of girls and women but also of boys and men themselves (Barker and Ricardo, 2005).

Direct causal relationships, linking cultural biases against girls and women to health outcomes, vary widely across regions and cultures, and over time. These biases include differential access to nutrition and health care for boys versus girls, and women versus men. Unequal control over income and productive resources, such as land and credit, can affect the value given to women's lives and health, and, hence, to health practices, health-seeking behaviors, and health access. Unequal burdens of work and responsibility, for the care of young and old, often means that women are expected to sacrifice their own rest, leisure, and health; women themselves internalize these values, which often mark who is seen to be a 'good' woman. Norms of masculinity vary, as do models of what represents perfect femininity. Idealized women in different cultures may be virgins, goddesses, sacrificing mothers, even sexual temptresses, but everywhere, the sexuality and reproductive capacity of the good woman is the property of her husband, family, clan, or community. Men, similarly, may be expected to be aloof, unemotional, aggressive, or emotional, etc., but everywhere, they are also expected to look after their female property and keep it in good order. The threat of violence, and violence itself, are central to the maintenance of the masculine–feminine order. This has obvious and serious consequences for the physical, emotional, and psychological health of women and of men.

Challenging Gender Stereotypes and how they Affect Health

Challenging gender norms, especially in the areas of sexuality and reproduction, touch the most intimate personal relationships, as well as one's sense of self and identity. No single or simple action or policy intervention can be expected, therefore, to provide a panacea for the problem. Targeting women and girls is a sound investment, but outcomes depend on integrated approaches and the protective umbrella of policy and legislative actions (Keleher and Franklin, 2008). Multilevel interventions are therefore needed. We identify three sets of actions.

The first is creating formal agreements, codes, and laws to change norms that violate women's human rights, and then implementing them. This may be easier said than done, especially if there is powerful organized opposition to gender equality. The cardinal rule is that there must be local groups of advocates, especially women's organizations or human rights groups who can play a strong role. In the meantime, capacity building among government officials, judges, and parliamentarians can be valuable against the day when change can happen (Sen et al., 2007).

Recent years have seen a number of legal changes in different countries. A milestone was the change in the personal status law in Tunisia beginning with a 1956 Personal Status Code outlawing repudiation and polygamy, establishing a minimum age for the marriage of girls, and providing for equal wages for men and women. Further reforms in 1993 concerned the marriage of minors, the mutual obligations of husband and wife, and domestic violence. This legislation has brought about a profound change in the norms regarding women's position in society and within marriage, characterized as moving "from sexual submission to voluntary commitment" (Labidi, 2001). In Egypt the revision in 2000 of the 1979 law on formal marriage contracts (the so-called Jihan al Sadat law) gave a woman much wider rights to ask for divorce, allowing her to obtain divorce unilaterally provided she is willing to renounce her financial rights. This formally gave women similar rights to divorce as men in Egypt, which thereby joined Tunisia, the only other Arab country to do this (Fargues, 2001). A remarkable combination of coalition politics, legal activism, and an intelligent reclaiming of Islam by women's rights advocates made this possible.

Yet another interesting example of legal change was the act against domestic violence in India. An example of poor formulation was the early draft in 2002 of India's Domestic Violence Bill, which left many loopholes. As a result of strong lobbying by women's groups, and effective redrafting by feminist lawyers, the draft was changed, and a considerably improved act has recently come into force as the Protection of Women from Domestic Violence Act 2005. The act uses a broad definition of violence, allows abused women to complain directly to judges instead of police, ensures the woman's right to stay in the family home regardless of whether or not she has legal title, and covers not only wives and live-in partners, but sisters, mothers, mothers-in-law, or any other female relation living with a violent man. As such, it is one of the most progressive pieces of legislation on this subject to date (Agnes, 2005).

However, passing a law is only the beginning of a process in many cases. Once laws are there, they need to be enforced and this requires that appropriate institutions and budgets be assigned for this. This is especially true when the constituencies of women who might benefit from the law are poor and low on voice and agency. Multilevel and multisectoral strategies are therefore a second area for priority actions to change inequitable gender norms (Keleher, this volume, Chapter 6). The former imply working at different levels within a given sector, while the latter means integrated interventions across sectors. Kim and Motsei (2002) in South Africa found that norms and values of health personnel regarding violence against women must be addressed through sensitizing workshops, before technical guidelines could be effectively taught, as health personnel have lived experiences that exemplify and replicate gender biases. Nonetheless, once sensitizing workshops that address values at the personal level succeed, they need to be matched with broader organizational and structural change in order for the new norms to be sustained. Technical guidelines or information alone will not change behavior if the values and social context of individuals are not changed.

One of the most thorough attempts to date to delineate a multilevel and multisectoral strategy for an important manifestation of unequal gender norms is in WHO's Report on Violence against Women (WHO, 2005), based on a multi-country study of violence against women. The 15 recommendations of the report together provide an excellent example for multilevel, multisectoral action.

Some norms may not respond well to legal changes but may require societal intervention. One such is female genital mutilation (FGM). WHO estimates that about 130 million girls and women in some 28 countries have undergone some form of FGM with the highest incidence found in parts of Africa. FGM is banned in 14 African countries, including Ethiopia, Uganda, Ghana, and Togo, but the practice is still carried out. Girls may undergo FGM from as young as three years old depending on local rituals and customs. Certainly, strong gender disparities within society lead to violations of women's rights but FGM appears to be part of a dense social and cultural fabric, from which the tradition can be extracted only with some difficulty and against tremendous resistance. Change appears to respond better to the crafting of community consensus. Multipronged education approaches have succeeded in changing attitudes and community-held norms in some cases. Examples of success include the Senegal project (spearheaded by the NGO Tostan) that is now a regional model endorsed by UNICEF. Its success involves public declaration of intent to abandon the practice; and slow but steady human rights education programs, which encourage villagers to make up their own minds about it. The model is being adopted in Guinea, Burkina Faso, Mali, and Somalia.

Particularly when attempting to change norms that violate human rights but are subject to significant conservative (including conservative religious) support, many methods may be needed to bring the issue out into the open. Fear, stigma, and shame prevent people, especially women, from speaking about the subject. This breeds misinformation as well as callousness and lack of public attention. One way that has been particularly used by women's organizations in such situations is to hold public tribunals with judges who have credibility. This helps to raise public awareness, build solidarity, and reduce misinformation.

The Polish Tribunal on Abortion Rights provides a useful example:

From 1956 until 1993, abortion in Poland was widely accessible on therapeutic and socioeconomic grounds. Terminations were performed free of charge in public hospitals, or could be obtained in private clinics for a relatively low fee. The 1993 Act on Family Planning, Human Embryo Protection and Conditions for Legal Pregnancy Termination, commonly known as the Polish Anti-Abortion Act, was adopted by the Polish Parliament following a systematic anti-abortion campaign by the Roman Catholic Church, supported by conservative political forces in the Solidarity movement and many in the medical profession.

In 2001 the Polish Federation for Women and Family Planning organized a Tribunal on Abortion Rights in Warsaw, to publicize the negative consequences of the criminalization of abortion in Poland. It provided compelling evidence that restrictive abortion laws make abortion unsafe by pushing it underground, endanger women's health, create a climate where even those services that are allowed by law become unavailable, and contravene standards set by international human rights law. The restrictive abortion law in Poland has not increased the number of births; it has only caused women and their families suffering. The Tribunal brought the issue of abortion into the media prior to an election campaign and galvanized Polish and other Eastern European women's groups to become more active in defense of abortion rights. (Girard and Nowicka, 2002)

Complementing legal changes and multilevel actions such as those exemplified earlier is the third action priority—working with boys and men towards male transformation. One of the major innovative ideas of the Cairo and Beijing conferences was the concept of male responsibility for the health of their partners as well as of themselves and their children. Since then, there has been a steady forward movement in understanding and experimentation with programs on the ground, as well as rethinking the ideas themselves. Barker (2006) argues that there are always some boys and men in each situation of gender inequity who will oppose inequitable norms. A closer look at these rather special boys and men revealed that typically they had observed and reflected about the injustice of gendered norms and had received positive reinforcement from family members or others. This research also confirmed the need to intervene: (a) at the level of individual attitude and behavior change, by engaging young men in a critical reflection to identify the costs of traditional versions of masculinity; and (b) at the level of social or community norms, including among parents, service providers, and others that influence these individual attitudes and behaviors (Barker, 2006).

Program H provides an interesting case. An innovative educational program that was pioneered by Latin American NGOs and has now spread to parts of Asia and Latin America, Program H, attempts to create a safe space in which young men can question manhood norms and learn alternatives through group activities and processes. A highly visible part of the program is social marketing involving the young men, to create positive messages about gender-sensitive men using youth culture. The 'cool' or 'hip' young man is portrayed as nonviolent and sensitive by popular and well-known youth icons.

Another example is provided by Stepping Stones in South Africa, a behavioral intervention that approaches HIV prevention and reduction in violence against women from the perspective of gender inequality, relationships and skills, and broader reproductive health concerns (Jewkes et al., 2007). Over the last decade, the intervention has been used in over 40 countries, adapted for at least 17 settings, and translated into 13 languages (Wallace, 2006). Stepping Stones has been subject to rigorous evaluation in South Africa and provides evidence of success in reducing sexually transmitted infections in women, changing men's sexual risk-taking behavior, and reducing their use of violence against women.

INTERMEDIARY FACTORS—DIFFERENTIAL EXPOSURES AND VULNERABILITIES

In a wide range of countries male survival at all ages is inferior to that of females and this is reflected in lower life expectancy for men. However, there are also a number of countries, such as Bangladesh, Tonga, Afghanistan, Nepal, Malawi, Benin, Botswana, Cameroon, Central African Republic, Kenya, Niger, Nigeria, Pakistan, Qatar, Tuvalu, and Zambia, where women's life expectancy is lower or equal to that of men (WHO, 2006). Even where men die earlier than women, most studies on morbidity from both high- and low-income countries show higher rates of illness among women. Thus, women's potential for greater longevity rarely results in their being or feeling healthier than men during their lifetimes (Östlin et al., 2001). This so-called 'gender paradox' (Danielsson and Lindberg, 2001) and the ways in which biological and social determinants interact to produce it have not yet been fully understood, but there is a growing body of evidence about health differences between men and women.

Some health conditions are determined primarily by biological sex differences.[8] Others are the result of how societies socialize women and men into gender roles supported by norms about masculinity and femininity, and power relations that accord privileges to men, but that adversely affect the health of both women and men.[9] However, many health conditions reflect a combination of biological sex differences and gendered social determinants. Gender differentials in exposure and vulnerability to health risks can arise for two main reasons: the interplay of biological sex with the social construction of gender, and the direct impacts of structural gender inequalities.

All biological differences between women and men are based on sex chromosome–linked differences—anatomical and physiological characteristics derived from the sex karyotypes 46, XX female and 46, XY male.[10] These inherited sex chromosomes cannot change, but other aspects of biological sex (sex hormones, reproductive organs, other secondary characteristics) can and do change through an individual's lifecycle (puberty, menopause), through their actions (sex change, hormone therapies, exercise), and through the environment to which they are exposed (environmental toxins). While individuals can have different biological and social exposures to health risks and conditions depending on both their sex karyotype and their social position, their vulnerability to health risks and conditions is determined socially, not biologically.

Vulnerability reflects an individual's capacity to avoid, respond to, cope, and/or recover from exposures. As such, one's ability to deflect or absorb exposures with differing health effects and social consequences depends on a range of normative and structural social processes. Snow (this volume, Chapter 2) argues that analyses of gender and health are currently undermined by conflation of sex and gender in much of the epidemiological and clinical literature, precluding meaningful reflection on the contributions of genetics versus gendered socialization to health vulnerabilities. The chapter distinguishes between vulnerabilities linked to XX or XY genotype and those due to gendered life experiences.

Biological differences are important, but they do not always have sufficient power to determine health outcomes on their own. Yet women's health concerns are often understood as being mainly determined by biology. One example is osteoporosis, which in women appears to be partly linked to hormonal changes at the time of menopause. However, a response focused on marketing hormone replacement therapies, while useful, is too narrow and overly medicalizes the problem. It tends to divert attention from other potentially more important social factors influencing women's vulnerability to osteoporosis and its complications, such as isolation among elderly women, poor public and private infrastructures, and possibly some features of traditional diets (Snow, 2002).

For malaria, pregnancy increases women's susceptibility by compromising their immunity (Rogerson et al., 2007; Shulman and Dorman, 2003), making them the main adult risk group in most malaria endemic areas (WHO/UNICEF, 2003). Despite this biological difference that increases their exposure, their vulnerability to malaria and its effects on pregnancy are predicated on a range of socially determined factors: access to malaria treatment during antenatal care; access to environments that protect against mosquitoes (bed nets, removal of stagnating water); good nutrition; and monitoring and treatment for anemia, a complication of malaria during pregnancy.

Similarly to malaria, tuberculosis increases poor health outcomes during pregnancy for both mother and child. Obstetric morbidity increases fourfold for pregnant women who have a late diagnosis of tuberculosis. For men, however, it is behavior in the form of smoking that influences disease progression. The male to female ratio in disease progression in a study population in south India reduced from 2.7 to 1.2 after excluding the men who were smokers and alcoholics (WHO, 2002a). An ecological study estimates that one-third of the gender differential in tuberculosis may be explained by male smoking (Watkins and Plant, 2006).

According to the most recent statistics (UNAIDS, 2006), out of 34 million adults (15+) living with HIV/AIDS, 17.3 million are women. The sex differences in adult HIV prevalence rates vary by region, reflecting different dominant modes of transmission and their social determinants. In sub-Saharan Africa, North Africa, the Middle East, and the Caribbean, the dominant mode of transmission is through heterosexual intercourse and there are more female than male HIV positive adults. In sub-Saharan Africa, 59% of adults with HIV are women, and young women aged 15 to 24 are more than three times as likely to be infected as young men. In unprotected heterosexual intercourse, females are about twice as likely as males to contract HIV from an infected partner.[11] The biological factors involved include: the nature of vaginal mucous membranes and reproductive lifecycles (Forrest, 1991); the infectiveness of semen (UNAIDS, 1999); and women's higher rates of sexually transmitted infections (STIs). However, most significant are the power relations that influence sexual behavior and constrain health-seeking behavior and social support. Increasingly, men at risk of HIV have been initiating sex with younger and younger female partners, and this places young girls at increasing risk (Brown et al., 2001). Heterosexual norms often reflect double standards for men and women in terms of awareness and agency. Heterosexual women are often stigmatized as 'sluts' or 'loose women' for daring to be aware about safe sex or attempting to negotiate safe sex, with social norms condoning violence against them as a means to discipline deviance. Dominant sexual norms for men encourage promiscuity, neglect poor or nonexistent condom use, and sanction violence against women and nonconforming minority men (WHO, 2003c; UNAIDS/UNFPA/UNIFEM, 2004; Rao Gupta et al., 1996).

At a policy level, women are also more vulnerable to HIV due to the conservative hierarchy of policy options that does not acknowledge women's realities or rights. An emphasis on abstinence and being faithful (the dominant emphasis of the ABC approach) fails to recognize that for many women being married and faithful in monogamous or polygamous marriages is their biggest risk factor for HIV, especially when their male partners refuse to use condoms (Kelly, 2006). Developing female-controlled methods of prevention has received limited support, in contrast to the enthusiasm with which male circumcision has been endorsed.

Another example is depression—women are two to three times more likely than men to be diagnosed with depression (Ustun et al., 2004; Bhugra and Mastrogianni, 2004; Desjarlais et al., 1995). Depression is also more likely to be medicalized in women than men (Russo, 1990). Women's experiences of depression often predate pregnancy or the onset of menopause (Piccinelli and Wilkinson, 2000; Bebbington, 1998). Social factors, like partner and social support, life events such as abuse during childhood and other victimization, the social experience of motherhood and infant temperament may play a more important role than biological factors (Astbury, 2002).

In addition, structural gender inequalities in legal frameworks governing control over resources, women's status and autonomy as subjects and citizens, the functioning of labor and other markets, access to social services, health care, education, *inter alia*, can have a powerful impact on differences in health risks for women and men. The consequences of gender inequality can be experienced by women as: differential vulnerability and exposure to illness, poor acknowledgment of women-specific health needs, and inequitable treatment of health problems across a wide spectrum of health—reproductive, occupational, environmental, infectious disease, to name only a few. Women's health has been beset by 'resounding silences' and 'misdirected or partial approaches' (Sen et al., 2002). These have affected such problems as: kitchen air pollution, risks of heart disease, mental health, reproductive tract infections, breast and cervical cancers, and depression, to give just a few examples.

In addition to the examples thus far where risks are determined by biological sex or by a combination of sex and gender, there are health risks and conditions that are determined primarily by gender structures and relations. For example, an outcome of masculinity norms as manifested through risk behavior is that globally, 2.7 times as many men as women die from road traffic injuries. Overall higher male risk is explained by greater exposure to driving, but it is also due to riskier forms of driving.[12] For instance, males are more likely than females to drive after they have been drinking (Stoduto et al., 1998; Snow, 2008; Oei and Kerschbaumer, 1990).

Violence against women is another consequence of macho male behavior and unequal power relationships between women and men (Garcia-Moreno, 2002). It includes domestic violence, trafficking of women, and forms of violence linked to traditions that are specific to certain countries, such as female infanticide, the deliberate neglect of girls, rape in war, dowry-related deaths, FGM, and honor killings. While causes of violence are multiple and interlinked, gender inequality and norms of masculine behaviors that sanction violence, poverty, low education, alcohol consumption, a history of witnessing abuse, and prior victimization are among those most commonly documented (Jewkes, 2002). Risk of violence is greatest in societies with accepted codes of social conduct that condone and even reward violence against women. The health consequences of violence against women are many: death and injuries ranging from cuts, bruises to permanent disabilities, STIs, HIV infection and AIDS, unwanted pregnancy, gynecological problems, miscarriage, stillbirth, chronic pelvic pain and pelvic inflammatory disease, depression, post-traumatic stress disorder, just to mention a few (WHO, 2005; ARROW, 2005; Campbell, 2002; Astbury, 2002; Gielen et al., 2000; Coker et al., 2000; Letourneau et al., 1999).

The workplace is a critical arena determining gendered health differentials. The gendered division of labor, exemplified by the allocation of specific tasks to men and women is extensive and pervasive in all countries, regardless of level of development, wealth, religious orientation, or political regime.[13] These factors negatively affect women's social position relative to men's and the resulting inequalities contribute to gender inequalities in health (Messing and Östlin, 2006; Östlin, 2002a, 2002b). Work-related fatalities are more common among men, due to the fact that men work in environments with greater risk for accidents, e.g., transportation, mining, fishing, and firefighting (Laflamme and Eilert-Petersson, 2001; Islam et al., 2001). Evidence mainly from high-income countries suggests that women more than men are engaged in work characterized by high demands and little control, with highly repetitive movements and awkward postures, often facing intense exposure to the public (Messing, 2004; Östlin, 2002a, 2002b). For example, women are the majority of those involved in lower levels of health care, which involves higher risks of infection (from biological agents in hospitals, needle injuries), violence, musculoskeletal injuries, and burnout (WHO, 2002b; Mayhew, 2003; Aiken et al., 2002; Josephson et al., 1997).

The few studies that exist for developing countries show that, for example, in *maquiladoras*[14] in Latin America, women are exposed to chemicals, ergonomic hazards, noise, and stress (Cedillo Becerril et al., 1997). Where access to safe water and sanitation does not exist, women are at higher risk of waterborne diseases when washing laundry and utensils in affected canals (Watts, 2004). Women cooking on open stoves not only are at risk of burns, but are at high risk of illness due to smoke pollution, as was found in India (Mishra et al., 1999) and Guatemala (Albalak et al., 2001). In developing countries, nearly two million poor women and children die annually from exposure to indoor air pollution caused by smoke from cooking fuels. Many more suffer from acute and chronic respiratory infection (Smith and Maeusezahl-Feuz, 2004).

Reducing the Health Risks of Being Women and Men

Where biological sex differences interact with social determinants to define different needs for women and men in health, policy efforts must address these different needs. Significant advocacy is required to raise attention and sustain support for other services that address the specific health needs of poor women, and those in low-income countries, thereby reducing their exposure and vulnerability to unfavorable health outcomes. Not only must neglected sex-specific health conditions be addressed, but sex-specific needs in health conditions that affect both women and men must be considered, so that treatment can be accessed by both women and men without bias. Two intertwined strategies to address social bias are: tackling the social context of individual behavior, and empowering individuals and communities for positive change. Strategies that aim at changing high-risk lifestyles would be more effective if combined with measures that could tackle the negative social and economic circumstances (e.g., unemployment, sudden income loss) in which the health-damaging lifestyles are embedded. Individual empowerment, linked to community-level dynamics, is also critical in fostering transformation of gendered vulnerabilities. For strategies to succeed they must provide positive alternatives that support individuals and communities to take action against the status quo.

Some examples include work in South Africa that combined micro-credit with gender and HIV awareness sessions into an integrated packaged for women, resulting in a 55% reduction in intimate partner violence over two years (Pronyk et al., 2006). Critical social mobilization efforts included setting up village rape and crime committees in association with the police; HIV education sessions in local schools, churches, burial societies, soccer clubs, and taxi ranks; and protests to improve local health clinics and against local bars serving alcohol to young men. As a result, household communication between partners and children improved and traditional gender norms were challenged among program participants (Pronyk et al., 2005). The Soul City intervention in South Africa operated at multiple, mutually reinforcing levels (individual, community, and sociopolitical) to address domestic violence by increasing knowledge about domestic violence and shifting perceptions of social norms on this issue. Evaluation suggests that the intervention played a role in enhancing women's and communities' senses of efficacy, enabling women to make more effective decisions around their health (Usdin et al., 2005; Goldstein et al., 2005). The loveLife campaign of South Africa is another example of a positive campaign to support alternative behaviors where billboards challenge gender assumptions of male dominance in sexual and romantic relationships among youth, and provide young people an alternative gender vision of balanced, equitable, negotiated partnerships.

INTERMEDIARY FACTORS—BIASED HEALTH SYSTEMS

The WHO defines health systems as "all the activities whose primary purpose is to promote, restore, or maintain health" (WHO, 2001). Given the broad social, cultural, and economic context in which health systems operate and the impact that factors external to the health system can have on health, health systems are not only "producers of health and health care," but also "purveyors of a wider set of societal norms and values" (Gilson, 2003).

While the traditional approach to health care systems tends to be management oriented, with focus on issues such as infrastructure, technology, logistics, and financing, the WGEKN looked at the human component of health care systems, and the social relationships that characterize service delivery. Evidence shows the different ways in which the health care system may fail gender equity from the perspective of women, as both consumers (users) and producers (caregivers) of health care services. Action priorities include supporting improvements in (especially poor) women's access to services, recognition of women's role as health care providers, and building accountability for gender equality and equity into health systems, and especially in ongoing health reform programs and mechanisms.

Women in most places need more health services than men but often have less access to them (Puentes-Markides, 1992; Thaddeus and Maine, 1994; Vlassoff, 1994) due to a series of barriers at the individual, familial, and community levels. These barriers are often manifestations of women's low social status and lack of autonomy and rights (Chatterjee, 1988). Women themselves, their families, and health care providers may not be *aware* of the existence of a health problem, and may treat chronic pain, depression, or reproductive tract infections, for instance, as normal states because they are so widely prevalent (Iyer, 2005). Even when women are aware of health problems, they may refuse to *acknowledge* them for fear of adverse reactions from the family, community, and health care providers. For example, adolescent girls in Koppal in India (Iyer, 2005) or young women with TB in Vietnam (Long et al., 2001; Johansson et al., 1999) do not publicly acknowledge their health problems because it would lead to poorer chances for marriage. If women and their families *acknowledge* the need for treatment, social and financial barriers may be encountered before health care can be utilized, and this may be influenced by gender-biased normative structures that govern households (Iyer, 2005). Women in some situations are reluctant to use health services because respect, privacy, confidentiality, and information about treatment options are not ensured by the often overworked, underpaid, and gender-insensitive health care providers (Bruce et al., 1998; George, 2007; Govender and Penn-Kekana, 2008; Vlassoff, 1994). The lack of female medical personnel—itself a reflection of gender bias in educational opportunity—is an important barrier to utilization of health services for many women (Zaidi, 1996).

Ironically, a majority of the health workforce is female, and the contributions of women to formal and informal health care systems are significant (George, 2008; Gupta et al., 2003; Joint Learning Initiative, 2004; Ogden et al., 2006; Schindel et al., 2006; WHO, 2006), but undervalued and unrecognized. Health systems tend to ignore women's crucial role as health providers, both within the formal health system (at its lower levels) and as informal providers and unpaid carers in the home. It is estimated that up to 80% of all health care and 90% of HIV/AIDS-related illness care is provided in the home (Uys, 2003; WHO, 2000). However, home carers remain unsupported and unrecognized by the health sector and policy makers. George (this volume, Chapter 8) examines the experiences of nurses, community health workers, and home carers in health systems. The major finding is that these female frontline health workers compensate for the shortcomings of health systems through individual adjustments, at times to the detriment of their own health and livelihoods.

Absence of effective accountability mechanisms for available, affordable, acceptable, and high-quality health services and facilities may seriously hinder women and their families in holding government and other actors accountable for violations of their human rights to health. Govender and Penn-Kekana (this volume, Chapter 7) argue that gender biases and discrimination occur at many levels of the health care delivery environment and affect the patient–provider interaction. Ensuring good interpersonal relationships between patients and providers—an important marker of quality of care—requires a broader approach of gender-sensitive interventions at multiple levels of policies and programs.

Health sector reforms can have fundamental consequences for gender equality and for people as patients in both formal and informal health care, as paid and unpaid care providers, as health care administrators, and as decision makers. The few existing gender analyses of health sector reform programs suggests that many of the reforms may affect women differently than men because of women's greater need for health care due to their reproductive functions, their greater social, cultural, and financial vulnerability, and their greater enrolment as health care providers both within the formal health care sector and the informal care system (Evers and Juárez, 2003; Ford Foundation, 2003; Mackintosh and Tibendebage, 2004; Neema, 2005; Onyango, 2001; Standing, 1997, 2000; Östlin, 2005).

Reforms in Africa included the introduction of new financing mechanisms such as user fees, revolving drug funds, and other community-run financing schemes as well as the use of essential drugs lists to ensure cost-effective use of resources. In the Americas, health sector reform is strongly focused on institutional change through decentralization, privatization, reform of social security systems, and the separation between financing and delivery of health services (Batthyany and Corrêa, this volume, Chapter 5). In Brazil, these reforms were implemented with strong involvement of civil society organizations but this is not true for all countries (Tajer, 2003). Reforms in South East Asia have focused on decentralization and improvement of financing mechanisms (Sharma, 2000). However, while health sector reforms have sometimes addressed their implications for the poor, consequences for gender equity in general and for health care specifically are seldom discussed or taken into consideration in planning (PAHO, 2001). Health sector reform strategies, policies, and interventions, introduced during the last two decades, have therefore had limited success in achieving improved gender equity in health.

Changing How We Care and Cure

Minimizing gender bias in health systems requires systematic approaches to building awareness and transforming values among service providers, steps to improve access to health services, and effective mechanisms for accountability.

The Health Workers for Change project is a departure from conventional training on interpersonal communication that does not take gender into account. It uses a participatory research and learning approach for bringing about improvements in quality of care with emphasis on the need for gender sensitivity in health services (Fonn and Xaba, 2001). It demonstrates the potential for improving health systems development by integrating gender considerations (Vlassoff and Fonn, 2001).

Transforming the medical curriculum is a key measure for building capacity of health care providers in gender analysis and responsiveness. The Gender and Health Collaborative Curriculum Project includes faculty and students from the six medical schools of Ontario as well as members of the Undergraduate Education and the Gender Issues Committees of the Council of Ontario Faculties of Medicine (COFM) working together to produce a resource focused on the role of gender in medical education. The project

aims to improve health care for both women and men through the development of a collaborative, Web-enabled medical curriculum that integrates
gender and health into all aspects of medical education. This integrated
curriculum will be a common provincial resource for use by all Ontario
medical schools (Ontario Women's Health Council, 2007).

Improving women's access to health care requires ensuring that user fees
are not collected at the point of access to the service. Upgrading local (vil-
lage-level) health centers, setting up systems for reliable emergency transport, and making it possible for women and their attendants to stay near
a health facility have yielded good results in countries such as Cuba, Sri
Lanka, Uganda, and, in the Matlab project, in Bangladesh. Many lives
could be saved through preventing and effectively taking care of complications during pregnancy and childbirth. This requires actions aimed at
improving access to a skilled attendant at delivery and to emergency obstetric care, and by improving the referral system to ensure that women with
complications can reach lifesaving emergency care in time.

Women- and adolescent-friendly services can take a range of forms: these
may include youth-only and men-only clinics, women-only services within
existing services, out-reach and community-based services, and different
hours of services in already existing services (Govender and Penn-Kekana,
2008). The Lady Health Workers initiate in Pakistan is the provision of
door-to-door services for women whose mobility and hence access to services is constrained, and has been effective in increasing the uptake of services, improved the adoption of contraceptives, and improved community
health (Douthwaite and Ward, 2005). The Kumar Warmi (Aymara for
'healthy woman') project in Bolivia illustrates how women-centered services, through educational processes, shared decision-making, and linking
with women's groups, can help women overcome negative perceptions of
the doctor–client relationship (Paulson et al., 1996).

Profamilia's Clinica Para El Hombre in Colombia represents one of the
most successful attempts to increase men's access to comprehensive reproductive health services through the introduction of men-only clinics. Quality of care and gender-sensitive patient–provider interactions are central to
the delivery of services. Staff are trained on personal and cultural beliefs
about masculinity, and are encouraged to reflect on their personal attitudes regarding gender and how gender impacts on their interactions with
patients.

INTERMEDIARY FACTORS—BIASED HEALTH RESEARCH

Gender discrimination and bias not only affect differentials in health
needs, health-seeking behavior, treatment, and outcomes, but also permeate the content and process of health research (Eichler et al., 1992; Sen et
al., 2002; Östlin et al., 2004; Theobald et al., 2006). Gender imbalances

in research content include the following dimensions: slow recognition of health problems that particularly affect women; misdirected or partial approaches to women's and men's health needs in different fields of health research; and lack of recognition of the interaction between gender and other social factors. Gender imbalances in the research process include: non-collection of sex-disaggregated data in individual research projects or larger data systems; research methodologies not sensitive to the different dimensions of disparity; methods used in medical research and clinical trials for new drugs that lack a gender perspective and exclude female subjects from study populations; gender imbalance in ethical committees, research funding, and advisory bodies; and differential treatment of women scientists. Mechanisms and policies need to be developed to ensure that gender imbalances in both the content and processes of health research are avoided and corrected.

The importance of having good quality data and indicators for health status, disaggregated by sex and age from infancy through old age, cannot be overstated. Gender-sensitive and human rights–sensitive country-level indicators are essential to guide policies, programs, and service delivery; without them, interventions to change behaviors, or increase participation rates, will operate in a vacuum.

Changing What We Know

Without sex-disaggregated data gender analysis of health is not possible. One good example of recording sex-disaggregated, gender-sensitive, and gender-specific health data comes from Malaysia. In 2000, the Asian-Pacific Resource and Research Centre for Women (ARROW) published *A Framework of Indicators for Action on Women's Health Needs and Rights after Beijing* (2000). This publication was developed as a tool for all government, nongovernment, and international organizations to use in monitoring implementation of the Beijing Platform for Action. Health Canada's Women's Health Indicators project is a research initiative led by the Bureau of Women's Health and Gender Analysis (WHB) to develop, validate, and evaluate a core set of indicators that takes gender and diversity into account. The aim is to improve the ways in which women's health is measured and to more accurately monitor changes in women's health status/outcomes (Colman, 2003). Another good practice comes from Sweden, where every year since 1994 the annual statement of the government policy has declared that a gender equality perspective must permeate all aspects of government policy (Swedish Institute, 2004). At the national level, one of the main measures that have been taken to integrate a gender perspective into every policy area, including health research, is that all official statistics have been disaggregated by sex.

Progress towards developing gender-sensitive indicators to monitor gender equity in health presents a mixed picture. At the international level, the normative role of the UN system coupled with the work of the UN Statistical Division and small innovative units (with large impact) such as the Human Development Report office at UNDP has advanced the availability of data and indicators regarding population health status at the national level. Some of this data, but not all, is disaggregated by sex; this reflects the quality of national data systems from which the UN system draws. Recently, the World Bank (Word Bank, 2007) has proposed strengthening the indicators base for tracking progress towards the MDGs.

In some countries, decennial censuses are supplemented by regular sample surveys that provide more detail and with greater disaggregation on different aspects of health status, behavior, and access to services.[15] To the extent that such data are disaggregated by income/expenditure quintiles, sex, age, location, or other socioeconomic characteristics, it makes possible more careful and nuanced analysis of the way in which different social stratifiers interact to produce gendered health outcomes. Demographic and Health Surveys (DHS) have generated useful data, especially on reproductive behavior but also on less common issues such as domestic violence and women's empowerment (Kishor, 2000). A single survey of this kind can sometimes have a powerful impact. For example, the information in India's second National Family Health Survey (NFHS) on the wide prevalence of domestic violence and attitudes towards it among both women and men catalyzed action to deal with the problem, culminating in the landmark Domestic Violence Act 2005.

The importance of having good quality data and indicators for health status disaggregated by sex and age from infancy through old age cannot be overstated. Surprisingly, in many situations data are not presented in a sex-disaggregated way even if they have been collected. Well-crafted gender-aware indicators can fulfill multiple functions, as "*signal* to all actors involved in the intervention, as *constant reminder* during the life of the intervention, as *measure of performance* in the achievement of gender-aware goals and objectives, and as a *tool* for analyzing shortfalls" (Kabeer and Subrahmanian, 1999, p. 352). The Women and Health Program of WHO's Centre for Health Development (Kobe, Japan) has produced a detailed evaluation of indicators for Gender Equity and Health that is an important resource in this area (WHO, 2003a).

Attention also needs to be paid to the possibility that data may reflect systematic gender biases due to inadequate methodologies that fail to capture women's and men's differential exposure to health risks and vulnerability to diseases (e.g., due to differential health-seeking behavior and insensitivity of diagnostic methodologies). The *BIAS FREE Framework* is an innovative tool designed to provide a unified approach to detect methodological and other types of biases that derive from *any and all* social hierarchies. The Framework identifies three major forms of bias—maintaining hierarchy, failing to recognize differences, and using double standards—and employs a set of 20 analytical questions to alert users to their presence in research (Eichler and Burke, 2006).

Although steps have been taken to include women in clinical trials and other health studies in appropriate numbers, a study by the US General Accounting Office reports that although women now are being adequately represented in clinical trials in the US, the data collected is not being analyzed by gender. Another study found that from 1994 to 1999, out of the 442 original articles including randomized, controlled trials published in the *New England Journal of Medicine*, only 120 met the inclusion criteria (enrolment of women with respect to disease state, funding source, site of trial performance, and use of gender-specific data analysis). On average, 24% women were enrolled and only 14% of the trials performed a gender-specific data analysis (Ramasubbu and Gurum, 2001).

To redress such foot-dragging, research-funding bodies should promote research that broadens the scope of health research and links biomedical and social dimensions, including gender considerations. Ethical and other review boards, editors, and editorial boards should include gender experts to ensure that gender dimensions of research projects are not missed. Medical and related journals should request that papers present data disaggregated by sex and explain observed differences adequately in terms of either sex or gender or both.

REMOVING ORGANIZATIONAL PLAQUE

Gender mainstreaming came to the forefront of gender equity and equality policies after the Beijing Conference on Women in 1995. Mainstreaming was clearly viewed at the time as a major advance, allowing forward movement beyond narrowly focused women's programs or patchwork gender equality legislation. It was understood generally to mean systematic integration of gender perspective at all relevant levels. A number of recent policy reviews have been critical of the progress made during the last decade in mainstreaming for gender equality (OECD/DAC, 2002; Aasen, 2006; Moser and Moser, 2005; AWID, 2006; Eyben, 2006; Mehra and Gupta, 2006; Reisen and Ussar, 2005; Rao and Keller, 2005; European Commission, 2005).

This is true, not only in developing countries but in countries in the European Union, many of which are global champions for women's human rights and gender equality and equity. Insufficient resources, weak organizational mechanisms, and poor political commitment have resulted in fragmented efforts, significant mismatches between stated gender policy and these efforts, and serious gaps between political rhetoric and actual practice. In their chapter on gender mainstreaming in health, Ravindran and Kelkar-Khambete (this volume, Chapter 10) argue that the gap between intention and practice is large. This can be attributed to depoliticization and delinking of gender mainstreaming from social justice agendas; top-down approaches;

hostility within the global policy environment to justice and equity concerns; as well as privatization and retraction of the state's role in health.

Many of the organizational structures of government, and other social and private institutions, through which gender norms have to be challenged and practices altered, have been in existence for decades, even centuries. Thickly encrusted with traditional (usually male-dominated) values, relationships, and methods of work, it has been a serious challenge to expect these same structures to deliver gender equality and equity. Working towards gender equality challenges long-standing male-dominated power structures, and patriarchal social capital (old boys' networks) within organizations. It crosses the boundaries of people's comfort zones by threatening to shake up existing lines of control over material resources, authority, and prestige. It requires people to learn new ways of doing things about which they may not be very convinced, and from which they see little benefit to themselves, and to unlearn old habits and practices. Resistance to gender-equal policies may take the form of trivialization, dilution, subversion, or outright resistance, and can lead to the evaporation of gender equitable laws, policies, or programs.

Despite this less than cheerful situation, positive examples do exist of effective policies. The main goal of gender mainstreaming in Sweden is to tackle the structural roots of gender equality in society at large. It involves taking gender relations into account in all activities by public, private, and voluntary organizations through systematic gender analysis in the design and delivery of all policies and services. Effective coordination and the use of external experts have generated a number of innovative methods for mainstreaming gender such as the 3-R method for analyzing gender-based differences in Representation and Resources, and the Reasons for these differences (European Commission, 2005, p. 106). A broad social consensus has been forged across the political spectrum that insulates gender mainstreaming to some extent from the vagaries of democratic politics.

Sweden's new public health policy, which came into force in 2003, is an excellent example of integrating gender within the framework of an existing equity-oriented public health policy (Östlin and Diderichsen, 2001). This policy is unique in many ways, including the fact that gender is integrally woven into the public health strategy. The policy document specifically highlights its commitment to a gender perspective and to reducing gender-based inequalities in health, alongside reductions in inequalities by socioeconomic groups, ethnic groups, and geographic regions. Gender is thus a crosscutting category within other dimensions of inequalities that the policy seeks to redress (Östlin and Diderichsen, 2001; Agren, 2003; Ravindran and Kelkar-Khambete, 2008).

Tackling this requires effective political leadership, well-designed organizational mandates, structures, incentives, and accountability mechanisms with teeth. It also requires actions to empower women and women's organizations, so that they can collectively press for greater accountability for gender equality and equity. In this volume, Murthy (Chapter 9) observes that four kinds of human rights, instruments, legislation, structures, and tools, have been used by citizens to press for accountability to gender and health. Among other things, the chapter recommends that accountability strategies should be extended to the private health sector and donors, that resources should be earmarked to respond to gender-specific health needs, and that mechanisms for enforcement of policies should be improved.

The Beijing Platform for Action had identified clearly the need for a dual focus on women's empowerment and gender mainstreaming. A detailed review of the links between empowerment and health improvements (Wallerstein, 2006) was done for WHO/EURO's Health Evidence Network. Based on evidence from interventions for youth empowerment, HIV/AIDS prevention, women's empowerment, and patient/family empowerment for health, the review concluded that "the most effective empowerment strategies are those that build on and reinforce authentic participation ensuring autonomy in decision-making, sense of community and local bonding, and psychological empowerment of the community members themselves" (p. 5).

While mainstreaming has been about policy structures, empowerment has typically focused on households and communities. Wallerstein's review concludes that improved education (including adult literacy) for women has clear positive effects for children's health, while income in women's hands through micro-credit or other means has the potential for better family nutrition and health. However, what is really needed for this potential to be realized are simultaneous increases in women's autonomy, mobility, decision-making authority, and power within the household. Without this, micro-credit may end up increasing women's work burdens without giving them greater authority or control. "A meta-analysis of 40 women's empowerment projects showed a wide range of quality of life improvements, including increases in women's advocacy demands and organizational strengths, enhanced services, and policy and government changes as a result of advocacy, with some organizations showing transformed economic conditions for the women" (Wallerstein, 2006, p. 13).

A different evaluation based on mobilization and organization by women sex workers in Sonagachi showed successful reduction in HIV infection and increased condom use (Jana et al., 2004). Its success has been based on "the use of peer outreach workers, broad community concern as the starting point of the project, leadership development of the women, support by health professionals, and the eventual ceding of leadership to a new sex worker association" (Wallerstein, 2006, p. 13). Similar experiences have been found in other parts of India as well.

A third set of experiences draws from the experiences of women community health workers. Meta-analysis of studies on health impact has shown improvements in health care utilization, in patient completion of health education programs, improved immunization coverage along with increased social support, leadership, and advocacy capacity of the health workers themselves. Wallerstein (2006) concludes that "interventions that have been most integrated with the economic, education, and/or political sectors have resulted in greater psychological empowerment, autonomy and authority, and have substantially affected a range of health outcomes" (p. 14).

THE WAY FORWARD

Gender relations of power exist both within and outside the health sector, and they exercise a pernicious influence on the health of people. This volume draws together some of the rapidly growing body of evidence that identifies and explains what gender inequality and inequity mean in terms of differential exposures and vulnerabilities for women versus men, and also how health care systems, and health research, reproduce these inequalities and inequities instead of resolving them. The consequences for people's health are not only unequal and unjust, but also ineffective and inefficient.

This volume also documents the growing numbers of actions by nongovernmental and governmental actors and agencies to challenge these injustices, and to transform beliefs and practices within and outside the health sector, in order to generate sustained changes that can improve people's health and lives. While there are still only a few countries that have taken comprehensive multisectoral actions backed by policies and legislation and supported by civil society actions, there are many smaller cases and examples from which all actors can learn, and which can be the basis for moving forward. We have pointed to a number of examples, some of which have been fully evaluated, and others of which are experimental and hold promise. These actions span a set of seven approaches that are essential for forward movement.

Seven Approaches that can Make a Difference

1. Address the essential structural dimensions of gender inequality

- Transform and deepen the normative framework for women's human rights and achieve them through effective implementation of laws and policies along key dimensions.
- Ensure that resources for and attention to access, affordability, and availability of health services are not damaged during periods of economic reforms, and that women's entitlements, rights, health, and gender equality are protected and promoted, because of the close connections between women's rights to health and their economic situation.
- Support through resources, infrastructure, and effective policies/programs for the women and girls who function as the 'shock absorbers' for families, economies, and societies through their responsibilities in

'caring' for people, and invest in programs to transform both male and female attitudes to caring work so that men begin to take an equal responsibility for such work.

- Expand women's capabilities particularly through education, so that their ability to challenge gender inequality individually and collectively is strengthened.
- Increase women's participation in political and other decision-making processes from household to national and international levels so as to increase their voice and agency.

2. Challenge gender stereotypes and adopt multilevel strategies to change the norms and practices that directly harm women's health

- Create, implement, and enforce formal international and regional agreements, codes, and laws to change norms that violate women's rights to health.
- Work with boys and men through innovative programs for the transformation of harmful masculinist norms, high-risk behaviors, and violent practices.

3. Reduce the health risks of being women and men by tackling gendered exposures and vulnerabilities

- Meet women's and men's differential health needs. Where biological sex differences interact with social determinants to define different needs for women and men in health, policy efforts must address these different needs.
- Tackle social biases that generate differentials in health-related risks and outcomes. Where no plausible biological reason exists for different health outcomes, policies and actions should encourage equal outcomes.
- Address the structural reasons for high-risk behavior. Strategies that aim at changing health-damaging lifestyles of men (or women) at the level of the individual are important but they can be much more effective if combined with measures to change the social environment in which these lifestyles and behaviors are embedded.
- Empower people and communities to take a central role in these actions. For strategies to succeed they must provide positive alternatives that support individuals to take action against the current status quo, which may be either gender blind or gender biased.

4. Transform the gendered politics of health systems by improving their awareness and handling of women's problems as both producers and consumers of health care, improving women's access to health care, and making health systems more accountable to women

- Provide comprehensive and essential health care, universally accessible to all in an acceptable and affordable way and with the participation of women: ensure that user fees are not collected at the point of access to the health service, and prevent women's impoverishment by enforcing rules that adjust user fees to women's ability to pay; offer care to women and men according to their needs, their time, and other constraints.
- Develop skills, capacities, and capabilities among health professionals at all levels of the health system to understand and apply gender perspectives in their work.
- Recognize women's contributions to the health sector, not just in the formal, but also through informal care.
- Strengthen accountability of health policy makers and health care providers in both private and nonprivate clinics to gender and health. Incorporate gender into clinical audits and other efforts to monitor quality of care.

5. Take action to improve the evidence base for policies by changing gender imbalances in both the content and the processes of health research

- Ensure collection of data disaggregated by sex, socioeconomic status, and other social stratifiers by individual research projects as well as through larger data systems at regional and national levels, and the classification and analysis of such data towards meaningful results and expansion of knowledge for policy.
- Women should be included in clinical trials and other health studies in appropriate numbers and the data generated from such research should be analyzed using gender-sensitive tools and methods.
- Research-funding bodies should promote research that broadens the scope of health research and links biomedical and social dimensions, including gender considerations.
- Strengthen women's role in health research. Redress the gender imbalances in research committees, funding, publication, and advisory bodies.

6. Take action to make organizations at all levels function more effectively to mainstream gender equality and equity and empower women for health by creating supportive structures, incentives, and accountability mechanisms

- Gender mainstreaming in government and nongovernment organizations has to be owned institutionally, funded adequately, and implemented effectively. It needs to be supported by an action-oriented gender unit with strong positioning and authority, and civil society linkages to ensure effectiveness and accountability.

- Effective interventions for women's empowerment need to build on and reinforce authentic participation ensuring autonomy in decision-making, sense of community, and local bonding.

7. Support women's organizations that are critical to ensuring that women have voice and agency, that are often at the forefront of identifying problems and experimenting with innovative solutions, that prioritize demands for accountability from all actors, both public and private, and whose access to resources has been declining in recent years

These seven approaches encompass a set of priority actions that need to be taken both within and outside the health sector, and need engagement and accountability from all actors—international and regional agencies, governments, the for-profit sector, civil society organizations, and people's movements. While health ministries nationally, and WHO and its regional organizations internationally, have a critical leadership role in mobilizing political will and energizing coalitions and alliances, no person or organization can be exempt from action to challenge the barriers of gender inequity. Only thus can the continuing vicious circles of health inequality, injustice, ineffectiveness, and inefficiency be broken.

NOTES

1. This chapter is based on the Final Report of the Women and Gender Equity Knowledge Network (Sen et al., 2007a) of the Commission on Social Determinants of Health.
2. The eight MDGs are: eradicating extreme poverty and hunger; achieving universal primary education; promoting gender equality and empowering women; reducing child mortality; improving maternal health; combating HIV/AIDS, malaria, and other diseases; ensuring environmental sustainability; and developing a global partnership for development.
3. The report uses the terms 'stratifiers' and 'stratification' to refer in a broad sense to the different dimensions along which societies are layered into hierarchies of power and control.
4. On February the 11th, the Andalusian Parliament had the representatives of Identidad de Genero as guests for the discussion of a motion introduced by the PSOE (Socialist Party) about transsexual people's rights. The motion was passed with no votes against (Euro-Letter, No 68, March 1999).
5. [T]he growth of selective primary health care approaches, rooted in cost-effectiveness analysis, in the 1980s was also led by international agencies. Although some, such as immunization, had positive impacts on child mortality, their impacts on health systems' ability to respond to the wider range of health problems it faces on a daily basis have been hotly contested. Past debates about selective vs. comprehensive approaches to health system development (Rifkin and Walt 1986) are now again on the agenda with the rise of the Global Health Initiatives, some targeting specific health problems and some particular services, that have brought enormous new levels of funding to health systems within LMICs (US$8.9 billion in 2006 for HIV/AIDS alone) An analysis of the policies, programmes and processes that govern the design and implementation of three Global Health Initiatives (PEPFAR, the

Global Fund and World Bank MAP) suggests that they can have negative effects on health systems and, specifically, gender equity, unless a stronger equity focus guides their future activities. (Hanefeld et al., 2007, cited in Gilson et al., 2007). See past debates in Rifkin and Walt (1986).

6. These include, among others, the UN Conference on Environment and Development (Rio de Janeiro, 1992), the UN Conference on Human Rights (The UN World Conference on Human Rights in Vienna, 1993), the International Conference on Population and Development (Cairo, 1994), the Social Summit (Copenhagen, 1995), the Fourth World Conference on Women (Beijing, 2005), and the International Conference against Racism (The UN World Conference against racism, racial discrimination, xenophobia and related intolerance in Durban, 2001).

7. See http://www.yogyakartaprinciples.org/docs/File/Yogyakarta_Principles_EN.pdf.

8. For example, hemophilia is expressed in men who have the recessive gene in their X chromosome. Some women can be carriers, but as they have two X chromosomes, the recessive gene is not expressed.

9. Examples are gendered health outcomes like violence against women (by definition targeted at women), road traffic accidents (disproportionately affecting men), and drowning, whether during natural disasters (disproportionately affecting women) or due to fishing (disproportionately affecting men).

10. Of the 46 chromosomes each human being has, only one (XX versus XY) differentiates females from males.

11. See http://www.unaids.org/en/Issues/Affected_communities/women.asp (accessed April 9, 2007).

12. In the US, when higher male exposure to driving is controlled for, their higher involvement in crashes disappears; however, this did not hold for male involvement in fatal crashes. The excess risk for fatal crashes among males is especially dramatic among the youngest drivers, and largely attributed to speed and alcohol (see Odero, 1998; Maio et al., 1997; MMWR, 1994).

13. Messing and Östlin (2006) found that women in general face unequal hiring standards, unequal opportunities for training, unequal pay for equal work, unequal access to productive resources, segregation and concentration in female sectors and occupations, different physical and mental working conditions, unequal participation in economic decision-making, and unequal promotion prospects.

14. A *maquiladora* (or *maquila*) is a factory that imports materials and equipment on a duty-free and tariff-free basis for assembly or manufacturing and then reexports the assembled product usually back to the originating country.

15. The National Sample Survey in India is a good example.

REFERENCES

Aasen, B. 2006. *Lessons from Evaluations of Women and Gender Equality in Development cooperation*. Oslo: Norwagian Agency for Development Cooperation (NORAD).

Abane, H. 2004. 'The girls do not learn hard enough so they cannot do certain types of work'—experiences from an NGO-sponsored gender sensitization workshop in a southern Ghanian community. *Community Development Journal* 39: 49–61.

Agnes, F. 2005. Women domestic violence act: A portal of hope. *Combat Law* 4 (6).

Agren, G. 2003. *Sweden's New Public Health Policy. National Public Health Objectives for Sweden*. Stockholm: Swedish National Institute of Public Health.

Aiken, L., S. Clarke, D. Sloane, J. Sochalski, and J. Silber. 2002. Hospital nurse staffing and patient mortality, nurse burnout, and job dissatisfaction. *Jama* 288: 1987–1993.

Albalak, R., N. Bruce, J.P. Mccracken, K.R. Smith, and T. De Gallardo. 2001. Indoor respirable particulate matter concentrations from an open fire, improved cookstove, and LPG/open fire combination in a rural Guatemalan community. *Environ Sci Technol* 35: 2650–2655.

ARROW. 2000. *A Framework of Indicators for Action on Women's Health Needs and Rights after Beijing.* Kuala Lumpur: ARROW.

———. 2005. *Monitoring ten years of ICPD implementation: The way forward to 2015, Asian Country Reports.* Kuala Lumpur: ARROW.

Ashcraft, K.L., and D.K. Mumby. 2004. *Reworking Gender: A Feminist Communicology of Organization.* Thousand Oaks, CA: Sage Publications.

Astbury, G. 2002. Mental health: Gender bias, social position, and depression. In *Engendering International Health: The Challenge of Equity,* edited by G. Sen, A. George, and P. Östlin. Cambridge: MIT Press: 143–166

AWID. 2006. *Where is the Money for Women's Rights? Assessing Resources and the Role of Donors in the Promotion of Women's Rights and the Support of Women's Organisations.* Toronto: Association for Women's Rights in Development.

Barker, G. 2006. Engaging boys and men to empower girls: Reflections from practice and evidence of impact. *Presented at United Nations Division for the Advancement of Women (DAW), in Collaboration with UNICEF, Expert Group Meeting: Elimination of all Forms of Discrimination and Violence Against the Girl Child, September 25–28.* Florence, Italy: UNICEF Innocenti Research Centre (EGM/DVGC/2006/EP.3).

Barker, G., and C. Ricardo. 2005. *Young Men and the Construction of Masculinity in Sub-Saharan Africa,* Washington, D.C.: World Bank.

Bebbington, P. 1998. Sex and depression. *Psychol Med* 28: 1–8.

Bhugra, D., and A. Mastrogianni. 2004. Globalisation and mental disorders. Overview with relation to depression. *Br J Psychiatry* 184: 10–20.

Birdsall, N., R. Levine, and A. Ibrahim. 2005. *Education and Gender Equality. Toward Universal Primary Education: Investments, Incentives, and Institutions.* London: Earthscan, for the UN Millennium Project Task Force on Education and Gender Equality.

Breen, N. 2002. Social discrimination and health: Gender, race, and class in the United States. In *Engendering International Health: The Challenge of Equity,* edited by G. Sen, A. George, and P. Östlin. Cambridge: MIT Press: 223–256.

Brown, A., S. Jejeeboy, I. Shah, and K. Yount. 2001. *Sexual Relations among Young People in Developing Countries: Evidence from WHO Studies.* Geneva: World Health Organization, Department of Reproductive Health Research.

Bruce, J., N. Haberland, K. Miller, and G. Fassihian. 1998. Unrealized quality and missed opportunities in family planning services. In *Clinic-Based Family Planning and Reproductive Health Services in Africa: Findings from Situation Analysis Studies,* edited by K. Miller, R. Miller, I. Askew, M.C. Horn, and L. Ndhlovu. New York: Population Council: 125–39.

Butler, J. 2005. *Undoing Gender.* New York: Routledge.

Campbell, J.C. 2002. Health consequences of intimate partner violence. *Lancet* 359: 1331–1336.

Cedillo Becerril, L.A., S.D. Harlow, R.A. Sanchez, and D.S. Monroy. 1997. Establishing priorities for occupational health research among women working in the Maquiladora Industry. *Int J Occup Environ Health* 3: 221–230.

Chatterjee, M. 1988. *Access to Health.* New Delhi: Manohar Publications.

Coker, A.L., P.H. Smith, L. Bethea, M.R. King, and R.E. Mckeown. 2000. Physical health consequences of physical and psychological intimate partner violence. *Arch Fam Med* 9: 451–457.

Colman,R.,and GPI Atlantic.2003.*A Profile of Women's Health Indicators in Canada*. www.hc-sc.gc.ca/hl-vs/women-femmes/indicators-indicateurs_e.html.

Crenshaw, K. 1991. Mapping the margins: Intersectionality, identity politics, and violence against women of color. *Stanford Law Review* 43: 1241–1299.

CSDH. 2007. The causes of the causes—a draft of the CSDH narrative values. *Paper Presented at the 7th Commissioners' Meeting, January 17–19*. Geneva.

Currah, P., R. Juang, and S. Price Minter, eds. 2006. *Transgender Rights*. Minneapolis: University of Minnesota Press.

Danielsson, M., and G. Lindberg. 2001. Differences between men's and women's health: The old and the new gender paradox. In *Gender Inequalities in Health. A Swedish Perspective*, edited by P. Östlin, M. Danielsson, F. Diderichsen, A. Härenstam, and G. Lindberg. Cambridge: Harvard University Press: 23–66.

deMesa, A.A., and V. Montecinos. 1999. The privatization of social security and women's welfare: Gender effects of the chilean reform. *Latin American Research Review* 34: 7–37.

Desjarlais, R., L. Eisenberg, and B. Good. 1995. *World Mental Health: Problems and Priorities in Low Income Countries*. Oxford: Oxford University Press.

Dewalt, D.A., N.D. Berkman, S. Sheridan, K.N. Lohr, and M.P. Pignone. 2004. Literacy and health outcomes: A systematic review of the literature. *J Gen Intern Med* 19: 1228–1239.

Dion, M. 2006. Women's welfare and social security privatization in Mexico. *International Studies in Gender, State and Society* 13: 400–426.

Douthwaite, M., and P. Ward. 2005. Increasing contraceptive use in rural Pakistan: An evaluation of the lady health worker programme. *Health Policy Plan* 20: 117–123.

Eichler, M., and M.A. Burke. 2006. The bias free framework: A new analytical tool for global health research. *Can J Public Health* 97: 63–68.

Eichler, M., A.L. Reisman, and E.M. Borins. 1992. Gender bias in medical research. *Women and Therapy* 12: 61–70.

European Commission. 2005. Gender-sensitive and women friendly public policies: A comparative analysis of their progress and impact. EQUAPOL Final Report. In *EU Research on Social Sciences and Humanities*, edited by M. Braitwaite. Brussels: European Commission: 1–115.

Evers, B., and M. Juárez. 2003. Understanding the links: Globalization, health sector reform, gender and reproductive health. In *Globalization, Health Sector Reform, Gender and Reproductive Health*. New York: Ford Foundation Reproductive Health Affinity Group: 5–8.

Eyben, R. 2006. The impact of global policies and international practices on pathways of women's empowerment. *Draft Discussion Paper for the Scoping Workshop at Dunford House of the Global Hub for the Research Programme Consortium*. Sussex: Institute for Development Studies.

Fargues, P. 2001. Terminating marriage. In *The New Arab family. Cairo: Papers in Social Science, 24 (1–2)*. Cairo and New York: American University in Cairo Press: 247–272.

Fausto-Sterling, A. 2000. *Sexing the Body: Gender Politics and the Construction of Sexuality*. New York: Basic Book.

Fazio, I. 2004. The family, honour and gender in Sicily: Models and new research. *Modern Italy* 9 (2): 263–280.

Fong, M.S., W. Wakeman, and A. Bhushan. 1996. Toolkit on gender in water and sanitation. In *World Bank Gender Toolkit Series 2*. Washington, DC: World Bank.

Fonn, S., and M. Xaba. 2001. Health workers for change: Developing the initiative. *Health Policy Plan* 16 (1): 13–18.

Ford Foundation. 2003. *Experts' Perspectives on Globalization, Health Sector Reform, Gender and Reproductive Health*. New York: Ford Foundation Reproductive Health Affinity Group.

Forrest, B.D. 1991. Women, HIV, and mucosal immunity. *Lancet* 337: 835–836.

Fried, S.T. 2007. *Women Won't Wait Campaign; Show Us the Money: Is Violence against Women on the HIV and AIDS Donor Agenda?* Washington, DC: Action Aid.

Fry, P.S. 2001. Predictors of health-related quality of life perspectives, self-esteem, and life satisfactions of older adults following spousal loss. An 18-month follow-up study of widows and widowers. *The Gerontologist* 41: 787–798.

Garcia-Moreno, C. 2002. Violence against women: Consolidating a public health agenda. In *Engendering International Health: A Challenge of Equity*, edited by G. Sen, A. George, and P. Östlin. Cambridge: MIT Press: 111-142.

Garcia-Moreno, C., H. Jansen, M. Ellsberg, L. Heise, C.H. Watts. 2006. Prevalence of intimate partner violence: Findings from the WHO multi-country study on women's health and domestic violence. *Lancet* 368: 1260–1269.

George, A. 2007. *The outrageous as ordinary: Primary health care workers' perspectives on accountability in Koppal district, Karnataka state, India*. Brighton: Institute of Development Studies, Sussex University.

———. 2008. Nurses, community health workers, and home carers: gendered human resources compensating for skewed health systems. *Global Public Health*, Supplement 1, 3 (2): 75–89.

Geronimus, A.T. 1992. The weathering hypothesis and the health of African-American women and infants: Evidence and speculations. *Ethn Dis* 2: 207–221.

———. 1996. Black/white differences in the relationship of maternal age to birth-weight: A population-based test of the weathering hypothesis. *Soc Sci Med* 42: 589–597.

Geronimus, A.T., M. Hicken, D. Keene, and J. Bound. 2006. "Weathering" and age patterns of allostatic load scores among blacks and whites in the United States. *Am J Public Health* 96: 826–833.

Geronimus, A.T, and J.P. Thompson. 2004. To denigrate, ignore, or disrupt: Racial inequality in health and the impact of a policy-induced breakdown of African American communities. *Du Bois Rev* 1: 247–279.

Gielen, A.C., K.A. Mcdonnell, J.G. Burke, and P. O'campo. 2000. Women's lives after an HIV-positive diagnosis: Disclosure and violence. *Matern Child Health J* 4: 111–120.

Gilson, L. 2003. Trust and the development of health care as a social institution. *Soc Sci Med* 56: 1453–1468.

Gilson L., J. Doherty, R. Loewenson, V. Francis, with inputs and contributions from the members of the Knowledge Network. 2007. *Final Report of the Health Systems Knowledge Network of the Commission on Social Determinants of Health*. Geneva: World Health Organization.

Girard, F., and W. Nowicka. 2002. Clear and compelling evidence: The polish tribunal on abortion rights. *Reprod Health Matters* 10: 22–30.

Global Campaign for Education. 2005. Girls can't wait: Why girls' education matters and how to make it happen now. *Reprod Health Matters* 13: 19–22.

Goldstein, S., S. Usdin, E. Scheepers, and G. Japhet. 2005. Communicating HIV and AIDS, what works? A report on the impact evaluation of Soul city's fourth series. *J Health Commun* 10: 465–483.

Gross, B., C. van Wijk, and N. Mukherjee. (2001) *Linking Sustainability with Demand, Gender and Poverty: A study in community managed water supply projects in 15 countries*. Washington D.C: UNDP-World Bank WSP and IRC International Water and Sanitation Centre.

Govender, V., and L. Penn-Kekana. 2008. Gender biases and discrimination: A review of health care interpersonal interactions. *Global Public Health*, Supplement 1, 3 (2): 90–103.

Grown C., G. Rao Gupta, and A. Kes. 2005a. Taking action: Achieving gender equality and empowering women. *Report of the UN Millennium Project Taskforce on Education and Gender Equality.* London and Virginia: Earthscan.

Grown, C., G.R. Gupta, and R. Pande. 2005b. Taking action to improve women's health through gender equality and women's empowerment. *Lancet* 365: 541–543.

Gupta, N., K. Diallo, P. Zurn, and M.R. Dal Poz. 2003. Assessing human resources for health: What can be learned from labour force surveys? *Hum Resour Health* 1: 5.

HDR. 2006. *Human Development Report 2006; Beyond Scarcity: Power, Poverty and the Global Water Crisis.* New York: UNDP.

Herz, B., and D. Sperling. 2004. *What Works in Girl's Education: Evidence and Policies from the Developing World.* New York: Council on Foreign Relations.

Hudson, V.M., and A.M. den Boer. 2004. *Bare Branches: The Security Implications of Asia's Surplus Male Population.* Cambridge: MIT Press.

Islam, S.S., A.M. Velilla, E.J. Doyle, and A.M. Ducatman. 2001. Gender differences in work-related injury/illness: Analysis of workers compensation claims. *Am J Ind Med* 39: 84–91.

Iyer, A. 2005. *Gender, Caste, Class, and Health Care Access: Experiences of Rural Households in Koppal District, Karnataka.* Trivandrum: Achutha Menon Centre for Health Science Studies, Sree Chitra Tirunal Institute for Medical Sciences and Technology.

———. 2007. *Gender, caste and class in health: compounding and competing inequalities in rural Karnataka, India.* Liverpool: Division of Public Health, University of Liverpool.

Iyer, A., G. Sen, and A. George. 2007. The dynamics of gender and class in access to health care: Evidence from rural Karnataka, India. *International Journal of Health Services* 37 (3): 537–554.

Iyer, A., G. Sen, and P. Östlin. 2008. The intersections of gender and class in health status and health care. *Global Public Health*, Supplement 1, 3 (2): 13–24.

Jana, S., I. Basu, M.J. Rotheram-Borus, and P.A. Newman. 2004. The Sonagachi project: A sustainable community intervention program. *AIDS Educ Prev* 16: 405–414.

Jewkes, R. 2002. Intimate partner violence: Causes and prevention. *Lancet* 359: 1423–1429.

Jewkes, R., M. Nduna, J. Levin, N. Jama, K. Dunkle, K. Wood, M. Koss, A. Puren, and N. Duvvury. 2007. *Evaluation of Stepping stones: A Gender Transformative Prevention Intervention. Policy Brief, March 2007.* South Africa: MRC.

Joekes, S. 1995. Gender and livelihoods in northern Pakistan. *IDS Bull* 26: 66–74.

Johansson, E., N.H. Long, V.K. Diwan, and A. Winkvist. 1999. Attitudes to compliance with tuberculosis treatment among women and men in Vietnam. *Int J Tuberc Lung Dis* 3: 862–868.

Joint Learning Initiative. 2004. *Human Resources for Health: Overcoming the Crisis.* Cambridge: Harvard University Press.

Josephson, M., M. Lagerstrom, M. Hagberg, and E. Wigaeus Hjelm. 1997. Musculoskeletal symptoms and job strain among nursing personnel: A study over a three year period. *Occup Environ Med* 54: 681–685.

Kabeer, N., and R. Subrahmanian. 1999. Following through the process: Implementation, monitoring and evaluation. In *Institutions, Relations and Outcomes: A*

Framework and Case Studies for Gender-Aware Planning, Edited by N. Kabeer, and R. Subrahmanian. New Delhi: Kali for Women: 339–360.

Keleher, H., and L. Franklin. 2008. Changing gendered norms about women and girls at the level of household and community: A review of the evidence. *Global Public Health*, Supplement 1, 3 (2): 42–57.

Kelly, L.M. 2006. Polygyny and HIV/AIDS: A health and human rights approach. *Journal for Juridical Science* 31: 1–38.

Kim, J., and M. Motsei. 2002. "Women enjoy punishment": Attitudes and experiences of gender-based violence among PHC nurses in rural South Africa. *Soc Sci Med* 54: 1243–1254.

Kishor, S. 2000. Empowerment of women in Egypt and links to the survival and health of their infants. In *Women's Empowerment and Demographic Processes: Moving beyond Cairo*, edited by H. Presser, and G. Sen. New York: Oxford University Press: 119–156.

Krieger, N., D.L. Rowley, A.A. Herman, B. Avery, and M.T. Phillips. 1993. Racism, sexism, and social class: Implications for studies of health, disease, and well-being. *Am J Prev Med* 9: 82–122.

Labidi, L. 2001. *From sexual submission to voluntary commitment: The transformation of family ties in contemporary Tunisia*. Cairo and New York: American University in Cairo Press.

Labonté R., C. Blouin, M. Chopra, K. Lee, C. Packer, M. Rowson, T. Schrecker, D. Woodward, and other contributors to the Globalization Knowledge Network. 2007. Towards health-equitable globalisation: Rights, regulation and redistribution. *Final Report of the Globalization Knowledge Network, World Health Organization Commission on Social Determinants of Health*. Globalization Knowledge Network. Ottawa: Institute of Population Health, University of Ottawa.

Laflamme, L., and E. Eilert-Petersson. 2001. Injury risks and socioeconomic groups in different settings. Differences in morbidity between men and between women at working ages. *Eur J Public Health* 11: 309–313.

Laurie, M., and R.P. Petchesky. 2008. Gender, health and human rights in sites of political exclusion. *Global Public Health*, Supplement 1, 3 (2): 25–41.

Letourneau, E.J., M. Holmes, and J. Chasedunn-Roark. 1999. Gynecologic health consequences to victims of interpersonal violence. *Womens Health Issues* 9: 115–120.

Long, N.H., E. Johansson, V.K. Diwan, and A. Winkvist. 2001. Fear and social isolation as consequences of tuberculosis in Vietnam: A gender analysis. *Health Policy* 58: 69–81.

Mackintosh, M., and P. Tibendebage. 2004. *Gender and Health Sector Reform: Analytical Perspective on African Experience*. Geneva: UNRISD.

Maio, R., F. Waller, F. Blow, E. Hill, and K. Singer. 1997. Alcohol abuse/dependence in motor vehicle crash victims presenting to the emergency department. *Academic Emergency Medicine* 4: 256–262.

Mayhew, C. 2003. Occupational violence: A neglected occupational health and safety issue? *Policy and Practice in Health and Safety* 1: 31–58.

Mehra, R., and R. Gupta. 2006. *Gender Mainstreaming: Making it Happen*. Washington, DC: International Center for Research on Women.

Messing, K. 2004. Physical exposures in work commonly done by women. *Can J Appl Physiol* 29: 639–656.

Messing, K., and P. Östlin. 2006. *Gender Equality, Work and Health: A Review of the Evidence*. Geneva: World Health Organization.

Mishra, V.K., R.D. Retherford, and K.R. Smith. 1999. Biomass cooking fuels and prevalence of tuberculosis in india. *Int J Infect Dis* 3: 119–129.

Misra, G., and R. Chandiramani, eds. 2005. *Sexuality, Gender and Rights. Exploring Theory and Practice in South and Southeast Asia*. New Delhi: Sage Publications.

MMWR. 1994. MMWR—Morbidity and mortality weekly report. *US Department of Health and Human Services*, June.

Monash, R., and J.T. Buerma. 2004. Orphanhood and childcare patterns in Sub-Saharan Africa: An analysis of national surveys from 40 countries. *AIDS* 18: S55–S65.

Moser, C., and A. Moser. 2005. Gender mainstreaming since Beijing: A review of success and limitations in international institutions. *Gender and Development* 13: 11–23.

Neema, S. 2005. *The impact of health policies and health sector reform on the readiness of health systems to respond to women's health needs, with special focus on reproductive health, reproductive rights and HIV/AIDS.* Paper prepared for the UN Division for Advancement of Women (DAW) Experts Group Meeting in Bangkok, Thailand. Document nr: EGM/WPD-EE/2005/EP.11, 3 November 2005.

Odero, W. 1998. Alcohol-related road traffic injuries in Eldoret, Kenya. *East African Medical Journal* 75: 708–711.

OECD/DAC. 2002. *Gender Equality in Sector Wide Approaches a Reference Guide.* Paris: Development Assistance Committee, OECD.

Oei, T.P., and D.M. Kerschbaumer. 1990. Peer attitudes, sex, and the effects of alcohol on simulated driving performance. *Am J Drug Alcohol Abuse* 16: 135–146.

Ogden, J., S. Esim, and C. Grown. 2006. Expanding the care continuum for HIV/AIDS: Bringing carers into focus. *Health Policy Plan* 21: 333–342.

Ontario Women's Health Council. 2007. Gender, and medical education toolkit. In *Gender and Health Collaborative Curriculum Project.* http://www.genderand-health.ca/en/modules/.

Onyango, C. 2001. *Gender and Equity in Health Sector Reform: A Review of Literature.* Washington, DC: PAHO/WHO.

Östlin, P. 2002a. Examining 'work' and its effect on health. In *Engendering International Health: The Challenge of Equity*, edited by G. Sen, A. George, and P. Östlin. Cambridge: MIT Press: 63–82.

———. 2002b. Gender inequalities in health: The significance of work. In *Gender and Socioeconomic Inequalities in Health*, edited by S.Wamala, and J. Lynch. Lund: Studentlitteratur: 43–61.

———. 2005. *What Evidence Is There about the Effects of Health Care Reforms on Gender Equity, Particularly in Health?* Geneva: World Health Organization, Regional Office, Health Evidence Network.

Östlin, P., and F. Diderichsen. 2001. Equity-oriented national strategy for public health in sweden: A case study. In *Policy Learning Curve Series*, Number 1, edited by Anna Ritsatakis. Brussels: European Centre for Health Policy, World Health Organization: 1–38.

Östlin, P., A. George, and G. Sen. 2001. Gender, health, and equity. The intersections. In *Challenging Inequities in Health: From Ethics to Action*, edited by T. Evans, M. Whitehead, F. Diderichsen, A. Bhuiya, and M. Wirth. New York: Oxford University Press: 175–189.

Östlin, P., G. Sen, and A. George. 2004. Paying attention to gender and poverty in health research: Content and process issues. *Bull World Health Organ* 82; 740–745.

PAHO. 2001. *Evaluating the Impact of Health Reforms on Gender Equity—A PAHO Guide.* Washington, DC: Pan American Health Organization

Parker, R., and P. Aggleton, eds. 2007. *Culture, Society and Sexuality.* New York: Routledge.

Paulson, S., M.E. Gisbert, and M. Quiton. 1996. *Case Studies of Two Women's Health Projects in Bolivia: Casa de la Mujer, Santa Cruz; CIDEM/Kumar Warmi, El Alto.* Research Triangle Park, NC: Family Health International.

Piccinelli, M., and G. Wilkinson. 2000. Gender differences in depression. Critical review. *Br J Psychiatry* 177: 486–492.

Pronyk, P.M., J.R. Hargreaves, J.C. Kim, L.A. Morison, G. Phetla, C. Watts, J. Busza, and J.D. Porter. 2006. Effect of a structural intervention for the prevention of intimate-partner violence and HIV in rural South Africa: A cluster randomised trial. *Lancet* 368: 1973–1983.

Pronyk, P.M., J.C. Kim, J.R. Hargreaves, M.B. Makhubele, L.A. Morison, C. Watts, and J.D.H. Porter. 2005. Microfinance and HIV prevention—emerging lessons from rural South Africa. *Small Enterprise Development* 16: 26–38.

Puentes-Markides, C. 1992. Women and access to health care. *Soc Sci Med* 35: 619–626.

Quisumbing, A.R., and J.A. Maluccio. 1999. Intrahousehold allocation and gender relations: New empirical evidence. In *Policy Research Report on Gender and Development, Working Paper Series, No. 2*, edited by The World Bank: Development Research Group/Poverty Reduction and Economic Management Network. Washington, DC: World Bank.

Raghupathy, S. 1996. Education and the use of maternal health care in Thailand. *Soc Sci Med* 43: 459–471.

Rahman, A., A. Mohamedani, E.M. Mirgani, and A.M. Ibrahim. 1996. Gender aspects and women's participation in the control and management of malaria in Central Sudan. *Soc Sci Med* 42: 1433–1446.

Ramasubbu, K., and H. Gurum. 2001. Gender bias in clinical trials: Double standards still apply? *Journal of Women's Health Based Medicine* 10: 757–764.

Rao, A., and D. Keller. 2005. The lack of sufficient analytical work to back it up has meant that, given the broadness of the definitions, gender mainstreaming suffers from the humpty-dumpty syndrome. *Gender and Development* 13: 57–69.

Rao Gupta, G., E. Weiss, and W. D. 1996. Gender and the global HIV/AIDS pandemic. In *The Gendered New World Order: Militarism, Development and the Environment*, edited by J. Turpin, and Lorentzen L.A. New York: Routledge: 147-160.

Ravindran, T.K.S. 1991. *Caste and the Agrarian Structure: A Study of Chingleput District, Tamil Nadu, South India*. Oxford: IBH Publishing Co.

Ravindran, T.K.S., and A. Kelkar-Khambete. 2008. Gender mainstreaming in health: Looking back, looking forward. *Global Public Health*, Supplement 1, 3 (2): 121–142.

Reisen, V.M., and M. Ussar. 2005. *Accountability Upside Down: Gender Equality in a Partnership for Poverty Reduction*. Brussels and Uruguay: Eurostep/Social Watch.

Rifkin, S.B., and G. Walt. 1986. Why health improves: Defining the issues concerning 'comprehensive primary health care' and 'selective primary health care. *Social Science Medicine* 23: 559–566.

Rogerson, S.J., L. Hviid, P.E. Duffy, R.F. Leke, and D.W. Taylor. 2007. Malaria in pregnancy: Pathogenesis and immunity. *Lancet Infect Dis* 7: 105–117.

Russo, N.F. 1990. Overview: Forging research priorities for women's mental health. *Am Psychol* 45: 368–373.

Schindel, J., D. Cherner, E. O'neil, K. Solomon, B. Immartino, and J. Santimauro. 2006. *Workers Who Care: A Graphical Profile of the Frontline Health and Health Care Workforce*. San Francisco: Robert Wood Johnson Foundation/Health Workforce Solutions LLC.

Schulz, A.J., and L. Mullings, eds. 2006. *Gender, Race, Class and Health: Intersectional Approaches*. San Francisco: Jossey-Bass.

Sen, G., A. George, and P. Östlin. 2002. Engendering health equity: A review of research and policy. In Engendering International Health—The Challenge of Equity, edited by G. sen, A. George, and P. Östlin. Cambridge: MIT Press: 1-34.

Sen, G., and P. Östlin. 2008. Gender inequity in health: Why it exists and how we can change it. *Global Public Health*, Supplement 1, 3 (2): 1–12.

Sen, G., P. Östlin, and A. George. 2007a. *Unequal, Unfair, Ineffective and Inefficient -Gender Inequity in Health: Why it exists and how we can change it. Final report of the Women and Gender Equity Knowledge Network to the WHO Commission on Social Determinants of Health.* Bangalore and Stockholm: Indian Institute of Management Bangalore and Karolinska Institutet.

Sen, G., A. Iyer, and A. George. 2007b. Systematic hierarchies and systemic failures: Gender and health inequities in Koppal district. *Economic and Political Weekly* XLII: 682–690.

Sharma, D.C. 2000. Who to support health reforms in South East Asian region. *Lancet* 356: 839.

Shulman, C.E., and E.K. Dorman. 2003. Importance and prevention of malaria in pregnancy. *Trans R Soc Trop Med Hyg* 97: 30–35.

Sibai, A.M., K. Sen, M. Baydoun, and P. Saxena. 2004. Population ageing in Lebanon: Current status, future prospects and implications for policy. *Bull World Health Organ* 82: 219–225.

Smith, K.M., and M. Maeusezahl-Feuz. 2004. Indoor air pollution from household use of solid fuels. In *Comparative Quantification of Health Risks: The Global and Regional Burden of Disease Due to Selected Major Risk Factors.* Geneva: World Health Organization: 1435–1494.

Snow, R. 2002. *Sex, Gender and Traffic Accidents: Addressing Male Risk Behavior.* Geneva: World Health Organization.

———. 2008. Sex, gender, and vulnerability. *Global Public Health*, Supplement 1, 3 (2): 58–74.

Standing, H. 1997. Gender and equity in health sector reform programmes: A review. *Health Policy Plan* 12: 1–18.

———. Standing, H. 2000. *Gender impacts of health reforms. The current state of policy and implementation.* Paper presented at Asociación Latinoamericana de Medicinia Social Meeting in Havana, Cuba.

Stiglitz, J.E., and A. Charlton. 2005. *Fair Trade for All. How Trade Can Promote Development.* Oxford: Oxford University Press.

Stoduto, G., Mann, R., Mitchell, B., Suurvali, H., Koski-Jannes, A., Room, R. & Harrison, S. (1998). *Existing Programs for Convicted Drinking Drivers in Canada.* Toronto: Addiction Research Foundation.

Swedish Institute. 2004. *Fact Sheets on Sweden: Equality between Women and Men.* Stockholm: Swedish Institute.

Tajer, D. 2003. Latin American social medicine: Roots, development during the 1990s, and current challenges. *Am J Public Health* 93: 2023–2027.

Thaddeus, S., and D. Maine. 1994. Too far to walk: Maternal mortality in context. *Soc Sci Med* 38: 1091–1110.

Theobald, S., B.N. Simwaka, and B. Klugman. 2006. Gender, health and development III: Engendering health research. *Progress in Development Studies* 6 (4): 337–342.

UNAIDS. 1999. *HIV/AIDS Prevention in the Context of New Therapies.* Geneva: UNAIDS.

UNAIDS. 2006. *Report on the Global AIDS Epidemic 2006.* Geneva: UNAIDS.

UNAIDS/UNFPA/UNIFEM. 2004. *Women and HIV/AIDS: Confronting the Crisis. A Joint Report.* Geneva: UNAIDS.

UNFPA. 2002. *State of World Population 2002—People, Poverty and Possibilities: Making Development Work for the Poor.* New York: United Nations Population Fund.

UNFPA. 2003. *State of World Population 2003. Making 1 Billion Count: Investing in Adolescents' Health and Rights.* New York: United Nations Population Fund.

UNFPA. 2006. *State of World Population 2006. A Passage to Hope Women and International Migration.* New York: United Nations Population Fund.

UNICEF. 2006. *The State of the World's Children: Excluded and Invisible.* New York: UNICEF.

United Nations. 1948. *Universal Declaration of Human Rights.* New York: United Nations.

United Nations. 1993. *The Report of the UN World Human Rights Conference in Vienna.* Vienna: United Nations.

United Nations. 1994. Report of the international conference on population and development. *United Nations International Conference on Population and Development (ICPD), September 5–13.* Cairo, Egypt.

United Nations. 1995. *Report of the fourth world conference on women. United Nations World Conference on Women,* September 4–15. Beijing, China. New York: United Nations.

United Nations. 2001. Report of the world conference against racism, racial discrimination, xenophobia and related intolerance. *World Conference against Racism, Racial Discrimination, Xenophobia and Related Intolerance, August 31–September 7.* Durban, South Africa.

United Nations. 2005. Taking action: Achieving gender equality and empowering women. *UN Millennium Project: Task Force on Education and Gender Equity.*

Usdin, S., E. Scheepers, S. Goldstein, and G. Japhet. 2005. Achieving social change on gender-based violence: A report on the impact evaluation of Soul city's fourth series. *Soc Sci Med* 61: 2434–2445.

Ustun, T.B., J.L. Ayuso-Mateos, S. Chatterji, C. Mathers, and C.J. Murray. 2004. Global burden of depressive disorders in the year 2000. *Br J Psychiatry* 184: 386–392.

Uys, L. 2003. Guest editorial: Longer-term aid to combat AIDS. *J Adv Nurs* 44: 1–2.

Vlassoff, C. 1994. Gender inequalities in health in the third world: Uncharted ground. *Social Science and Medicine* 39: 1249–1259.

Vlassoff, C., and S. Fonn. 2001. Health workers for change as a health systems management and development tool. *Health Policy Plan* 16: 47–52.

Wallace, T. 2006. *Evaluating Stepping Stones. A Review of Existing Evaluations and Ideas for Future M&E Work.* London: ActionAid International.

Wallerstein, N. 2006. *What is the evidence on effectiveness of empowerment to improve health?* Report for the Health Evidence Network. Copenhagen: Regional Office for Europe, World Health Organization.

Watkins, R.E., and A.J. Plant. 2006. Does smoking explain sex differences in the global tuberculosis epidemic? *Epidemiol Infect* 134: 333–339.

Watts, S. 2004. Women, water management and health. *Emerg Infect Dis* 10: 2025–2026.

WHO. 2000. *Fact Sheets on HIV/AIDS for Nurses and Midwives.* Geneva: World Health Organization.

WHO. 2001. *World Health Report.* Geneva: World Health Organization.

WHO. 2002a. *Gender and Tuberculosis.* Geneva: World Health Organization, Department of Gender and Women's Health.

WHO. 2002b. *The World Health Report 2002. Reducing Risks, Promoting Healthy Life.* Geneva: World Health Organization.

WHO. 2003a. *Comparative Evaluation of Indicators for Gender Equality and Health.* Kobe, Japan: Women and Health Programme, Centre for Health Development, World Health Organization.

WHO. 2003b. *Gender, health and ageing. Fact Sheet.* Geneva: Department of Gender and Women's Health and Unit of Ageing and Life Course, World Health Organization.

WHO. 2003c. *Integrating Gender into HIV/AIDS Programmes: A Review Paper.* Geneva: World Health Organization, Gender and Women's Health Department.

WHO. 2005. *WHO's Multi-Country Study on Women's Health and Domestic Violence against Women*. Geneva: World Health Organization.

WHO. 2006. *The World Health Report—Working Together for Better Health*. Geneva: World Health Organization.

WHO/UNICEF. 2003. *The Africa Malaria Report 2003*. Geneva: World Health Organization/UNICEF.

Wildsmith, E.M. 2002. Testing the weathering hypothesis among Mexican-origin women. *Ethn Dis* 12: 470–479.

World Bank. 2007. Promoting gender equality and women's empowerment. In *Global Monitoring Report, Millennium Development Goals: Confronting the Challenges of Gender Equality and Fragile States*, edited by World Bank. Washington, DC: World Bank: 105–148.

Yount, K.M., and E.M. Agree. 2005. Differences in disability among older women and men in Egypt and Tunisia. *Demography* 42: 169–187.

Yount, K.M., E.M. Agree, and C. Rebellon. 2004. Gender and use of health care among older adults in Egypt and Tunisia. *Soc Sci Med* 59: 2479–2497.

Zaidi, S.A. 1996. Gender perspectives and quality of care in underdeveloped countries: Disease, gender and contextuality. *Soc Sci Med* 43: 721–730.

Zwane, P.A., and M. Kremer. 2007. *What works in fighting diarrheal diseases in developing countries? A critical review*. The World Bank Research Observer Advance Access published online on May 4, 2007, The World Bank Research Observer, doi:10.1093/wbro/lkm002.

2 The Social Body
Gender and the Burden of Disease

Rachel Snow

INTRODUCTION

Gender is a particularly complex social determinant of health because it interacts with, and is closely identified with, biologic dimensions of vulnerability. Research efforts to understand 'what gender does' to health are challenging for several reasons, including the fact that sex and gender are frequently conflated in the epidemiologic and medical literature. While a growing number of health studies claim to include an analysis of gender, they use the terms *sex* and *gender* interchangeably, and go no further than including sex/gender as one bivariate category in their analysis. By using the terms *gender* and *sex* interchangeably, the public health literature implicitly endorses the notion that gender is an extension of sex. Recent studies offer us disaggregated data by sex, but such data alone does little to further our understanding of whether observed sex differentials are attributable to underlying chromosomal sex differences, to gender experience, or a combination of factors.

Why would this matter? Because our approach to interventions could be different depending on the answer—sex-linked vulnerabilities attributable to *gendered experience* open room for debate about prevailing gender norms, and whether gendered expectations may be leading to more harm than good. An acknowledgment that certain aspects of gendered behavioral expectations are harmful to health, or even potentially fatal, begs a discussion of whether re-visioning gender may be warranted for public health purposes.

In this chapter I compare the 2002 global disability adjusted life years (DALYs) for males and females, and illustrate how biologic differences in sex chromosomes contribute to a subset of these differentials through intrinsic vulnerabilities (for example, birth asphyxia among males, glaucoma among females). I describe how a further subset of health conditions with large differentials by sex are more directly attributable to gendered patterns of work and social experience (e.g., road traffic accidents among males, trachoma among females). With a third list of health conditions, I illustrate how sex and gender vulnerabilities may be overlaid on one another in ways that can exacerbate sex differences in outcome (e.g., the female excess in blindness), or mitigate risks. A residual group of health outcomes that disproportionately affect one sex remain mystifying (e.g., the high burden of gout among males, the high burden of depression among females), because our current understanding of causality is incomplete.

In the second part of the chapter I argue that gender effects on health are characterized by a capacity to change rapidly over time and space, in response to fashion, media, or public policy. As such, they invite the possibility for interventions that directly target gender-based health risks. Yet even when the impact of gender on health is substantial, and appears amenable to intervention, such efforts to intervene have been limited. This hesitation to intervene when gendered socialization and gender discrimination harm, suggests an abiding unwillingness to design policies or programs that might instrumentally challenge gendered identities. A more open reflection on gender interventions is called for in the interest of health.

DEFINITIONS

Before proceeding, let me affirm the definitions used in this chapter. The term *biologic sex* refers to the developmental differentiations in anatomy and physiology that are a direct consequence of the inherited composition of sex chromosomes (46 XX versus 46 XY karyotypes). It is this difference in sex chromosomes that leads to differentiation of the gonads, steroid production, and, eventually, secondary sex characteristics. The cascade of differentiating events is well underway in the unborn fetus at 20 weeks, and accelerates once again at puberty. Both before birth and after puberty it is the dramatic quantitative differences in the production of hormones (i.e. androgens and estrogens) that serve as the intermediaries between the sex genotype (i.e., the inherited sex chromosomes) and the manifestation of physical characteristics observed in postpubertal males and females (Federman, 2006).

It is the phenotype of sex,[1] or whether an individual is judged to *look* male or female by others, that evokes a constellation of *gendered social expectations*, *responsibilities*, and *obstacles*; such a gendered experience incurs health risks unrelated to chromosomal sex itself.

SEX DIFFERENCES IN HEALTH

To conduct a review of sex, gender, and vulnerability, one must have sex-disaggregated data. Such data is increasingly available in the health field, but not in all countries or international databases. The aggregate data used for this analysis are taken from the World Health Organization's (WHO) original Global Burden of Disease (GBD) 2002 estimates of DALYs by age, sex, and cause, *without age-weighting or discounting* (DALYs [0,0]). DALYs provide an aggregate measure of healthy years of life lost due to premature death or disability. These estimates are extremely rough, as they reflect the many extant gaps in regional, and thereby global, epidemiologic data. Epidemiologic data itself may be subject to systematic biases, including intrinsic sex and gender biases (Sundby, 1997; Hanson, 2002). For example, select conditions are known to be underreported by one sex or another due to gender-based fears of stigma and discrimination, e.g., infertility or domestic violence among females, sexual dysfunction among males. In select regions of northwest India, China, and South Korea, child health data may be more accurate for male children, given persistent evidence of son-preference (Das Gupta et al., 2003), and discrimination against health-seeking for girl children (Chen et al., 1981; Das Gupta, 1987; Das Gupta et al., 2003).

Furthermore, the estimation of DALYs requires the generation of disability weights, i.e., subjective estimations of how 'burdensome' a given illness is for a human life. These estimations have been found to vary substantially depending on the local culture and professional status of those undertaking the estimations (Sadana, 1998; Jelsma et al., 2000). In Zimbabwe and Cambodia, for example, nonprofessionals weighted infertility as substantially more burdensome than did the Burden of Disease experts. Other conditions affecting marriage prospects for women, such as vitiligo, were also ranked higher by local evaluators in Cambodia, leading to criticism that disability weights reflect the gender biases of elite male health professionals.[2]

Substantial criticism has also been raised over the use of age-weighting and discounting in the DALY, but use of these adjustments is optional, and the present analysis makes use of DALYs *without* weighting or discounting [DALYs 0,0]. While a full account of the arguments against age-weighting and discounting are beyond the scope of this chapter, the rationale for age-weighting, i.e., an *a priori* assumption that a given year of life at different ages has greater or lesser value to society, is persuasively rejected by Anand and Hanson (1997). With regard to discounting, it is sufficient to quote Beermann (1999): "Ethical criteria become relevant to this question, because, health (or life-years) is a basic aspect of life, so that correspondingly there exists a basic right to health. The *specific* ethical problem in this context is the problem of justice between generations and the general answer to the problem is that current and future generations must be treated equally."

Acknowledging the underlying weaknesses in epidemiologic coverage of the DALY, and possibilities for systematic underreporting for the poor and for women's conditions, these estimates still remain the best available source on the *relative* global status of health outcomes, especially if used *without* age-weighting or discounting, as provided here.

Based on the 2002 global data for all ages combined, the 10 leading causes of lost DALYs among females and males are listed in Table 2.1. The first three leading causes are similar for males and females; at least when viewed in large aggregate ICD-10[3] categories: lower respiratory conditions, HIV, and diarrheal disease top the list for both sexes. Thereafter, sex differences of relative magnitude emerge, with ischemic heart disease, low birth weight, malaria, cerebrovascular disease, and birth trauma on both lists, but with differences in absolute numbers of DALYs, as well as relative rank order. The overall greater DALY burden among males worldwide is evident in the absolute numbers of DALYs lost in the top 10 conditions, e.g., the tenth ranked condition for males is still accounting for 44 million DALYs worldwide; females, on the other hand, have two conditions on their list that contribute less than 35 million DALYs.

The top 10 lists are also distinct in telltale ways, i.e., in the appearance of two injury-related categories on the male list, i.e., unintentional injury and road traffic accidents, and the appearance of unipolar depressive disorders on the female list. The relative and absolute importance of accident and injury to men's health emerges under many separate conditions in the GBD statistics. Alcohol contributes to road traffic accidents, especially fatal accidents. A cluster of health outcomes that include substance abuse (alcohol or drug) and their direct or indirect consequences (such as traffic accidents) are consistently in excess among males (see further discussion in the following pages).

Table 2.1   Top 10 Causes of Disease or Disability for Males and Females, Based on the Number of Total Global DALYS Lost at all Ages—Data Based on DALYs [0,0] Published in 2002 (GBD 2002)

Males (all ages)		*Females (all ages)*	
Cause	*DALYs*	*Cause*	*DALYs*
1 Lower respiratory infections	99,057,981	Lower respiratory infections	97,801,108
2 HIV	78,020,596	HIV	73,516,955
3 Diarrheal diseases	71,883,930	Diarrheal diseases	67,296,145
4 Ischemic heart disease	64,504,498	Malaria	52,646,469
5 Low birth weight	58,925,647	Low birth weight	51,321,438
6 Other unintentional injuries	49,236,025	Ischemic heart disease	50,082,860
7 Malaria	47,184,421	Cerebrovascular disease	47,623,180
8 Cerebrovascular disease	46,437,060	Other infectious diseases	45,068,486
9 Road traffic accidents	45,112,383	Birth asphyxia and birth trauma	34,940,346
10 Birth asphyxia and birth trauma	44,068,687	Unipolar depressive disorders	32,507,673

Women's apparent vulnerability to unipolar depression in the top 10 list is echoed by excess female DALYs for a range of other psychiatric conditions, including panic disorder, post-traumatic stress disorder, and obsessive compulsive disorder; the excess female DALYs for these outcomes is found in many national and cross-national studies (Hallstrom, 2001; Angst et al., 2002; Hopcraft and Bradley, 2007). Several authors have highlighted possible gender biases in current diagnostic instruments that would lead to underdiagnosis of male depression (Rutz, 1999; Bech, 2001; Moeller Leimkuehler et al., 2007). The feminist community, in fact, has questioned assumptions that women are inherently vulnerable to mental illness for some time (Chessler, 1972), and the diagnosis and gendered causes of depression may receive more concerted attention given growing interest in male depression (van Grootheest et al., 1999; Han et al., 2006; Moeller Leimkuehler et al., 2007).

A more compelling perspective on male–female sex differences is provided by looking at conditions for which there are large disparities in DALYs by sex. Tables 2.2 and 2.3 list all conditions for which males or females, respectively, have a 25% or greater excess in overall DALYs.

ATTRIBUTING HEALTH OUTCOMES TO SEX OR GENDER

Among the conditions listed in these tables one can start to parse out a subset of outcomes that are intrinsically linked to an XX or XY genotype and sex-linked differences in function (and vulnerability). For others, vulnerabilities are clearly associated with specific types of jobs and social exposures that are socially divided between the sexes. A further group of conditions are impossible to classify as attributable to sex or gender, either because both dimensions are involved in complex ways, or because the level of fundamental understanding (and corresponding basic research) is inadequate.

Differences in health outcome that are linked to an XX or XY karyotype (Table 2.4) include the risk of hemophilia among XY karyotypes, and the vulnerability to testicular and prostate cancers made possible by the karyotypes encoding the growth and development of a prostate and testes; likewise, corresponding XX karyotypes allow the development of a cervix and ovaries. Male fetal lung development is also distinct from that of females in utero, such that male pulmonary function matures more slowly, contributing to more respiratory distress syndromes and lung-related injuries among male newborns. The male excess of 35–50% for a wide range of respiratory-related causes of death in the newborn, including infant respiratory distress syndromes (IRDS), sudden infant death syndrome (SIDS), upper respiratory infections, and asphyxia (Stevenson et al., 2000), are increasingly theorized to reflect an X-linked recessive allele, i.e., a sex-linked chromosomal vulnerability (Mage and

Table 2.2   Select Health Conditions for which Global DALYs [0,0] Lost to Males Are at Least 25% Above Those Lost to Females (GBD 2002)

Condition	Male DALYs	Female DALYs	Male DALYS / Female DALYS
War	9,306,296	1,131,676	8.223
Gout	4,246,359	572,741	7.414
Alcohol Use Disorders	14,810,111	2,662,637	5.562
Road and Traffic Accidents	45,112,383	9,532,961	4.732
Violence	27,470,156	6,810,306	4.034
Other Intentional Injuries	496,974	126,953	3.915
Drug Use Disorders	6,006,662	1,616,742	3.715
Lymphatic Filariasis	6,248,138	2,056,275	3.039
Mouth and Propharynx Cancers	4,751,823	1,991,476	2.386
Lung Cancer (Trachea & Bronchus)	15,232,399	6,687,840	2.278
Liver Cancer	9,409,480	4,208,880	2.236
Drowning	13,983,352	6,795,333	2.058
Bladder Cancer	1,913,556	964,949	1.983
Anorectal Atresia	49,504	25,843	1.916
Hepatitis B	2,645,774	1,408,635	1.878
Poisoning	8,927,574	5,011,169	1.782
Esophagus Cancer	5,266,748	3,049,496	1.727
Trypanosomiasis	1,741,306	1,043,857	1.668
TB	37,298,748	22,944,907	1.626
Peptic Ulcer Disease	4,574,045	2,939,246	1.556
Stomach Cancer	9,576,685	6,171,105	1.552
Schistosomiasis	1,025,505	666,404	1.539
Other Unintentional Injuries	49,236,025	32,020,194	1.538
Falls	14,429,845	9,532,961	1.514
Cirrhosis of the Liver	14,613,849	9,734,719	1.501
Renal Agenesis	104,192	69,973	1.489
Self-Inflicted Injuries	21,665,217	15,201,138	1.425
Leprosy	198,328	142,864	1.388
Leishmaniasis	1,970,613	1,462,594	1.347
Onchocerciasis	355,411	264,327	1.345
Other Malignant Neoplasm's	9,324,018	6,993,333	1.333
Inflammatory Heart Disease	5,650,277	4,387,989	1.288

continued

Table 2.2 continued

Appendicitis	359,687	281,805	1.276
Benign Prosthetic Hypertrophy	3,747,386		
Prostate Cancers	3,254,128		

Table 2.3 Select Health Conditions for which Global DALYs [0,0] Lost to Females Are at Least 25% Above Those Lost to Males (GBD 2002)

Condition	Female DALYs	Male DALYs	Female DALYs / Male DALYs
Breast Cancer	11,733,351	44,483	263.772
Gonorrhea	2,888,421	264,196	10.933
Chlamydia	2,888,421	264,196	10.933
Trachoma	2,475,721	811,980	3.049
Migraine	8,802,838	3,146,812	2.797
Post-Traumatic Stress Disorder	1,883,391	720,628	2.614
Rheumatoid Arthritis	4,259,468	1,672,682	2.546
Panic Disorder	3,594,381	1,844,713	1.948
Alzheimer and Other Dementias	12,818,790	7,213,869	1.777
Osteoarthritis	15,629,274	9,149,400	1.708
Other Musculoskeletal Disorders	3,518,880	2,093,852	1.681
Fires	12,768,433	8,223,566	1.553
Unipolar Depressive Disorders	32,507,673	21,133,650	1.538
Iron-Deficiency Anemia	9,025,199	6,077,808	1.485
Other Oral Diseases	95,088	65,503	1.452
Insomnia (Primary)	1,894,676	1,362,610	1.390
Multiple Sclerosis	1,000,898	722,796	1.385
OCD	2,330,821	1,705,743	1.366
Other Intestinal Diseases	88,928	65,128	1.365
Cataracts	21,454,199	15,729,865	1.364
Rheumatic Heart Disease	6,184,772	4,548,016	1.360
Vision Disorders, Age-Related	12,714,330	9,413,331	1.351
Glaucoma	3,304,452	2,464,786	1.341
Other Genitourinary Systems Diseases	3,668,296	2,842,889	1.290
Japanese Encephalitis	658,357	522,117	1.261
Other Maternal Conditions	15,062,497		

continued

Table 2.3 continued

Maternal Sepsis	8,688,660
Maternal Hemorrhage	7,602,986
Cervix Uteri Cancer	6,322,294
Abortion	5,967,628
Obstructed Labor	4,851,864
Hypertensive Disorders	3,889,105
Ovary Cancer	3,174,156
Corpus Uteri Cancer	2,075,423

Donner, 2004), contributing to the 'newborn male disadvantage' in low birth weight as well.[4] On the other hand, differences in the biology of male and female lungs also suggest that that an equivalent exposure to tobacco smoke leads to a greater risk of molecular aberrations (i.e., mutations) in female lungs (Patel et al., 2004). While the sex genotype does not *cause* these outcomes, it is a necessary precondition to the outcome, distinguishing a sex-linked vulnerability, i.e., a vulnerability not experienced by members of the opposite sex. Health outcomes such as testicular cancer or low birth weight, for example, may be caused by environmental risks or poverty, respectively, but they also reflect sex-specific vulnerabilities.

Gendered expectations imposed on members of each sex impact health in a variety of ways. Divisions of labor between the sexes underlie some of the most obviously gendered differences in health outcome, such as the greater risk of drowning among males worldwide because of their roles as fishermen and boatmen, and by contrast, the greater number of

Table 2.4   Sex-Specific Vulnerabilities

XY Vulnerabilities	*XX Vulnerabilities*
Hemophilia	Breast Cancer
Prostate Cancer	Ovarian Cancer
Testicular Cancer	All Maternal Causes
Birth Asphyxia and Trauma	Chlamydia
Low Birth weight	Rheumatoid Arthritis
Acute Starvation	Osteoarthritis
Renal Agenesis	Glaucoma
	Cataracts (in part)

burnings among women due to their responsibility for cooking and fire-tending (Table 2.5).

But gendered differences in occupational health risk are only the tip of the iceberg. Gendered leisure activities and ways of coping with life stress, shaped by social messaging about what leisure activities a male or female should undertake, result in differential rates of cigarette smoking, alcohol and drug use, and a cascade of associated health risks. Cigarette smoking continues to be more common among men in much of the world, contributing not only to lung, mouth, and bladder cancer (Meisel, 2002), but also to an estimated one-third of the male excess in reported tuberculosis (TB) cases (Watkins and Plant, 2006).

Differential gendered obligations to children, the sick, and community affect exposure to infections (e.g., trachoma, influenza), and the structure and responsiveness of the health system itself biases care. For example, there is evidence of more renal transplantation for males than females, controlling for medical need and patient interest (Alexander and Sehgal, 1998), and fewer referrals of women than men for angiography, despite identical clinical characteristics (Schulman et al., 1999). The literature provides substantial documentation of gendered divisions in health care experience (see Doyal, 1995; Annandale and Hunt, 2000; Östlin et al., 2001; Sen et al., 2002, among others).

One of the challenges in studying how gender affects health is the near-ubiquitous assumption that sex-linked genetic differences in biologic capabilities (e.g., women's ability to give birth and breast-feed, men's upper body strength), justify professional and social exclusions that, in turn, come with certain health risks. It is tempting to treat sex and gender as if the latter is a natural extension of the former, especially for health conditions that result from women's role in homemaking (e.g., fires), and childrearing (e.g., trachoma), or men's work in heavy labor (e.g., falls, drowning). This extends to subtle (and deeply problematic) assumptions about the hormonal or genetic basis of interpersonal violence among males, i.e., that males are genetically motivated to protect or control their interests by force. Use of the terms 'gender' and 'sex' interchangeably endorses such a perspective, implying that gendered behaviors and vulnerabilities are an organic consequence of genetic sex; there is much support for such an approach among social conservatives, rationalized as a division of labor rooted in nature, or divine intent.

The excess incidence of depressive and other mental health difficulties among females begs research on the relative contributions of sex chromosome–linked vulnerabilities versus gendered experience, or the possibility that the relevant diagnostic criteria are themselves gender biased, leading to overdiagnosis of women, or underdiagnosis of men (Moeller Leimkuehler et al., 2007). Astbury comments, "notions of women's biologically based vulnerability or proneness to [mental] disorder have proved rather resistant to change," while not subjected to empirical investigation (Astbury, 2002).

Table 2.5   Gendered Vulnerabilities

Male gender vulnerabilities	Female gender vulnerabilities
Falls	Fires
Drowning	Trachoma
Road traffic accidents	Cataracts (in part)
Self-inflicted injuries	? Panic disorders
Lung cancer	? Depressive disorders
Drug use disorders	? Post-traumatic stress disorders
Alcohol use disorders	? Insomnia
Cirrhosis of the liver	? Migraine
Bladder cancer (in part)	
TB (in part)	

Rising interest in men and depression will certainly heighten the attention to possible gender biases in diagnoses, but more analysis is warranted on at least two other questions: whether there are social advantages (for men) in constructing women as vulnerable to mental illness, and, on the other hand, whether the world is organized in ways that so limit women's options, and so heighten their fears, that depression (and panic disorder) are a reasonable outcome.

Men's greater vulnerability to alcohol-related disorders has been commented on by Astbury (2002, also citing Kessler, 1994), as possibly exaggerated by reporting bias, i.e., a consequence of women selectively underreporting alcohol problems. While this cannot be ruled out in particular cases, regions, or even subpopulations, the aggregate global DALYs for alcohol-related outcomes including cirrhosis, gout, and road traffic accidents are consistently higher among males, strongly suggesting more alcohol abuse by men than women, even if women underreport their drinking.

Traffic accidents are not only one of the 10 highest causes of global DALYs for males, but they offer a potent area for gendered analysis of cause and debates over policy. The following case draws on a paper by this author prepared for the WHO in 2002 (Snow, 2002). Globally, males sustain approximately 70% of all traffic accident deaths, and over 70% of all traffic-related DALYs per year. Much of the male excess in traffic accidents can be attributed to men's greater access to vehicles and their roles as drivers. In general, males have more experience than females in driving all types of vehicles, and socialization of males emphasizes mastery over motorized transport of all kinds. Therefore, does the excess male involvement in traffic accidents simply reflect more (gendered) driving time? US data allows an analysis of crashes adjusted for the total vehicle miles traveled; when controlling for males' excess exposure, the sex difference in crash involvement disappears. But the same adjustment fails to account for excess male involvement *in fatal crashes*. The excess risk for fatal crashes among males is especially dramatic among the youngest drivers, and largely attributable to speed and alcohol (Maio et al., 1997; Odero, 1998). Males are not only more likely than females to drive after they have been drinking, but when simulated driving was evaluated among 18-year-olds who had their blood alcohol raised experimentally, girls drove more cautiously as they got drunker, while boys became more reckless (Oei Tian and Kerschbaumer, 1990).

To what extent is such risk-taking encouraged as part of masculine identity, i.e., a way of 'doing' male gender, or a sex-linked predisposition of the genotype? Investigations of the biologic basis of male risk-taking have been largely inconclusive. Small, complex studies of twins find more sensation-seeking behavior among those with greater in utero exposure to androgens (Daitzman et al., 1978; Resnick et al., 1993), but the magnitude of the effects are small, and variations in childrearing cannot be excluded. Even in the event of a sex-linked genetic predisposition to risk-taking among males, we also have powerful social and media messages that promote risk-taking as a signature means of demonstrating masculinity. Courtenay (2000) argues that dismissing risks in general is a crucial means by which males construct their gender. Recognizing that some degree of risk-taking has positive value in modern life, the outstanding question may be whether and how risk-taking tendencies might be shaped or regulated to avoid endangering males, and society more generally (Snow, 2002).

For a range of health outcomes with large differences between the sexes, sex and gender vulnerabilities may both be operative, compounding, or mitigating one another. The challenge here is to undertake a careful desegregation of measured affects that may be caused by sex or gender, often in the midst of other independent causes.

Blindness offers a compelling example of a health outcome attributable to a combination of sex and gendered causes that heighten female risk, resulting in almost 150 blind women for every 100 blind men in the world. This example draws on the research of Courtright, Lewallen, and colleagues, who have undertaken a model effort to disentangle sex and gendered causes of blindness (see Abou-Gareeb et al., 2001; Courtright and Lewallen, 2002; Lewallen and Courtright, 2002).

Women bear approximately two-thirds of the global burden of blindness; results of a meta-analysis suggest a pooled age-adjusted odds ratio of 1.43 (95% CI 1.33–1.53) (Abou-Gareeb et al., 2001). This reflects several dimensions of heightened risk for women: a 10–15% greater incidence of cataracts, the leading cause of global blindness, which Courtright and Lewallan propose is due to sex-linked inherent risks for women (2002). To this is added a 2.5–3 times greater risk of trachoma-related blindness among adult women than men. As the proportion of active infections is similar among boys and girls, the greater number of active infections among adult women is attributed to their greater contact with infected children. These disparities in vulnerability are compounded by men's greater access to cataract surgery in many parts of the developing world. Hence, the global excess of female blindness is attributed to a (hypothesized) sex-linked vulnerability to cataract, a gendered risk of trachoma, and a gendered distribution of eye-care services. This analysis is particularly helpful in that the authors have identified gendered dimensions that, by definition, are amenable to intervention, such as delivering more cataract surgical services to women.

IMPLICATIONS FOR RESEARCH AND POLICY

The causal factors responsible for many of the sex differences in health listed in Tables 2.2 and 2.3. remain poorly understood, including those causing TB, depression, osteoarthritis, Alzheimer's and dementia, migraine, and gout. TB and depression deserve special concern, due to the magnitude of global DALYs lost to these two conditions.

The higher proportion of male cases of reported TB may reflect underlying sex-based genetic vulnerabilities, or cultural and service barriers that limit case-reporting among women, or some combination of both (Thorson et al., 2004; Weiss et al., 2006). Given the high global burden of TB for both sexes, there should be sustained efforts to explore all social vulnerabilities, including those attributable to gender. Better understanding of systematic biases in diagnosis, willingness to screen, or access to care would shed light on male and female vulnerabilities alike, furthering TB control for all patients. Recent data from Malawi, Bangladesh, India, and Colombia found women more likely than men to drop out of care during TB diagnosis, while men were less likely than women to complete treatment once diagnosed (Weiss et al., 2006). The way that gender interacts with stigma to affect compliance with care can differ significantly by locale, depending on local confidence about TB treatment, and gendered aspects of the marriage and job markets (Weiss et al., 2006; Thorson et al., 2004). A cautionary lesson from the emerging data on gender and TB is the apparent local mutability of how gender affects health-seeking. In the case of TB at least, generalizations seem difficult. Variations don't preclude national or even regional interventions, but they do call for robust specification of *how* gender impacts health-seeking in a given setting.

With regard to depression, substantial gender biases in diagnosis cannot be excluded. Some diagnostic scales include questions about frequent crying or irritability, behaviors that are already laden with gender implications. It's tempting to parallel the female DALYs lost to depression, panic disorder, and post-traumatic stress with the excess of male DALYs lost to negative coping behaviors such as alcohol or drug use, violence, or risk-taking. The possibility that depression and panic disorder in women, and alcohol, drug use, and risk-taking (and even interpersonal violence) in men are gendered ways of reacting to similar underlying distress has been raised previously (Bech, 2001; Rutz, 1999; Moeller Leimkuehler et al, 2007). The ages at which these conditions peak and decline are more or less the same for males and females, with highest numbers of DALYs lost in young adulthood. The numbers of DALYs lost to panic disorder, post-traumatic stress disorder, unipolar depression, violence, drug use, and alcohol use disorders by males or females at different ages are shown in Figures 2.1–2.7.

DALYs lost to panic disorder peak abruptly in young adulthood (15–29 years) for both sexes, with little reporting before or after. But while the peak age for experiencing (or receiving a diagnosis of) panic disorder is the same, females lose almost twice as many DALYs to panic disorder as males. Similar patterns follow for post-traumatic stress disorder (PTSD) and drug use disorders, with peak DALYs lost to both sexes at ages 15–29 years, but these conditions have broader peaks and decline more gradually with age. The big distinctions lie in the numbers of DALYs lost to each condition: females lose 2.6 as many DALYs to PTSD as males, while males lose 3.7 times more DALYs to drug use disorders. For unipolar depression DALYs are already being lost in children under 15, and this increases in the years between ages 15 to 29 for both sexes, but females lose even more DALYs to depression between ages 30 to 44 years, while male DALYs lost to depression decline after age 30 (albeit gradually). Males over age 30, on the other hand, are losing far more DALYs to drug use disorders and alcohol disorders, when these conditions have become negligible for women, and males over 30 are just entering their peak years for lung cancer and others cancers due to smoking.

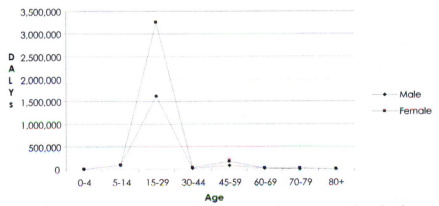

Figure 2.1   Sex differences in global DALYs [0,0] lost to panic disorder, by age (GBD 2002).

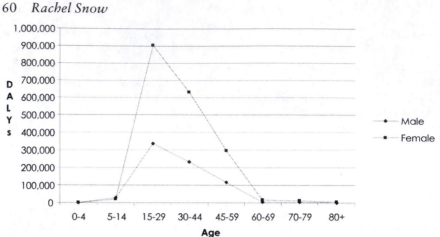

Figure 2.2   Sex differences in global DALYs [0,0] lost to post-traumatic stress disorder (PTSD), by age (GBD 2002).

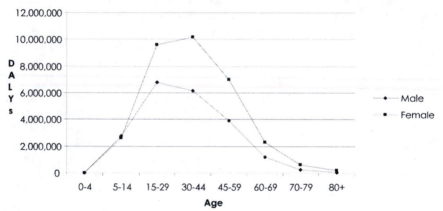

Figure 2.3   Sex differences in global DALYs [0,0] lost to unipolar depressive disorder, by age (GBD 2002).

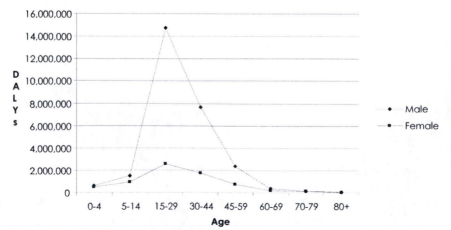

Figure 2.4   Sex differences in global DALYs [0,0] lost to violence, by age (GBD 2002).

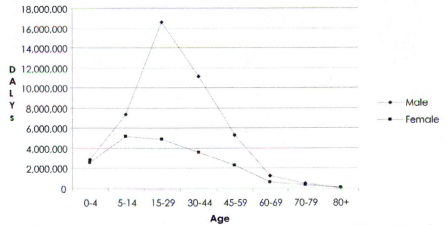

Figure 2.5 Sex differences in global DALYs [0,0] lost to road traffic accidents, by age (GBD 2002).

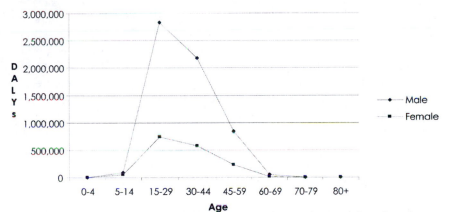

Figure 2.6 Sex differences in global DALYs [0,0] lost to drug use disorders, by age (GBD 2002).

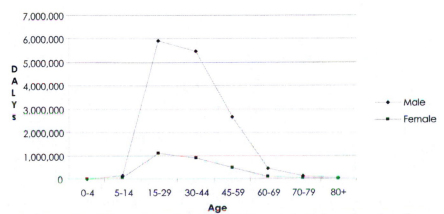

Figure 2.7 Sex differences in global DALYs lost to alcohol use disorders, by age (GBD 2002).

A notable distinction of Figure 2.4 and Figure 2.5 is the sheer magnitude of global DALYs lost to violence and road traffic accidents among males (27,470,156 and 45,112,383, respectively), and the male to female ratios for each (4 to 1 for violence, 4.7 to 1 for road traffic accidents). While sex differentials may be greater for other conditions (e.g., war, alcohol, chlamydia, gout), these conditions lead to substantially fewer lost DALYs (see Tables 2.2 and 2.3); and while other conditions lead to high lost DALYs (e.g., unipolar depression, TB, other injuries), the sex differences are not as great. The plausible genetic or social bases for these sex-specific losses deserve special attention.

THE MUTABILITY OF GENDER

Pollack (1998) argues that current cultural standards in the West trap boys into a 'boy code' of macho, self-negating behaviors that emphasize bravado, extreme daring, and attraction to violence, and it remains an active social norm to shame boys who fail to comply with such behaviors. Pollack argues that such codes lead to loneliness and distress for a large proportion of boys, putting them at social risks throughout life. Such theories are supported by evidence that males progress to depression after periods of aggression and alcohol abuse that are not observed in females (Bech, 2001), and by evidence that depressed men are more likely than women to cope by increasing their sports activity and alcohol consumption (Angst et al., 2002). The social or genetic determinants of these differences warrant much closer scrutiny. In the event that gender socialization itself contributes substantially to depression or negative coping, public information (at the least) and possibly regulation warrant consideration.[5]

If one agrees that gendered behaviors are subject to socialization, then at least theoretically the DALYs attributable to gendered behaviors that endanger people should be responsive to intervention. Recent history suggests that gendered health behaviors can change in response to marketing, fashion, or public legislation. In the case of smoking, both the percentage of smokers and the incidence of lung cancer in many high-income countries like the US have shifted towards equity, even as overall rates of smoking have declined. In the US, for example, the proportion of adult males who smoke has dropped by 55% in the past 40 years, from just over half of all adult males in 1965 to fewer than a quarter in 2004 (American Lung Association, 2006).

While the data suggest that an impressive proportion of US males no longer look to smoking as a requisite accessory of masculinity, women's relationship to smoking seems fraught by contradictory trends. On one hand, women have always smoked less than males; in fact, smoking was a means of doing 'maleness' because it was something most women did *not* do. But therefore women's smoking has been associated with rebellion from restrictive gender norms, and effectively marketed by the cigarette companies as a symbol of female liberation[6] (Brown, 2000). The decline in female smokers since 1965 has been less than that observed among males (about 45%), leaving the current percentage of adult male and female smokers in the US closer to equity than ever before (e.g., 23.4% of males and 18.5% of females currently smoke) (American Lung Association, 2006).

In middle- and low-income countries there is typically a much larger gap in smoking behavior between the sexes; the percentages of male and female smokers, respectively, are 51% and 18% in Mexico, 40% and 7% in Zambia, 22% and 2% in Iran, and 29% and 2% in India (Pampel, 2006). In many countries, female smoking continues to be regarded as immodest and unfeminine, and is strongly discouraged in all but elderly women. Given that similar social constraints on Western women's smoking gradually lifted as women moved into public and professional roles, there is understandable concern that women's emerging autonomy in poorer countries may also lead to increased smoking (Patel et al., 2004; Pampel, 2006), aided by the cigarette companies efforts to sell smoking as an attractive attribute of modern femininity.

While cigarette companies have readily promoted change in gender norms to sell smoking, public health advocacy has made only a few concerted attempts to explicitly address gendered imagery to promote health. One such program that targeted female smoking was undertaken by the Irish National Health Promotion Strategy 2000–2005, with a campaign that concentrated on the unattractiveness of smoking to challenge media images of female smoking as fashionable. Following the campaign the percentage of young women 18–35 who smoked dropped by an average of 4%, with proponents encouraged that the gender-targeted approach was a contributing factor.

A much more expanded and long-term effort was initiated in Sweden two decades ago to promote healthy gender norms. The Swedish government initiated educational policies in the 1980s that explicitly sought to end stereotyped gender patterns in society, with curricula that are required to challenge traditional gender messages. These policies were extended to Swedish preschools in 1998 (LPFÖ, 1998), and both Sweden and France now claim that their preschools avoid war toys or fashion dolls such as Barbies. The long-term impact of these efforts deserves scrutiny, not the least for how they impact health behaviors and outcomes.

In the African context, anti-HIV campaigns explicitly challenge aspects of gender identity that endanger young people. The loveLife billboards in South Africa question gendered assumptions about male control in sexual and romantic relationships, and provide young people (and all viewers) with an alternative gender vision of equitable, negotiated partnerships. LoveLife is not alone, but perhaps more innovative in their messaging than others. Social marketing firms such as New Start promote condom use, HIV testing, and family planning with ads that incorporate images of a new responsible male. The longer-term impact of such messages is largely untested and warrants evaluation, and it would be particularly worthwhile to examine how such expanded messaging efforts may evoke behavior change in nonreproductive and nonsexual domains. What, for example, might be the impact on female depression, or men's negative coping behaviors? The health and social costs of gender stereotyping warrant more systematic enquiry and more quantitative evaluation.

POLICY IMPLICATIONS OF THE GENETIC/ SOCIALIZATION DEBATES

In the West, most sex-specific restrictions on men's or women's behavior (e.g., employment or mobility) have now been disallowed in the interest of gender equity, with the exception of restricting pregnant women's exposure to occupational hazards. Yet the magnitude of the global DALYs lost to road traffic accidents among males (and the acknowledged impact of restrictive licensing), might warrant another exception. Licensing laws and punishments for driving under the influence (DUI) are sex neutral. But automobile insurance companies have long differentiated between the sexes and their differential risks with driving, compensating for the excess male risk of traffic accidents through sex-disaggregated premium scales and closer scrutiny of risky behavior among young males. An intervention looking for high impact on sex-specific DALYs might entertain sex-specific policies of graduated licensing, a higher age for licensing males, a higher age for legal consumption of alcohol by males, or a policy of zero-tolerance for male drinking and driving.

Gender equality legislation in the US currently prohibits any such sex-specific regulations *unless sex-specific risk behaviors are proven to be genetically or biologically based* (Kommers and Finn, 1998). Occupational restrictions of pregnant women are allowed under this exception, for example, because only females become pregnant. In the case of dangerous masculine behavior such as drinking and driving, the logical extension of the legislative requirement is that anyone who argues that male risk-taking is genetically/hormonally programmed (i.e., 'in their genes'), are, in fact, supporting a rationale for sex-specific restrictions.

Arguments that such behaviors are socialized, on the other hand, would limit any legal chance at regulation (at least in the US). But such arguments will also place the DALYs due to men's risk-taking (or interpersonal violence, or any dimension of negative coping) directly on our social doorstep, as a public pathology that we've created and are responsible to change.

If it's not in our genes, then trials of interventions that reduce gender stereotyping of males as risk-takers, or promote doing gender in less dangerous ways, are plausible at a significant scale. Likewise, if the excess in female depression, panic disorder, or OCD is 'all in her genes,' then special protections may be called for—protections only recently discarded for equity reasons. If instead these female DALYs are a consequence of gendered experience, then we're pressed to examine how the social conditions of women's lives lead to such outcomes. For containing the cost of health care alone, we need to reexamine the risks and benefits of gendered life, and ask what's making men so prone to alcohol, drug use, and risk-taking, and what's making women so depressed?

Some elements of the loveLife campaign already offer a radical challenge to female vulnerability—identifying romantic female subservience as fatal and encouraging self-regard. It's notable that the campaign has been controversial, with accusations of using 'overly intellectual' or 'obscure' messages. In a world of highway billboards that routinely sell images of male sexual power and female subordination, messages that digress from these norms stand out and can momentarily confuse. Our expectations of how gender is going to be portrayed in modern marketing are so entrenched that any innovation takes us by surprise. Legal theorists like Catherine MacKinnon (1987) have challenged the free-speech defense of sexist media imagery on the principle that such 'speech' endangers women. Without discounting the severity of women's suffering, one can argue that sexist 'speech' endangers men as well. But to date even violently sexist images remain protected in much of the world, and regulation standards seem to be eroding rapidly. And the focus of debate is more often on sexual imagery, rather than the more ubiquitous gender-stereotyping imagery that ultimately promotes erotic response. Such debates over gender imagery in the media might be strengthened and enriched by greater regard for the extent to which masculine and feminine stereotyping endangers the health of *both* women and men.

CONCLUSION

While long-standing academic and activist discourse has emphasized that gender stereotypes and discrimination are harmful to women's health, the global DALYs underscore negative health effects of gender for both males and females. In the various treatments of gender and health to date, there has been far too little attention given to the potential public health impact of interventions that offer alternative gender images for both males and females. To accommodate our struggles with complexity, sex and gender continue to be conflated and used interchangeably, and examined as if the latter is simply the extension of the former. But our widening exposure to historical change and variations across different societies underscores the fact that gender identity is mutable and amenable to social messaging.

To the extent that chromosomal sex dictates human capability, it would appear to provide an impressive array of options for 'doing gender,' suggesting that our species, at the least, is highly adaptive and amenable to experimentation and adoption of new habits. Given the extent of psychiatric conditions leading to lost DALYs among females, and the extent of male DALYs lost to negative coping, one has to wonder at the paucity of larger-scale efforts to examine how these health costs might be mitigated by a concerted effort at alternative social messaging about gender. Interventions that would explore and promote affirming ways of 'doing gender' may ultimately constitute 'best buys' for health and society.

ACKNOWLEDGMENTS

With considerable thanks to Piroska Östlin and Gita Sen and members of the Women and Gender Equity Network Hub for encouraging this chapter, and providing many valuable suggestions on an early draft. The chapter has been much improved by further comments from anonymous peer reviewers.

NOTES

1. Phenotype is the observable physical characteristics of an organism, or the appearance of an organism resulting from the interaction of genotype and the environment. At birth, infants are typically identified as being male or female based on the appearance (i.e., phenotype) of their external genitalia; a minority of infants have 'ambiguous' genitalia and require genotyping to identify their chromosomal sex as male or female.
2. Others have criticized the very notion of characterizing an 'every-person's' response to any given illness, because the true human burden of disability is so affected by social context (Sundby, 1997).
3. ICD-10, i.e., the International Statistical Classification of Diseases and Related Health Problems, 10th Revision.
4. Which includes, in this coding, an unspecified proportion of premature births in which the maturation of the lungs informs survival.
5. One can anticipate that legislation to restrict gender imagery in the media would spark debate along lines already drawn over the regulation of pornography and other violence.
6. For example, the Virginia Slims ad copy that read . . . *You've come a long way baby!*

REFERENCES

Abou-Gareeb, I., S. Lewallan, K. Bassett, and P. Courtright. 2001. Blindness and gender: A meta-analysis of published surveys. *Ophthalmic Epidemiology* 8: 39–56.
Alexander, G.C., and A.R. Sehgal. 1998. Barriers to cadaveric renal transplantation among Blacks, women and the poor. *JAMA* 280: 1148–1152.
American Lung Association. 2006. *Trends in Tobacco Use*. American Lung Association Epidemiology and Statistic Unit, Research and Program Services.

Anand, S., and K. Hanson. 1997. Disability-adjusted life years: A critical review. *Journal of Health Economics* 16: 685–702.

Angst, J., A. Gamma, M. Gastpar, J.P. Lepine, J. Mendlewicz, and A. Tylee. 2002. Gender differences in depression. *European Archives of Psychiatry and Clinical Neuroscience* 252: 201–209.

Annandale, E., and K. Hunt, eds. 2000. *Gender Inequalities in Health*. Buckingham: Open University Press.

Astbury, J. 2002. Mental health: Gender bias, social position and depression. In *Engendering International Health: The Challenge of Equity*, edited by G. Sen, A. George, and P. Östlin. Cambridge: MIT Press: 143–166.

Bech, P. 2001. Male depression: Stress and aggression as pathways to major depression. In *Depression—Social and Economic Timebomb*, edited by A. Dawson and A. Tylee. London: British Medical Journal Books: 63–66.

Beermann, W. 1999. Discounting in health economics: An ethical approach. *Paper Presented at the Workshop of Measuring Health and Disability, July*. University of Heidelberg.

Brown, C. 2000. "Judge me all you want": Cigarette smoking and the stigmatization of smoking. *Paper Presented at the Society for the Study of Social Problems*. Santa Cruz.

Chen, L., E. Huq, and S. D'Souza. 1981. Sex bias in the family allocation of food and health care in rural Bangladesh. *Population and Development Review* 7 (1): 55–70.

Chessler, P. 1972. *Women and Madness*. New York: Four Walls Eight Windows.

Courtenay, W. 2000. Constructions of masculinity and their influence on men's well-being: A theory of gender and health. *Social Science and Medicine* 50: 1385.

Courtwright, P., and S. Lewallen. 2002. Sex, gender and blindness, eye disease and use of eye care services. *Paper Presented at a World Health Organization Conference*. Geneva: WHO.

Daitzman, R., M. Zuckerman, O. Sammelwitz, and V. Ganjam. 1978. Sensation-seeking gonadal hormones. *Journal of Biosocial Science* 10: 401–408.

Das Gupta, M. 1987. Selective discrimination against female children in rural Punjab, India. *Population and Development Review* 13 (1): 77–100.

Das Gupta, M., J. Zhenghua, L. Bohua, X. Zhenming, W. Chung, and B. Hwa-Ok. 2003. Why is son preference so persistent in East and South Asia? A cross-country study of China, India and the Republic of Korea. *Journal of Development Studies* 40 (2): 153–187.

Doyal, L. 1995. *What Makes Women Sick: Gender and the Political Economy of Health*. New Brunswick: Rutgers University Press.

Federman, D.D. 2006. The biology of human sex differences. *New England Journal of Medicine* 354: 1507.

Hallstrom, T. 2001. Gender differences in mental health. In *Gender Inequalities in Health*, edited by P. Östlin, M. Danielsson, F. Diderichsen, A. Härenstam, and G. Lindberg. Boston: Harvard School of Public Health: 117–135.

Han. H.-R., M.T. Kim, L. Rose, C. Dennison, L. Bone, and M. Hill. 2006. Effects of stressful life events in young black men with high blood pressure. *Ethnicity and Disease* 16: 64–70.

Hanson, K. 2002. Measuring up: Gender, burden of disease, and priority setting. In *Engendering International Health: The Challenge of Equity*, edited by G. Sen, A. George, and P. Östlin. Cambridge: MIT Press: 313–345.

Hopcraft, R.L., and D.B. Bradley. 2007. The sex difference in depression across 29 countries. *Social Forces* 85 (4): 1483–1507.

Jelsma, J., V. Chivaura, K. Mhundwa, W. De Weerdt, and P. de Cock. 2000. The global burden of disease disability weights. *The Lancet* 355: 2079–2080.

Kommers, D.P., and J.E. Finn. 1998. *American Constitutional Law.* Belmont: Wadsworth Publishing.

Lewallen, S., and P. Courtright. 2002. Gender and use of cataract surgical services in developing countries. *Bulletin of the World Health Organization* 80: 300–303.

LPFÖ 98. 1998. *Curriculum for the Pre-School Lpfö 98. National Agency for Education (SKOLFS 2006:22).* Stockholm: Fritzes Kundservice.

MacKinnon, C.A. 1987. *Feminism Unmodified: Discourses on Life and Law.* Cambridge: Harvard University Press.

Mage, D.T., and E.M. Donner. 2004. The fifty percent male excess of infant respiratory mortality. *Acta Pediatrica* 93: 1210–1215.

Maio, R., F. Waller, F. Blow, E. Hill, and K. Singer. 1997. Alcohol abuse/dependence in motor vehicle crash victims presenting to the emergency department. *Academic Emergency Medicine* 4: 256–262.

Meisel, P. 2002. Letter to the editor: Cancer, genes and gender. *Carcinogenesis* 23: 1087–1088.

Moeller Leimkuehler, A.M., J. Heller, and N. Paulus. 2007. Subjective well-being and 'male depression' in male adolescents. *Journal of Affective Disorders* 98: 65–72.

Odero, W. 1998. Alcohol-related road traffic injuries in Eldoret, Kenya. *East African Medical Journal* 75: 708–711.

Oei Tian, P.S., and D.M. Kerschbaumer. 1990. Peer attitudes, sex, and the effects of alcohol on simulated driving performance. *American Journal of Drug and Alcohol Abuse* 16: 135–146.

Östlin, P., M. Danielsson, F. Diderichsen, A. Harenstam, and G. Lindberg, eds. 2001. *Gender Inequalities in Health: A Swedish Perspective.* Boston: Harvard School of Public Health.

Pampel, F.C. 2006. Global patterns and determinants of sex differences in smoking. *International Journal of Comparative Sociology* 47: 466–487.

Patel, J.D., P.B. Bach, and M.G. Kris. 2004. Lung cancer in US women. *JAMA* 291 (14): 1763–1768.

Pollack, W. 1998. *Real Boys: Rescuing our Sons from the Myths of Boyhood.* New York: Random House.

Resnick, S., I. Gottesmann, and M. McGue. 1993. Sensation seeking in opposite-sex twins: An effect of prenatal hormones? *Behavioral Genetics* 23: 323–329.

Rutz, W. 1999. Improvement of care for people suffering from depression: the need for comprehensive education. *International Clinical Psychopharmacology* 14: 27–33.

Sadana, R. 1998. A closer look at the WHO/World Bank Global Burden of Disease Study's methodologies: How do poor women's values in a developing country compare with international public health experts? *Conference Presentation at the Public Health Forum, Reforming Health Sectors.* London: London School of Hygiene and Tropical Medicine.

Schulman, K.A., J.A. Berlin, W. Harless, J.F. Kerner, S. Sistrunk, and B.J. Gersh. 1999. The effect of race and sex on physicians' recommendations for cardiac catheterization. *New England Journal of Medicine* 340: 618–626.

Sen, G., P. Östlin, and A. George, eds. 2002. *Engendering International Health: The Challenge of Equity.* Cambridge: MIT Press.

Snow, R.C. 2002. Sex, gender and traffic accidents: Addressing male risk behaviour. *Paper Presented at a Conference for the World Health Organization.* Geneva: WHO.

Stevenson, D.K., J. Verter, A.A. Fanaroff, W. Oh, R.A. Ehrenkranz, S. Shankaran, E.F. Donovan, et al. 2000. Sex differences in outcomes of very low birthweight infants: The newborn male disadvantage. *Archives of Disease in Childhood. Fetal and Neonatal Edition* 83: 182–185.

Sundby, J. 1997. A gender perspective on disability adjusted life years and the global burden of disease. *Paper Presented at a Conference for the World Health Organization.* Geneva: WHO.

Thorson, A., N.P. Hoa, N.H. Long, P. Allebeck, V.K. Diwan. 2004. Do women with tuberculosis have a lower likelihood of getting diagnosed? Prevalence and case detection of sputum smear positive pulmonary TB, a population based study from Vietnam. *Journal of Clinical Epidemiology* 57: 398–402.

van Grootheest, D.S., A.T.F. Beekman, M.I. Broese van Groenou, and D.J.H. Deeg. 1999. Sex differences in depression after widowhood. Do men suffer more? *Social Psychiatry and Psychiatric Epidemiology* 34: 391–398.

Watkins, R.E., and A.J. Plant. 2006. Does smoking explain sex differences in the global tuberculosis epidemic? *Epidemiology and Infection* 134: 333–339.

Weiss, M.G., C. Auer, D. Somma, and A. Abouihia. 2006. Gender and tuberculosis: Cross-site analysis of a multi-country study in Bangladesh, India, Malawi and Columbia. World Health Organization, TDR/SDR/SEB/RP/06.1.

3 Inequalities and Intersections in Health

A Review of the Evidence

Aditi Iyer, Gita Sen, and Piroska Östlin

INTRODUCTION

Social relations of power based on gender, class, caste, race, and ethnicity structure women's and men's exposure and vulnerability to ill-health, their access to health protective resources, and the consequences to them of disease, disability and violence (Lynch and Kaplan, 2000; Östlin, 2002). Since the 1990s, feminist theorists have increasingly argued that these axes of power are intertwined as processes that construct and are constructed by the other (Collins, 1998; Davis, 2008; McCann and Kim, 2003). The interrelationships occur in—and affect—individual lives, social practices, institutional arrangements and cultural ideologies (Davis, 2008).

Crenshaw (1989, 1991) used the metaphor of intersecting roads to depict how race and gender can lead to multilayered discrimination, especially for women of color. Collins (2000, cited by Dhamoon, 2008) identified *intersectionality* as the micro processes that determine how individuals and groups occupy certain social positions within a macro system of what she termed *interlocking* oppressions. Razack (1998, cited by Dhamoon, 2008) viewed race, gender and class as *interlocking systems* that need and secure each other, making it impossible to extract relations based on one type of inequality from the others. Other conceptualizations of the interrelations—viz., *discrimination within discrimination* (Kirkness, 1988), *multiple jeopardy* and *multiple consciousness* (King, 1988), *translocational positionality* (Anthias, 2001), and *multiplex epistemologies* (Phoenix and Pattynama, 2006)—and applications of intersectional approaches in diverse disciplines (Brewer et al., 2002; Burman, 2004; Davis, 2008; Phoenix and Pattynama, 2006; Schulz and Mullings, 2006) point to the presence of a lively and growing literature.

Intersectional analyses are used to examine identities of marginalized individuals or social groups, categories of difference, processes of subject formation and differentiation (radicalization, gendering), and systems of domination (Dhamoon, 2008). Empirical work employing intersectional approaches has begun, in recent years, to also yield new insights about the social determinants of health and the social patterning of health inequalities. Authors reviewing existing research in health from an intersectional perspective have begun to question dominant discourses of sexuality and vulnerability guiding public health and have offered insights that can usefully feed into policies and programs (Bredstrom, 2006; Dworkin, 2005; Reddy, 2005). However, these analyses and insights have still not fully entered the mainstream of health equity research and policy-making.[1]

Many who work on health equity view the sources of inequity as primarily linked to economic class differentials, but this often leaves a number of crucial questions unanswered. For example, the standard work on gradients, gaps and medical poverty traps tells us easily enough that the poor are worse off, in terms of both health care access and health outcomes, than those who are economically better off. But it does not tell us whether the burden of this inequity is borne equally by different castes or racial groups among the poor. Nor does it tell us how the burden of health inequity is shared among different members of poor households. Are women and men (girls and boys), income earners and nonearners, equally vulnerable to ill-health in poor households? Are they equally at risk in rich households? Are women, men, widows, and income-earning youths equally trapped by medical poverty? Are they treated alike in the event of catastrophic illness or injury? When health costs go up significantly, as they have in many countries in recent years, do households tighten their belts equally for women and men? And are these patterns similar across different income quintiles?

If the answers to such questions are in the negative, it poses a challenge for policies to ensure not only equity across, but also, and simultaneously, within households. Consequently, both theoretical and empirical work on the intersections and their impact on health are necessary for the advancement of social theory, for effective feminist politics, for better empirical science, and for appropriate social and health policies.

Annandale and Hunt (2000) hypothesize that these intersections could be such that the impact on health of one type of inequality can be confounded by others, leading to unpredictable outcomes. In other words, similar inequalities along one given dimension can sometimes render men and women equally vulnerable to ill-health and, at other times, produce differential effects, depending on the presence of—and interaction with—other dimensions. The intersections can also result in wide differences among women and among men. It is important, therefore, to study different dimensions of inequality simultaneously, e.g., class differences among men and women, and gender differences by class (Macintyre and Hunt, 1997); and also, to analyze differences along the entire social gradient, not just at the two extremes (Sen et al., 2009, 2002a). According to Weber and Parra-Medina (2003, p. 222):

> intersectional approaches complicate the traditional models of health and illness by incorporating more dimensions, situationally specific interpretations, group dynamics and an explicit emphasis on social change. On the other hand, they provide a powerful alternative way

of addressing questions about health disparities that traditional approaches have been unsuccessful in answering.

Our objective in this chapter is to highlight, from existing empirical studies, what insights can be gained if multiple inequalities are treated as intersecting, not separable, processes.

SEARCH STRATEGIES

The review is based on a search for the relevant literature on inequalities in health status and health care in high- and low-income countries. Electronic journals and databases, including Medline, PubMed, JStor, Science Direct, and Ingenta Connect, were accessed through the University of Liverpool (UK), Karolinska Institutet (Sweden), and Harvard University (US). Additional literature was identified from Listservs, such as PAHO—Equidad. The searches were limited to English. Library searches were also conducted at the University of Liverpool (UK) and at the Indian Institute of Management Bangalore, Institute for Social and Economic Change, Centre for Development Studies and the Achutha Menon Centre for Health Sciences (India).

INTERSECTING INEQUALITIES IN HEALTH STATUS

We first summarize, and then critically question, the findings of studies that analyze gender, class, race, ethnicity and caste as separable sources of inequality. We then discuss the findings and implications of studies that analyze their intersections and impact on health.

With regard to gender inequalities in health, studies have long since established that women live longer but report more ailments than men, although this pattern applies to certain types of illnesses and at certain life stages (Annandale, 1998; Macintyre et al., 1996; Östlin et al., 2001). Such studies do not tell us, however, whether gender differentials are similar in different economic groups. Analysis of British survey data reveals that the gender gap in the prevalence of self-reported morbidity varies by both class and ethnicity, being wider among the professional and managerial class than among manual workers (Drever et al., 2004); and significant among Black Caribbean, Indian and Pakistani adults, but not among white adults (Cooper, 2002). Gender differences in self-rated health, functional limitations, and life-threatening medical conditions also vary by both race and ethnicity in the US (Read and Gorman, 2006), a finding that is reflected in another study in the US of adolescents attending high school (Almgren et al., 2009). Gender differences in self-rated health were miniscule among first- or second-generation Vietnamese and Cambodian youngsters compared to other racial/ethnic groups (whites, blacks, Hispanics, American

Indians, Filipinos, and East Asians). Patterns of gender differentials in self-assessed health also vary across 13 countries in Europe differentiated by 'regime type' and by socioeconomic status (Bambra et al., 2009). While there were no gender differences in "Corporatist" countries (Germany, Belgium, France); there were wide differences in Finland and the UK where men were more likely to report worse self-assessed health; and in Social Democratic countries (Denmark, Sweden, Norway, Holland) and Southern welfare states (Italy, Spain, Portugal), where women were more likely to do so. In Italy, Sweden and Portugal, the most educated women were in fact more likely to report worse self-assessed health.[2]

Studies with a gender focus often do not examine whether there are social differences among women or among men in the ways in which they experience, recognize and articulate illness symptoms, and may therefore presume greater within-sex similarity than is warranted. A Canadian study showed, on the contrary, that women tended to experience mental health problems differently depending on their socioeconomic status, ethnicity, family structure, quality of family relationships, and nature of participation in the labor market (Walters, 1993). Another study revealed that different familial and parental roles among British and Finnish women created significant differences in perceived general health and limiting long-standing illness through accompanying socioeconomic factors (Lahelma et al., 2002). Considerable differences were also evident among black, white, and Latina women in the US in the extent and ways in which embodied femininity (the way femininity is physically constructed) and weight concerns resulted in symptoms suggestive of depression (Bay-Cheng et al., 2002). Women in south India assessed their health differently depending on both economic status and caste (Mohindra et al., 2006).

Studies analyzing class inequalities without reference to gender, race, ethnicity or caste are equally limited. For instance, investigations in the nineteenth century in Paris, Upper Silesia and England (Lynch and Kaplan, 2000), and studies carried out in the 1970s and 1980s in Britain (Townsend et al., 1992) and the US (Feinstein, 1993; Navarro, 2002), consistently revealed that mortality rates were higher among the poor compared to the rich. Morbidity rates were also higher among persons in lower socioeconomic groups, in a comparative study of 11 countries in Western Europe (Machenbach et al., 2002). These early studies did not ask whether the impact of socioeconomic position on health varied by gender, or by other dimensions of inequality. However, subsequent empirical evidence from high-income countries suggests that it does.[3]

Studies in the US and Canada indicate that the strength of the association between social class and ill-health is stronger among women than among men (Mei Tang and Krewski, 2003; Thurston et al., 2005), within different race/ethnic groups (Loucks et al., 2007b), and especially in certain age intervals (Loucks et al., 2007a). In the US, both childhood and adult class positions influence class gradients in women's health (Krieger et al., 2001).

Other studies in Europe reveal mixed results. While the socioeconomic gradients of chronic conditions and poor perceived general health were stronger among men than women in the Netherlands (Stronks et al., 1995), the gradients in the incidence of stroke, its recurrence and case fatality were sharper among Swedish women relative to men, and there were further differences by subtype (Li et al., 2008). Studies in Britain point to the fact that class inequalities are not of the same magnitude among men and women (Drever et al., 2004; Emslie et al., 1999; Matthews et al., 1999). Moreover, a study in Sweden describes how the lived experience of social class, in the form of stress associated with insecure incomes, adverse material conditions in the home and excessive workloads, gets filtered through the gender system (Ahnquist et al., 2007).

Christensen and others (2006) found variations by gender in the magnitude and direction of the social class effects on strategies adopted to cope with musculoskeletal pain. Whereas there was no correlation between social class and "avoidant coping"[4] among Danish women; there was a significant increase in the use of "avoidant coping" with decreasing social class among the men. Further, whereas there was a significant decrease in the use of "problem-solving coping" with decreasing social class among women, there was no correlation between "problem-solving coping" and social class among men.

In addition to gender, the effects of socioeconomic class on health also differ by race (Farmer and Ferraro, 2005; Kahn and Fazio, 2005), ethnicity (Bhopal et al., 2002; Kimbro et al., 2008), and caste (Mohindra et al., 2006) for a number of possible reasons.

First, these differences can at least partly emanate from the choice of indicator. For example, conventional indicators of socioeconomic status can have different meanings for ethnic groups, depending on how the many dimensions of ethnicity (viz., migration, language, religion, experience of racism and family formation) interlink (Davey Smith et al., 2000). This is probably why analysis of survey data in the US reveals that education is not an acceptable proxy for income in ethnically diverse populations: treating it as one can result in greater socioeconomic status misclassification of women of color (except American Indians/Alaskan Natives) than of European/Middle Eastern women (Braveman et al., 2001). Another study in the US found that conclusions about whether cumulative disadvantage explains racial differences in health over a life-course can vary depending on which indicator of socioeconomic status is analysed (Shuey and Willson, 2008). *Second*, economic class interacting with caste can either buffer the adverse health consequences of low economic class status for upper caste individuals, or magnify its effects for lower caste individuals, as indicated by a study in south India (Mohindra et al., 2006). *Third*, the phenomenon of 'diminishing returns'—the fact that black Americans consistently derive lower returns from improvements in socioeconomic status than white Americans—results in flatter gradients among blacks relative to whites, and in a racial gap that is widest at highest levels of income and occupational prestige (Farmer and Ferraro, 2005). In other words, the same amount of income can have a more protective effect for whites than for African Americans (Kahn and Fazio, 2005). Other evidence from the US suggests that socioeconomic status may provide unequal returns to health by both gender and race (Cummings and Jackson, 2008).[5]

Krieger and others (1999) found that the socioeconomic gradients in the incidence of cancer in the US differed in magnitude and direction by race/ ethnicity *and*, where applicable, by gender. For example, the incidence of both breast and lung cancer increased as socioeconomic status improved among Hispanic women, whereas for Asian and Pacific Islanders, blacks and whites, lung cancer incidence increased as socioeconomic status worsened. Cervical cancer incidence increased with socioeconomic deprivation among all four racial/ethnic groups (the trend being strongest among white women), but colon and prostate cancer incidence was inconsistently associated with socioeconomic position.

The studies cited so far complicate our understanding of the social patterning of health inequalities. They point to the inaccuracies that occur when conclusions are drawn about the inequalities based on one axis of power alone. They challenge the idea that social groups (male–female, rich–poor) are homogeneous entities and suggest that the distribution of power within each group along any single dimension can be uneven. They reveal patterns of inequalities in health outcomes that are more complex and unexpected, and consequently yield additional empirical evidence from which theoretical insights can usefully be drawn.

Studies focus on the differential effects of change over time on the patterning of health inequalities (Cummings and Jackson, 2008; Krieger et al., 2008, 2006; Luchenski et al., 2008). A study from Canada found that the health of men and women was not differentially affected by declines or improvements in socioeconomic position (Luchenski et al., 2008). Another from the US found strong evidence to the contrary, of differential change in the socioeconomic gradients in breast cancer (Krieger et al., 2006). The study revealed a highly heterogeneous pattern wherein changes in the magnitudes of the socioeconomic gradients were relatively small among white non-Hispanic and black women (who had the highest overall rates of breast cancer), but marked among Asian and Pacific Islander and Hispanic women. Another study found that between 1960 and 2002, as rates of premature mortality and infant death declined in the US, socioeconomic and racial/ ethnic inequities in premature mortality and infant death (both relative and absolute) shrank between 1966 and 1980, especially for US populations of color. Thereafter, relative health inequities widened even as absolute differences barely changed in magnitude (Krieger et al., 2008).

Three groups of studies explore the way in which different axes might overlap. The *first* group analyzing the extent to which socioeconomic factors account for gender, racial, and ethnic disparities in health concludes that they cannot do so fully or uniformly across all divisions. Cooper (2002) found that socioeconomic factors (indicated by material deprivation, educational attainment, employment and occupational status) accounted for a sizeable proportion of the racial/ethnic inequalities in self-assessed health in Britain. However, they did not alter gender differences in health within nonwhite ethnic groups: Black Caribbean, Indian, and Pakistani women were significantly more likely to report poor health than white adults were. Farmer and Ferraro (2005) found that in the US, racial differences in morbidity, functional impairment/disability, and self-rated health and well-being persisted even after controlling for socioeconomic factors. However, Kahn and Fazio (2005) found an inconsistent pattern in the US wherein racial differences in self-rated health and functional impairment were completely explained by education, wealth, and income, but remained strong and significant in the number of fatal conditions and health symptoms, even after controlling for socioeconomic factors. Other evidence from the US (Almgren et al., 2009) showed that racial/ethnic disadvantage in self-rated health disappeared for all adolescents—other than adolescent males of South East Asian origin—after controlling for the influence of social class (viz., parental education).

The *second* group that asks whether socioeconomic factors contribute to racial differences over a life course concludes that they do. Li and Robert (2008) found that both individual and neighborhood socioeconomic status explained why black older adults had greater declines in (self-rated) health over time than white older adults. Individual and neighborhood socioeconomic status also served to perpetuate health disparities at older ages. Walsemann and others (2008) found a widening health disparity in adulthood between individuals who had greater educational advantages in youth and those who had few advantages or none. Among individuals with few educational advantages, blacks experienced a greater health burden as they aged compared to whites and Hispanics. An older study that explored the contribution of social class to the phenomenon of the "racial crossover" in breast cancer rates in the US (wherein the rate among women over 40 years is higher among whites than blacks, but lower among white women under age 40) found that these patterns applied only to a certain socioeconomic group within each cohort (Krieger, 1990). Whereas the higher rates among white women (over 40) applied only to the working class, the higher rates among black women (under 40) applied only to the nonworking class.

The *third* group of studies found evidence of the phenomenon of *double* and *triple jeopardy* when each of the intersecting inequalities reinforced the other(s). A prospective study of adolescents in the US showed that unlike boys, girls from households with the lowest socioeconomic status were doubly jeopardized in terms of an increased risk for poor mental health outcomes, which were defined in terms of a clustering of depressive, anxiety, somatic, and withdrawal symptoms. Not only were their levels of mental ill-health higher at follow-up, levels of severe symptoms were maintained from baseline to follow-up (Mendelson et al., 2008).

A number of other studies confirm that risk factors influence health outcomes for individuals differently depending on their social position: the same level of exposure can have differential impacts on different groups, or different levels of exposure can have differential impacts. However, as social position itself is multidimensional, the processes and pathways leading to social inequalities in health can be complex, and cannot be predicted along a single dimension of power and inequality.

A study of different aspects of mental health (Griffin et al., 2002) found that among British civil servants, both men and women with low control, either at work or at home, had an increased risk of developing depression and anxiety, but women were more at risk for depression, while men were more prone to anxiety. Women in the lowest or middle employment grades, who also reported low control at work or home, were at most risk for depression and anxiety. Men in the middle grade, with low work control, were at risk for depression, while those in the lowest grade were at risk for anxiety. Men in the middle and highest grades were at greatest risk for both outcomes if they reported low control at home.

Studies in Canada show that the determinants of health—e.g., structural (including socioeconomic factors) versus behavioral (including lifestyle factors)—varied by type and by relative importance among men and women (Denton et al., 2004; Denton and Walters, 1999). A study in the US found that gender moderated the relationship between racial discrimination and anxiety symptoms: African-American women were more likely to report experiencing anxiety symptoms overall and in association with everyday discrimination compared to African-American men (Banks et al., 2006). Another study in the US found that general life events, chronic strains, and systemic stressors (in the economic, job, and domestic spheres) that were conditioned by racial stratification accounted for much of the variation in vulnerability to depressive symptoms and major depressive disorders for black men and black women (Dinwiddie, 2006). However, whereas all blacks were exposed to higher levels of social stress compared to whites, black women were the ones who experienced the most stressors compared to all other groups.

Differences in the risks for poor health among men and women are linked to differences in their exposures to the factors that cause or prevent disease. These exposures are, in turn, structured by the process and consequences of gendering, which are embedded within a web of power relations emanating from multiple sources. Thus, gender relations (including norms, values, behavior, and practices) across and within caste, race, class, and ethnicity-based groups are important drivers of differences in the patterning of risk factors and their consequent influence on health.

Studies that employ qualitative methodologies reveal the intricate web of relationships that structure women's vulnerability and exposure. For example, Collins and others (2008) show how multiple stigmatizing identities (based on having a mental illness, being a member of an ethnic minority group, being an immigrant, being poor, and being a woman who does not live up to gendered expectations) intersect to influence women's sexuality and HIV risk. From firsthand accounts, they showed how 24 Latina women living with severe mental illness in New York City sought identities that opposed the stigmatizing label of *loca* (meaning "crazy" in Spanish) while bestowing respect and dignity. The women identified with faith and religion ("church ladies") and upheld more traditional gender norms ("good girls") but engaged in sexual relationships that left them feeling both unsatisfied and disempowered, and that additionally increased their HIV risk.

Studies employing quantitative methodologies cannot match the richness of qualitative studies, but usefully provide precision and clarity about the significance or otherwise of hypothesized relationships.[6] For example, a study among British civil servants in the UK pointed out that low control at home, resulting from lack of material and psychological resources to cope with excessive household and family demands, predicted coronary heart disease (CHD) among women, but not among men; and explained part of the association between social position and CHD among women (Chandola et al., 2004). Another study in Catalonia, Spain (Borrell et al., 2004), found that, among men, the association between social class position and self-reported health status was explained by work organization exposures, including physical and psychosocial working conditions and job insecurity. Among women, the association between poor health and working-class position was accounted for not only by hazardous forms of work organization, but also by material well-being at home, and excessive amounts of uncompensated household labor.

Another Catalonian study (Artazcoz et al., 2001) showed that the prevalence of limiting long-standing illness, chronic conditions, and poor mental health was significantly higher among women, in both manual and nonmanual worker categories. However, the magnitude of gender differences in mental health was much higher among manual workers than among nonmanual workers. The relationship between family demands and health was influenced by both gender and social class. Among nonmanual workers (both men and women), none of the indicators of family demands were associated with any health indicator. Among manual workers, on the other hand, there were differences in the family demands that exerted an impact on the health of men and women. Among male manual workers, living with children less than 15 years of age was positively associated with limiting long-standing illness. Among women manual workers, household size affected their workloads and, thus, had a significant adverse effect on self-perceived health status, limiting long-standing illness, and chronic conditions.

A later study (Artazcoz et al., 2004) found that while unemployment resulted in poor mental health for Catalonian men and women, its impact was greater on men than on women. This gender difference was related to family responsibilities and social class. Unemployed men who were manual workers in their last job were at higher risk of poor mental health than men who were nonmanual workers, and marriage only increased that risk, especially if they were not receiving unemployment benefits. For women, being unemployed and not receiving benefits was associated with poor mental health only if they were married, had no children, and were nonmanual workers.

The quantitative studies cited here indicate, without specifying how, the process of gendering across caste, class, racial, and ethnic divisions can have differing consequences for health. However, a wide literature indicates how these processes operate in the realm of identity formation, risk-taking, health behaviors, lifestyle choices, violence and violations of dignity, work burdens, mobility, workplace-related and other types of discrimination, and opportunities for health care (Chakravarti, 2002; Rosen et al., 2003; Townsend, 2008 among others). More research is required from an intersectional perspective to understand the specific linkages between differential processes of gendering and health outcomes.

INTERSECTING INEQUALITIES IN ACCESS TO HEALTH CARE

Women generally need more health services than men do, due to their role in reproduction, but also due to excess female health problems not caused by reproductive morbidity. In high-income countries, women take more medication and visit physicians more often than men, largely due to their use of preventive services for contraceptives, cervical screening, and other diagnostic tests (Gijsbers van Wijk et al., 1996). In low-income countries, although reproductive problems and other chronic diseases play a large role in explaining gender differences in health status, women often have less access to health care services than men (Vlassoff, 1994), due to barriers located at the individual, familial, community, and health system levels.

In this section, we discuss the intersections between gender, class, and other inequalities in access to health care. We review the evidence from countries that do not have nationalized health systems, many of which are undergoing structural reforms in the direction of greater privatization and liberalization. Wherever possible, we contrast the findings with evidence from countries that do have nationalized systems assuring universal access to care.

Class inequality in access to health care, in market-driven health systems, stems from differences in the ability to pay. An extensive literature indicates that although the poor suffer greater ill-health, their ability to access care is less than that of the rich. Levels of nontreatment are substantially higher among the poor compared to the rich, even though the magnitude of the differences may vary. Analysis of inequalities in utilization of health care in eight developing countries—several in Africa—found that the rich were more likely to obtain care when sick, to be seen by a qualified doctor, and to receive medicines than the poor were (Makinen et al., 2000). These trends were also evident in different parts of Asia, such as Vietnam, China (Huong et al., 2007; Luong et al., 2007), and India (George, 1997; National Sample Survey Organisation, 2006); and in Central and Eastern Europe, such as Kosovo (World Bank, 2001, cited in Walters and Suhrcke, 2005) and Poland (Lewis, 2000, p. 25, cited in Walters and Suhrcke, 2005). Sick persons in low-income households tended to normalize and ignore health problems in Chad, and keep debilitating symptoms at bay with intermittent or suboptimal therapies that provide temporary reprieve but no cure (Leonard, 2005). As backward and remote regions of India have fewer (qualified) health care providers than better-off regions (Nandraj and Duggal, 1997), the poor have to travel longer distances to obtain care from qualified providers. Consequently, physical accessibility, reputation of the provider, and cost were important considerations for low-income rural households in eastern India (Ager and Pepper, 2005). Finally, while the rich may spend more on treatment in absolute terms, in most instances the poor are the ones who pay substantially more relative to household incomes or consumption expenditure, as shown by studies in Africa (Makinen et al., 2000), India (George, 1997), and Vietnam (Luong et al., 2007; Segall et al., 2002). In 2001–2002, the total cost of an inpatient stay in Vietnam was equal to seven months of per capita income for poor households versus under four months for nonpoor households (Huong et al., 2007).

Health reforms supporting privatization or liberalization have pushed up health care costs significantly and worsened inequalities in access to care, given greater burdens of out-of-pocket payments, especially for the poor. For example, in 2003, expenditure on a single inpatient episode in China was equivalent to 42 months of per capita income for the poorest households, compared with nine months for the richest ones; these ratios were almost double those of 1993 (Huong et al., 2007). The percentage of rural people reporting illness but not using services—ambulatory and inpatient—also increased substantially since 1993, the rates of nontreatment being much higher among the poor than among the rich. The opposite trend was found in Uganda after removal of user fees: there was a greater increase in utilization for curative outpatient care among the poor than for other socioeconomic categories (Nabyonga et al., 2005).

Households respond to growing economic pressure by rationing health care among their members. Evidence from Peru (Oths, 1994), Ghana (Asenso-Okyere et al., 1998), Vietnam (Segall et al., 2002, 2000), and India (Iyer, 2007) suggests that individuals within households curtailed expenditure by denying care, relying on self-care, delaying formal care, taking fewer tablets than required, making fewer visits to the health provider, or switching to less expensive providers. At times, they stretched resources at hand to obtain health care and in the process put their household economies under considerable strain. This was evident in both Vietnam (Segall et al., 2000) and Sri Lanka (Perera et al., 2007; Perera and Gunatilleke, 2006; Russell, 2001), although the latter has a widely accessible public health system. To cope with illness and the lump-sum expenditures required for its treatment, households in Uganda (Lucas and Nuwagaba, 1999), Ethiopia (Russell and Abdella, 2002), China (Wilkes et al., 1997), and rural Cambodia (Kenjiro, 2005), among others, adopted cost management and labor substitution strategies. They cut back on essential spending on food and education, borrowed at high rates of interest in informal credit markets or from community-based credit societies, engaged in distress sales of productive assets (land or livestock), mortgaged a crop, or sought help in terms of labor. The poor may also have differed from the rich in terms of their ability to access resources, including cheap credit, through social networks (Russell, 2001; Wilkes et al., 1997). In consequence, unaffordable health care has led, in many instances, to medical impoverishment in countries as diverse as China (Liu et al., 2003), Vietnam (Wagstaff and Van Doorslaer, 2003), India (Krishna et al., 2003; Krishna 2003, 2006), Bangladesh (Sen, 2003), and Kenya (Krishna et al., 2004), among others (Xu et al., 2007, 2003). Nonpoor households are pushed into poverty or forced into deeper poverty and destitution when confronted with substantial medical expenses and a simultaneous loss of household income due to ill-health (McIntyre et al., 2006; Whitehead et al., 2001).

The poor fare less well than the rich, even in high-income countries such as Canada and the UK where access does not hinge upon the ability of households to pay, apart from Australia and New Zealand (Blendon et al., 2002), although the gradients may be less steep and the impact in terms of household impoverishment less striking. A study measuring inequity in the utilization of general practitioners and medical specialists by income in OECD countries found physician utilization favoring better-off patients in about half of the countries. The degree of pro-rich inequity in doctor use was highest in the United States and Mexico, followed by Finland, Portugal, and Sweden. After controlling for differences in health needs, people with higher incomes in all countries for which data were available, were significantly more likely to see a specialist, and more frequently, than were people with lower incomes (Van Doorslaer et al., 2006).

The studies just cited raise compelling issues that demand policy interventions. However, while the bulk of the literature focuses on class-based inequalities, other evidence points to the fact that class inequalities do not operate singly, without reference to other dimensions of power. An analysis of inequalities in access to health care in India during the 1990s, after the economy was liberalized, showed that class inequalities in access differed by gender before and after economic liberalization; furthermore, class inequalities among men increased in the 1990s, in terms of untreated sickness and their use of hospitals (Sen et al., 2002b). Thus, class barriers are differentiated by gender, for a number of reasons.

Women tend to have poorer access to and control over resources within households, communities, and credit markets; are tied to gendered divisions of labor that leave them with little time or opportunity for health-seeking and may be restricted in their mobility. In low-income countries, not only is nontreatment higher among women than among men, women are also more likely to self-treat, or to receive treatment from informal health providers, or for shorter durations than men (Russell and Abdella, 2002; Sen et al., 2007). They incur lower expenditures than men do in India (Sen et al., 2002b), or spend amounts that entail lower financial and social burdens for the household (Iyer, 2007). In Bangladesh, women tend to have poor access to preventive and curative care, as they are economically dependent on their husbands, or on male heads of household, who may be unwilling to spend money on them (Schuler et al., 2002). Lower value placed on the well-being of girls and women also results in their receiving lower support when ill and unable to carry out daily chores, as shown by a study in a poor district in north India (Sama—Resource Group for Women and Health, 2005). Moreover, when health care has to be purchased out of pocket, or through private insurance, women are particularly hard-hit (Doyal, 2003; Falkingham, 2004; Östlin, 2005; Ravindran and Maceira, 2005). They are forced to alter normal health-seeking behavior, to seek less treatment, or to delay treatment, with adverse health consequences ranging from recurring or prolonged morbidity to untimely death.

The preceding studies indicate that responses to unaffordable health care vary by gender and class location of sick individuals and their households, but they raise a further set of questions. Are economic burdens shared more equally between men and women (boys and girls) in rich households or in poor households? What happens to gender relations as households accrue class privilege? Do gender inequalities in access to care reduce or disappear if there are no financial barriers? These questions are multidimensional and suggest more complex intersections.

A 16-month longitudinal study in rural northern Bangladesh (Rousham, 1996) revealed no apparent gender bias in child growth and nutritional status for those in farming and trading/employee households (which were nonpoor). However, in landless households, girls had significantly poorer height-for-age and weight-for-age than boys. During a natural disaster, being a girl in a landless household was more detrimental to nutritional status than being a girl *per se*, or simply belonging to a landless household. Interestingly, while differences by gender were statistically significant in landless households during the disaster, they became insignificant when local conditions improved.

Another study (Iyer et al., 2007) probed how economic class, caste, and gender affect treatment seeking for long-term ailments in a poor rural area in south India, where health services are sparse and of doubtful quality, and health care costs are high and rising. The study used a simple but powerful method to test for the significance of differences along the entire span of the social spectrum, not just between the extremes (Sen et al., 2009). It found, on the basis of a large sample, that caste did not significantly predict the likelihood of treatment, but gender and economic class were highly significant. Health care was affordable for only one out of three households, wherein affordability was defined as expenditures incurred without associated indebtedness or sale of assets and social burdens (Iyer, 2007). Individuals and households responded to long-standing health needs by rationing treatment seeking (through lack of any care or discontinuing care) according to both class and gender. Gender differences were observed in all economic classes of households, but were larger in poorer households due to the effect of rationing. There were also significant class-based differences in the likelihood of nontreatment, but these differences were limited to women. Thus, apparent class differences could only be understood through a gender analysis.

The interplay between gender and class can be important in relation to access to health care, even in high-income countries with universal health insurance. For example, a study in Sweden revealed significant effects of discrimination and socioeconomic disadvantage on nonseeking of medical treatment by women, but not by men (Wamala et al., 2007). The authors associated these findings with "vulnerable exposures of gendered discrimination in relation to social divisions premised on power and authority", and concluded that adverse discrimination based on race/ethnicity, gender, and age are relevant, even in more egalitarian societies, such as Sweden.

Gender- and race-based differences can be important in the uptake of free preventive services, as shown by a study in the US (Middleman, 2004), where participation and completion rates in a school-based hepatitis B vaccination program varied by race with black and Hispanic potential enrollees participating more frequently than white and Asian potential enrollees. Gender differences were significant among blacks and Hispanics, wherein girls were significantly more likely to complete the vaccination series than boys, but differences were nonsignificant among white and Asian children.

Another study in Pakistan (Mumtaz and Salway, 2005, 2007) found that the quality of a woman's interpersonal ties, particularly with her mother-in-law and husband, were important in terms of her ability to access resources, including antenatal care. Her education was also important, as were family finances. Pregnant woman who were wealthy and enjoyed high-status could circumvent more easily gendered proscriptions against their mobility while pregnant, and suffered fewer consequences in doing so. Their higher unaccompanied mobility did not become an excuse for male exploitation, and nor did it lead to a loss of familial status; whereas poor women's higher unaccompanied mobility was associated with a loss of familial prestige and increased their susceptibility to sexual violence.

Apart from gender and class, race, ethnicity and caste are other barriers that impinge upon access to health care. For example, a review of research suggests that the prevalence of mental disorders is higher among blacks than among whites, probably due to the nexus of race and socioeconomic factors that affect both the quality and adequacy of mental health care received (Nelson, 2006). Factors contributing to poorer access to care among blacks include a general mistrust of medical health professionals, cultural barriers, co-occurring disorders, socioeconomic factors, and primary reliance on family and the religious community during times of distress. However, there is little by way of evidence in the published literature on intersectionality: a number of studies consider multiple axes of power but view them simply as separable processes (Adamson et al., 2003; Campbell et al., 2001; Malat et al., 2006).

Ethnic, caste, and race-based differences may become particularly evident when access to care does not primarily depend on the ability to pay (economic class). For example, a study in India showed that caste was a significant source of inequality in the uptake of schooling when affordability was not the binding constraint. But it was not a significant predictor of inequalities in access to curative care, which was a function of purchasing power in the first instance, and not cultural bias (Iyer, 2007). A study on differences in health-seeking for children in a tea estate in India (where income and levels of access to medical facilities do not vary by caste) discovered that low caste households were more likely to treat their children in expensive facilities outside the estate, consequently spending more on treatment than the upper castes (Luke and Munshi, 2007). Moreover, these expenditures did not vary by gender within each caste. These findings run counter to what one would expect to find elsewhere in the country.

Studies conducted in Bangladesh, in areas serviced by BRAC where differences by economic status are believed to be less stark than elsewhere in the country, reveal that gender differences in treatment seeking persist despite socioeconomic development over time (Ahmed et al., 2000, 2003). However, another study conducted in the same area comparing the health-seeking behavior among the old with that among the young (Ahmed et al., 2005) found no significant difference in health expenditures by gender and age once they controlled for economic class. More in-depth research would be required to make sense of these contrasting patterns.

The studies discussed here highlight the need to consider class and gender simultaneously, together with race, caste, and ethnicity, as they reveal important social processes from which theoretical and policy relevant insights can be drawn. The study from rural south India (Iyer et al., 2007) shows that class is a gendered phenomenon that hits women first before affecting men. This finding is important for predictions of the likely results of rising health care costs: they are likely to be much more severe for women (and girls). Indeed, the ability of men (and boys), to hold on to health care in hard times may even be at the expense of the women in their households. This finding has significant implications for policies.

CONCLUSION

This chapter reviewed existing research on the intersections between different social axes of power (viz., gender, class, race, ethnicity, and caste), and their impacts on health status and access to health care. Evidence on intersectionality and its implications for health is relatively new and growing, since the problem itself has only recently begun to be examined in-depth. The bulk of the studies identified for this chapter focus on intersecting inequalities in health status; the evidence in relation to access to health care is by comparison extremely limited, and even these studies mainly pertain to countries with market-oriented health systems. The issues, however, are crucial from a policy perspective, since intersecting stratification processes can significantly alter the impacts of any one dimension of inequality taken by itself. Gender differences in health vary by race, ethnicity, caste, and class; and differences by race, ethnicity, caste, and class vary by gender, or by a number of other combinations.

The studies complicate our understanding of the social patterning of health inequalities and reveal additional insights from which policy-relevant lessons can be drawn. They confirm that socioeconomic status measures cannot fully account for gender, racial, ethnic, and caste-based inequalities in health. The effects of socioeconomic class on health can vary in magnitude and direction by race/ethnicity and by gender. Moreover, changes in socioeconomic position over time can result in differential effects and changing patterns of inequalities in health.

A number of studies point out that as social position is multidimensional, the influence of risk factors and their impact in terms of health inequalities can be complex and cannot be predicted satisfactorily along a single dimension of power. The relative importance of risk factors for health outcomes often differs for men and women in different socioeconomic and racial groups, and in different contexts. Indeed, gender (including norms, values, behavior, and practices) across and within caste, race, class, and ethnicity-based groups, is an important driver of differences in the patterning of risk factors and their consequent influence on health.

Other studies indicate that responses to unaffordable health care often vary by the gender and class location of sick individuals and their households. They strongly suggest that economic class should not be analyzed by itself, and that apparent class differences can be misinterpreted without gender analysis. The burden of economic pressures on the household, and responses to disasters, can be disproportionately borne by girls and women. They are the ones more likely to be trapped by medical poverty.

Insufficient attention to intersectionality in much of the health literature has had, we believe, significant human costs, because those affected most negatively tend to be those who are poorest and most oppressed by gender and other forms of social inequality. The program and policy costs are also likely to be high, in terms of poorly functioning programs, ineffective poverty alleviation and social and health policies that often target along a single dimension, such as income. In particular, antipoverty programs, intended to counter rising health care costs, must specifically support women's access. This can be done through a combination of universal systems (of provisioning or health insurance) coupled with forms of targeting, or other mechanisms, to ensure that they actually reach women and girls within households.

ACKNOWLEDGMENTS

We would like to thank Linda Rydberg at the Karolinska Institutet for assisting us with the search for relevant literature included in this review.

NOTES

1. Several studies do consider multiple axes of social inequality, but continue to treat them as separable processes (Dransfield et al., 2006; Green et al., 2004; Krause and Broderick, 2004; Lacey and Walters, 2003; McGrath et al., 2006).
2. The findings from all the studies cited have to be qualified with the caveat that self-reports of morbidity reveal a mix of objective illness and subjective willingness to acknowledge or claim illness. Consequently, self-reported illness is not equivalent to clinically diagnosed disease.
3. Recent analysis of employment data in Sweden refutes the argument that socioeconomic gradients in health among men and women can be due to possible misclassification of socioeconomic position among women (Ljung and Hallqvist, 2007).
4. The authors use the terms "avoidant coping" and "problem-solving coping" to distinguish between the actions that do not actively confront the problem of musculoskeletal pain from those that do. For example, actions grouped under "avoidant coping" include using stronger medicine, being less physically active, staying in bed most of the time, and contacting a medical doctor. Actions termed "problem-solving coping" include being in contact with a medical doctor, receiving and following treatment suggested by a chiropractor, physiotherapist, or other therapist, asking the advice of others who have similar experiences of pain, demanding changes in work environment and residence, and making changes in daily life.
5. The limitation of this study is that being descriptive, it does not adequately explain complex patterns—the explanations are post hoc and will require further study (Lynch, 2008). Further:

   there are grounds for reservation about the conclusions drawn from the model specification and estimation. *First*, the dependent variable, viz. self-assessed health status, is an ordinal variable on a discrete scale of 1 to 4. However, the model treats it as a continuous variable in order to apply the classical Ordinary Least Square (OLS) method of estimation. Though the sample size is reasonably large (1500), it does not ensure that the model assumption of normal distribution of the error term is valid, which is required for the subsequent tests of significance. *Second*, the conclusions are drawn from simple comparisons of the estimated coefficients without testing. Standard tests of significance could be applied for the purpose, provided of course the residuals passed the diagnostics tests for the assumption as stated earlier. (Sen et al., 2009, p. 413)

6. Although intersectionality is a topic for which there is growing interest and evidence, several questions remain unanswered, in part because of limitations in the quantitative methods used, even though the techniques used to analyze health inequalities as separable processes can be sophisticated. Sen and others (2009) develop a quantitative methodology applicable to large data sets that is able to rigorously compare and test for the significance of differences along the entire multidimensional and intersecting social scale in a relatively economical way.

REFERENCES

Adamson, J., Y. Ben-Shlomo, N. Chaturvedi, and J. Donovan. 2003. Ethnicity, socio-economic position and gender—do they affect reported health-care seeking behaviour? *Social Science and Medicine* 57 (5): 895–904.

Ager, A., and K. Pepper. 2005, Patterns of health service utilization and perceptions of needs and services in rural Orissa. *Health Policy and Planning* 20 (3): 176–184.

Ahmed, S.M., A.M. Adams, M. Chowdhury, and A. Bhuiya. 2000. Gender, socio-economic development and health-seeking behaviour in Bangladesh. *Social Science and Medicine* 51 (3): 361–371.

———. 2003. Changing health-seeking behaviour in Matlab, Bangladesh: Do development interventions matter? *Health Policy and Planning* 18 (3): 306–315.

Ahmed, S.M., G. Tomson, M. Petzold, and Z.N. Kabir. 2005. Socioeconomic status overrides age and gender in determining health-seeking behaviour in rural Bangladesh. *Bulletin of the World Health Organization* 83 (2): 109–117.

Ahnquist, J., P. Fredlund, and S.P. Wamala. 2007. Is cumulative exposure to economic hardships more hazardous to women's health than men's? A 16-year follow-up study of the Swedish Survey of Living Conditions. *Journal of Epidemiology and Community Health* 61 (4): 331–336.

Almgren, G., M. Magarati, and L. Mogford. 2009. Examining the influences of gender, race, ethnicity, and social capital on the subjective health of adolescents. *Journal of Adolescence* 32 (1): 109–133.

Annandale, E. 1998. *The Sociology of Health and Medicine: A Critical Introduction*. Cambridge and Oxford: Polity Press in association with Blackwell Publishers Ltd.

Annandale, E., and K. Hunt. 2000. Gender inequalities in health: Research at the crossroads. In *Gender Inequalities in Health*, edited by E. Annandale and K. Hunt. Buckingham and Philadelphia: Open University Press: 1–35.

Anthias, F. 2001. Beyond feminism and multiculturalism: Locating difference and the politics of location. *Women's Studies International Forum* 25 (3): 275–286.

Artazcoz, L., J. Benach, C. Borrell, and I. Cortes. 2004. Unemployment and mental health: Understanding the interactions among gender, family roles and social class. *American Journal of Public Health* 94 (1): 82–88.

Artazcoz, L., C. Borrell, and J. Benach. 2001. Gender inequalities in health among workers: The relation with family demands. *Journal of Epidemiology and Community Health* 55 (9): 639–647.

88   *Aditi Iyer, Gita Sen, and Piroska Östlin*

Asenso-Okyere, W.K., A. Anum, I. Osei-Akoto, and A. Adukonu. 1998. Cost recovery in Ghana: Are there any changes in health care seeking behaviour? *Health Policy and Planning* 13 (2): 181–188.

Bambra, C., D. Pope, D. Stanistreet, A. Roskam, A. Kunst, and A. Scott-Samuel. 2009. Gender, health inequalities and welfare state regimes: A cross-national study of 13 European countries. *Journal of Epidemiology and Community Health* 63 (1): 38–44.

Banks, K.H., L.P. Kohn-Wood, and M. Spencer. 2006. An examination of the African American experience of everyday discrimination and symptoms of psychological distress. *Community Mental Health Journal* 42 (6): 555–570.

Bay-Cheng, L.Y., A.N. Zucker, A.J. Stewart, and C.S. Pomerleau. 2002. Linking femininity, weight concern, and mental health among Latina, black and white women. *Psychology of Women Quarterly* 26 (1): 36–45.

Bhopal, R., L. Hayes, M. White, N. Unwin, J. Harland, S. Ayis, and G. Alberti. 2002. Ethnic and socio-economic inequalities in coronary heart disease, diabetes and risk factors in Europeans and South Asians. *Journal of Public Health* 24 (2): 95–105.

Blendon, R.S., C. Schoen, C.M. DesRoches, R. Osborn, K.L. Scoles, and K. Zapert. 2002. Inequities in health care: A five-country survey. *Health Affairs* 21 (3): 182–190.

Borrell, C., C. Muntaner, J. Benach, and L. Artazcoz. 2004. Social class and self-reported health status among men and women: What is the role of work organisation, household material standards and household labour? *Social Science and Medicine* 58 (10): 1869–1887.

Braveman, P., C. Cubbin, K. Marchi, S. Egerter, and G. Chavez. 2001. Measuring socioeconomic status/position in studies of racial/ethnic disparities: Maternal and infant health. *Public Health Reports (1974–)* 116 (5): 449–463.

Bredstrom, A. 2006. Intersectionality: A challenge for feminist HIV/AIDS research? *European Journal of Women's Studies* 13 (3): 229–243.

Brewer, R.M., C.A. Conrad, and M.C. King. 2002. The complexities and potential of theorizing gender, caste, race, and class. *Feminist Economist* 8 (2): 3–17.

Burman, E. 2004. From difference to intersectionality: Challenges and resources. *European Journal of Psychotherapy, Counselling and Health* 6 (4): 293–308.

Campbell, J.L., J. Ramsay, and J. Green. 2001. Age, gender, socioeconomic, and ethnic differences in patients' assessments of primary health care. *Quality in Health Care* 10 (2): 90–95.

Chakravarti, U. 2002. Through another lens: Men, women and caste. In *Translating Caste*, edited by T. Basu. New Delhi: Katha: 198–218.

Chandola, T., H. Kuper, A. Singh-Manoux, M. Bartley, and M. Marmot. 2004. The effect of control at home on CHD events in the Whitehall II study: Gender differences in psychosocial domestic pathways to social inequalities in CHD. *Social Science and Medicine* 58 (8): 1501–1509.

Christensen, U., L. Schmidt, C.Ø. Hougaard, M. Kriegbaum, and B.E. Holstein. 2006. Socioeconomic position and variations in coping strategies in musculoskeletal pain: A cross-sectional study of 1287 40- and 50-year old men and women. *Journal of Rehabilitation in Medicine* 38 (5): 316–321.

Collins, P.H. 1998. It's all in the family: Intersections of gender, race, and nation. *Hypatia* 13 (3): 62–82.

———. 2000. *Black Feminist Thought: Knowledge, Consciousness and the Politics of Empowerment*. Boston: Unwin Hyman.

Collins, P.Y., H. von Unger, and A. Armbrister. 2008. Church ladies, good girls, and locas: Stigma and the intersection of gender, ethnicity, mental illness, and sexuality in relation to HIV risk. *Social Science and Medicine* 67 (3): 389–397.

Cooper, H. 2002. Investigating socio-economic explanations for gender and ethnic inequalities in health. *Social Science and Medicine* 54 (5): 693–706.

Crenshaw, K. 1989. Demarginalizing the intersection of race and sex: A black feminist critique of antidiscrimination doctrine, feminist theory and antiracist politics. *University of Chicago Legal Forum* 14: 538–554.

———. 1991. Mapping the margins: Intersectionality, identity politics, and violence against women of color. *Stanford Law Review* 43 (6): 1241–1299.

Cummings, J.L., and P.B. Jackson. 2008. Race, gender, and SES disparities in self-assessed health, 1974–2004. *Research on Aging* 30 (2): 137–168.

Davey Smith, G., K. Charsley, H. Lambert, S. Paul, S. Fenton, and W. Ahmad. 2000. Ethnicity, health and the meaning of socio-economic position. In *Understanding Health Inequalities*, 1st ed., edited by H. Graham. Maidenhead, Berkshire, and Philadelphia: Open University Press: 25–37.

Davis, K. 2008. Intersectionality as buzzword: A sociology of science perspective on what makes a feminist theory successful. *Feminist Theory* 9 (1): 67–85.

Denton, M., S. Prus, and V. Walters. 2004. Gender differences in health: A Canadian study of the psychosocial, structural and behavioural determinants of health. *Social Science and Medicine* 58 (12): 2585–2600.

Denton, M., and V. Walters. 1999. Gender differences in structural and behavioral determinants of health: An analysis of the social production of health. *Social Science and Medicine* 48 (9): 1221–1235.

Dhamoon, R. 2008. Considerations in mainstreaming intersectionality as an analytic approach. *Paper Presented at Workshop on Intersectionality in Theory and Practice: An Interdisciplinary Dialogue, April 17–18*. Vancouver: Simon Fraser University.

Dinwiddie, G.Y. 2006. The social antecedents of stress exposure: Implications for status variations and social disparities for mental health. *PhD Dissertation.* Philadelphia: University of Pennsylvania.

Doyal, L. 2003. *Gender and Health Sector Reform: A Literature Review and Report from a Workshop at Forum 7.* Geneva: Global Forum for Health Research.

Dransfield, M.T., J.J. Davis, L.B. Gerald, and W.C. Bailey. 2006. Racial and gender differences in susceptibility to tobacco smoke among patients with chronic obstructive pulmonary disease. *Respiratory Medicine* 100 (6): 1110–1116.

Drever, F., T. Doran, and M. Whitehead. 2004. Exploring the relation between class, gender, and self rated general health using the new socioeconomic classification. A study using data from the 2001 census. *Journal of Epidemiology and Community Health* 58 (7): 590–596.

Dworkin, S.L. 2005. Who is epidemiologically fathomable in the HIV/AIDS epidemic? Gender, sexuality, and intersectionality in public health. *Culture, Health and Sexuality* 7 (6): 615–623.

Emslie, C., K. Hunt, and S. Macintyre. 1999. Problematizing gender, work and health: The relationship between gender, occupational grade, working conditions and minor morbidity in full-time bank employees. *Social Science and Medicine* 48 (1): 33–48.

Falkingham, J. 2004. Poverty, out-of-pocket payments and access to health care: Evidence from Tajikistan. *Social Science and Medicine* 58 (2): 247–258.

Farmer, M.M., and K.F. Ferraro. 2005. Are racial disparities in health conditional on socioeconomic status? *Social Science and Medicine* 60 (1): 191–204.

Feinstein, J.S. 1993. The relationship between socioeconomic status and health: A review of literature. *The Milbank Quarterly* 71 (2): 279–322.

George, A. 1997. *Household Health Expenditure in Two States. A Comparative Study of Districts in Maharashtra and Madhya Pradesh.* Pune/Mumbai: Foundation for Research in Community Health.

Gijsbers van Wijk, C.M.T., K.P. van Vliet, and A.M. Kolk. 1996. Gender perspectives and quality of care: Towards appropriate and adequate health care for women. *Social Science and Medicine* 43 (5): 707–720.

Green, C.R., S.K. Ndao-Brumblay, A.M. Nagrant, T.A. Baker, and E. Rothman. 2004. Race, age, and gender influences among clusters of African American and white patients with chronic pain. *The Journal of Pain* 5 (3): 171–182.

Griffin, J.M., R. Fuhrer, S.A. Stansfeld, and M. Marmot. 2002. The importance of low control at work and home on depression and anxiety: Do these effects vary by gender and social class? *Social Science and Medicine* 54 (5): 783–798.

Huong, D.B., N.K. Phuong, S. Bales, C. Jiaying, H. Lucas, and M. Segall. 2007. Rural health care in Vietnam and China: Conflict between market forces and social need. *International Journal of Health Services* 37 (3): 555–572.

Iyer, A. 2007. Gender, caste and class in health: Compounding and competing inequalities in rural Karnataka, India. *PhD Thesis*. Liverpool: University of Liverpool, Division of Public Health.

Iyer, A., G. Sen, and A. George. 2007. The dynamics of gender and class in access to health care: Evidence from rural Karnataka, India. *International Journal of Health Services* 37 (3): 537–554.

Kahn, J.R., and E.M. Fazio. 2005. Economic status over the life course and racial disparities in health. *Journals of Gerontology Series B: Psychological Sciences and Social Sciences* 60 (2): S76–S84.

Kenjiro, Y. 2005. Why illness causes more serious economic damage than crop failure in rural Cambodia. *Development and Change* 36 (4): 759–783.

Kimbro, R.T., S. Bzostek, N. Goldman, and G. Rodriguez. 2008. Race, ethnicity, and the education gradient in health. *Health Affairs* 27 (2): 361–372.

King, D.K. 1988. Multiple jeopardy, multiple consciousness: The context of a black feminist ideology. *Signs: Journal of Women in Culture and Society* 14 (1): 42–72.

Kirkness, V. 1988. Emerging native women. *Canadian Journal of Women and Law* 2 (2): 408–415.

Krause, J.S., and L. Broderick. 2004. Outcomes after spinal cord injury: Comparisons as a function of gender and race and ethnicity. *Archives of Physical Medicine and Rehabilitation* 85 (3): 355–362.

Krieger, N. 1990. Social class and the black/white crossover in the age-specific incidence of breast cancer: A study linking census-derived data to population-based registry records. *American Journal of Epidemiology* 131 (5): 804–814.

Krieger, N., J.T. Chen, and J.V. Selby. 2001. Class inequalities in women's health: Combined impact of childhood and adult social class—a study of 630 US women. *Public Health* 115 (3): 175–185.

Krieger, N., J.T. Chen, P.D. Waterman, D.H. Rehkopf, R. Yin, and B.A. Coull. 2006. Race/ethnicity and changing US socioeconomic gradients in breast cancer incidence: California and Massachusetts, 1978–2002 (United States). *Cancer Causes and Control* 17 (2): 217–226.

Krieger, N., C. Quesenberry, T. Peng, P. Horn-Ross, S. Stewart, S. Brown, K. Swallen, T. Guillermo, D. Suh, L. varez-Martinez, and F. Ward. 1999. Social class, race/ethnicity, and incidence of breast, cervix, colon, lung, and prostate cancer among Asian, black, Hispanic, and white residents of the San Francisco Bay Area, 1988–1992 (United States). *Cancer Causes and Control* 10 (6): 525–537.

Krieger, N., D.H. Rehkopf, J.T. Chen, P.D. Waterman, E. Marcelli, and M. Kennedy. 2008. The fall and rise of US inequities in premature mortality: 1960–2002. *PLoS Med* 5 (2), e46: 0227–0241.

Krishna, A. 2003. Falling into poverty: Other side of poverty reduction. *Economic and Political Weekly* XXXVIII (6): 533–542.

———. 2006. Pathways out of and into poverty in 36 villages of Andhra Pradesh, India. *World Development* 34 (2): 271–288.

Krishna, A., P. Kristjanson, M. Radeny, and W. Nindo. 2004. Escaping poverty and becoming poor in 20 Kenyan villages. *Journal of Human Development* 5 (2): 211–226.

Krishna, A., M. Kapila, M. Porwal, and V. Singh. 2003. Falling into poverty in a high-growth state: Escaping poverty and becoming poor in Gujarat villages. *Economic and Political Weekly* XXXVIII (49): 5171–5179.

Lacey, E.A., and S.J. Walters. 2003. Continuing inequality: gender and social class influences on self perceived health after a heart attack. *Journal of Epidemiology and Community Health* 57 (8): 622–627.

Lahelma, E., S. Arber, K. Kivela, and E. Roos. 2002. Multiple roles and health among British and Finnish women: The influence of socioeconomic circumstances. *Social Science and Medicine* 54 (5): 727–740.

Leonard, L. 2005. Where there is no state: Household strategies for the management of illness in Chad. *Social Science and Medicine* 61 (1): 229–243.

Lewis, M. 2000. *Who Is Paying for Health Care in Eastern Europe and Central Asia?* Washington, DC: The World Bank, Europe and Central Asia Region, Human Development Sector Unit.

Li, C., B. Hedblad, M. Rosvall, F. Buchwald, F.A. Khan, and G. Engstro. 2008. Stroke incidence, recurrence, and case-fatality in relation to socioeconomic position: A population-based study of middle-aged Swedish men and women. *Stroke* 39 (8): 2191–2196.

Liu, Y., K. Rao, and W.C. Hsaio. 2003. Medical expenditure and rural impoverishment in China. *Journal of Health, Population and Nutrition* 21 (3): 216–222.

Li, Y., and S.A. Robert. 2008. The contributions of race, individual socioeconomic status, and neighborhood socioeconomic context on the self-rated health trajectories and mortality of older adults. *Research on Aging* 30 (2): 251–273.

Ljung, R., and J. Hallqvist. 2007. Misclassification of occupation-based socioeconomic position and gender comparisons of socioeconomic risk. *Scandinavian Journal of Public Health* 35 (1): 17–22.

Loucks, E.B., K.T. Magnusson, S. Cook, D.H. Rehkopf, E.S. Ford, and L.F. Berkman. 2007a. Socioeconomic position and the metabolic syndrome in early, middle, and late life: Evidence from NHANES 1999–2002. *Annals of Epidemiology* 17 (10): 782–790.

Loucks, E.B., D.H. Rehkopf, R.C. Thurston, and I. Kawachi. 2007b. Socioeconomic disparities in metabolic syndrome differ by gender: Evidence from NHANES III. *Annals of Epidemiology* 17 (1): 19–26.

Lucas, H. A. Nuwagaba. 1999. Household coping strategies in response to the introduction of user charges for social service: A case study on health in Uganda. *IDS Working Paper* 86. Brighton, Sussex: Institute of Development Studies.

Luchenski, S., A. Quesnel-Vallee, and J. Lynch. 2008. Differences between women's and men's socioeconomic inequalities in health: Longitudinal analysis of the Canadian population, 1994–2003. *Journal of Epidemiology and Community Health* 62 (12): 1036–1044.

Luke, N., and K. Munshi. 2007. Social affiliation and the demand for health services: Caste and child health in South India. *Journal of Development Economics* 83 (2): 256–279.

Luong, D.H., S. Tang, T. Zhang, and M. Whitehead. 2007. Vietnam during economic transition: A tracer study of health service access and affordability. *International Journal of Health Services* 37 (3): 573–588.

Lynch, J., and G. Kaplan. 2000. Socioeconomic position. In *Social Epidemiology*, edited by L.F. Berkman and I. Kawachi. Oxford and New York: Oxford University Press: 13–35.

Lynch, S.M. 2008. Race, socioeconomic status, and health in life-course perspective: Introduction to the special issue. *Research on Aging* 30 (2): 127–136.

Machenbach, J.P., M.J. Bakker, A.E. Kunst, and F. Diderichsen. 2002. Socioeconomic inequalities in health in Europe: An overview. In *Reducing Inequalities in Health: A European Perspective*, edited by J.P. Machenbach and M.J. Bakker. London and New York: Routledge: 3–24.

Macintyre, S., and K. Hunt. 1997. Socio-economic position, gender and health: How do they interact? *Journal of Health Psychology* 2 (3): 315–334.

Macintyre, S., K. Hunt, and H. Sweeting. 1996. Gender differences in health: Are things really as simple as they seem? *Social Science and Medicine* 42 (4): 617–624.

Makinen, M., H. Waters, M. Rauch, N. Almagambetova, R. Bitran, L. Gilson, D. McIntyre, S. Pannarunothai, A.L. Prieto, G. Ubilla, and S. Ram. 2000. Inequalities in health care use and expenditures: Empirical data from eight developing countries and countries in transition. *Bulletin of the World Health Organization* 78 (1): 55–65.

Malat, J.R., M. Van Ryn, and D. Purcell. 2006. Race, socioeconomic status, and the perceived importance of positive self-presentation in health care. *Social Science and Medicine* 62 (10): 2479–2488.

Matthews, S., O. Manor, and C. Power. 1999. Social inequalities in health: Are there gender differences? *Social Science and Medicine* 48 (1): 49–60.

McCann, C.R., and S.K. Kim. 2003. Theorizing intersecting identities: Introduction. In *Feminist Theory Reader: Local and Global Perspectives*, edited by C.R. McCann and S.K. Kim. New York and London: Routledge: 148–162.

McGrath, J.J., K.A. Matthews, and S.S. Brady. 2006. Individual versus neighborhood socioeconomic status and race as predictors of adolescent ambulatory blood pressure and heart rate. *Social Science and Medicine* 63 (6): 1442–1453.

McIntyre, D., M. Thiede, G.R. Dahlgren, and M. Whitehead. 2006. What are the economic consequences for households of illness and of paying for health care in low- and middle-income country contexts? *Social Science and Medicine* 62 (4): 858–865.

Mei Tang, Y.C., and D. Krewski. 2003. Gender-related differences in the association between socioeconomic status and self-reported diabetes. *International Journal of Epidemiology* 32 (3): 381–385.

Mendelson, T., L.D. Kubzansky, G.D. Datta, and S.L. Buka. 2008. Relation of female gender and low socioeconomic status to internalizing symptoms among adolescents: A case of double jeopardy? *Social Science and Medicine* 66 (6): 1284–1296.

Middleman, A.B. 2004. Race/ethnicity and gender disparities in the utilization of a school-based hepatitis B immunization initiative. *Journal of Adolescent Health* 34 (5): 414–419.

———. 2002. Economic transition should come with a health warning: The case of Vietnam. *Journal of Epidemiology and Community Health* 56 (7): 497–505.

Mohindra, K.S., S. Haddad, and D. Narayana. 2006. Women's health in a rural community in Kerala, India: Do caste and socioeconomic position matter? *Journal of Epidemiology and Community Health* 60 (12): 1020–1026.

Mumtaz, Z., and S. Salway. 2005. 'I never go anywhere': Extricating the links between women's mobility and uptake of reproductive health services in Pakistan. *Social Science and Medicine* 60 (8): 1751–1765.

———. 2007. Gender, pregnancy and the uptake of antenatal care services in Pakistan. *Sociology of Health and Illness* 29 (1): 1–26.

Nabyonga, J., M. Desmet, H. Karamagi, P.Y. Kadama, F.G. Omaswa, and O. Walker. 2005. Abolition of cost-sharing is pro-poor: Evidence from Uganda. *Health Policy and Planning* 20 (2):100–108.

Nandraj, S., and R. Duggal. 1997. *Physical Standards in the Private Health Sector: A Case Study of Rural Maharashtra*. Mumbai: Centre for Enquiry into Health and Allied Themes.

National Sample Survey Organisation. 2006. *Morbidity, Health Care and the Condition of the Aged. (NSS 60th round: January–June 2004), 507 (60/25.0/1).* New Delhi: Ministry of Statistics and Programme Implementation, Government of India.

Navarro, V. 2002. A historical review (1965–1997) of studies on class, health and quality of life: A personal account. In *The Political Economy of Social Inequalities: Consequences for Health and Quality of Life*, edited by V. Navarro. Amityville, NY: Baywood Publishing Company, Inc: 13–32.

Nelson, C.A. 2006. Of eggshells and thin-skulls: A consideration of racism-related mental illness impacting Black women. *International Journal of Law and Psychiatry* 29 (2): 112–136.

Östlin, P. 2002. Gender perspective on socioeconomic inequalities in health. In *Reducing Inequalities in Health: A European Perspective*, edited by J.P. Machenbach and M.J. Bakker. London and New York: Routledge: 315–324.

———. 2005. *What Evidence Is There About the Effects of Health Care Reforms on Gender Equity, Particularly in Health?* Denmark: World Health Organisation Regional Office for Europe.

Östlin, P., A. George, and G. Sen. 2001. Gender, health and equity: The intersections. In *Challenging Inequities in Health: From Ethics to Action*, edited by T. Evans et al. Oxford and New York: Oxford University Press: 174–189.

Oths, K.S. 1994. Health care decisions of households in economic crisis: An example from the Peruvian highlands. *Human Organization* 53 (3): 245–254.

Perera, M., and G. Gunatilleke. 2006. Affordability and accessibility of health care for non-communicable diseases in Sri Lanka: Synopsis of the Sri Lanka case study in the Affordability Ladder Programme. *Marga Journal (Burden of Disease and Equity)* (April): 1–43.

Perera, M., G. Gunatilleke, and P. Bird. 2007. Falling into the medical poverty trap in Sri Lanka: What can be done? *International Journal of Health Services* 37 (2): 379–398.

Phoenix, A., and P. Pattynama. 2006. Intersectionality. *European Journal of Women's Studies* 13 (3): 187–192.

Ravindran, T.K.S., and D. Maceira. 2005. Health financing reforms. In *The Right Reforms? Health Sector Reforms and Sexual and Reproductive Health*, edited by T.K.S. Ravindran and H. de Pinho. Parktown, South Africa: Women's Health Project: 26–89.

Razack, S. 1998. *Looking White People in the Eye: Gender, Race, and Culture in Courtrooms and Classrooms.* Toronto: University of Toronto Press.

Read, J.G., and B.K. Gorman. 2006. Gender inequalities in US adult health: The interplay of race and ethnicity. *Social Science and Medicine* 62 (5): 1045–1065.

Reddy, G. 2005. Geographies of contagion: Hijras, Kothis, and the politics of sexual marginality in Hyderabad. *Anthropology and Medicine* 12 (3): 255–270.

Rosen, A.B., J.S. Tsai, and S.M. Downs. 2003. Variations in risk attitude across race, gender, and education. *Medical Decision Making* 23 (6): 511–517.

Rousham, E.K. 1996. Socio-economic influences on gender inequalities in child health in rural Bangladesh. *European Journal of Clinical Nutrition* 50: 560–564.

Russell, S. 2001. *Can Households Afford to Be Ill? The Role of the Health System, Material Resources and Social Networks in Sri Lanka. PhD Thesis* London: University of London, London School of Hygiene and Tropical Medicine, Department of Public Health and Policy, Health Policy Unit.

Russell, S., and K. Abdella. 2002. *Too Poor to Be Sick: Coping with the Costs of Illness in East Hararghe, Ethiopia.* London: Save the Children.

Sama—Resource Group for Women and Health. 2005. *The Interrelationship between Gender and Malaria among the Rural Poor in Jharkhand.* Trivandrum:

Sree Chitra Tirunal Institute for Medical Science and Technology, Achutha Menon Centre for Health Science Studies.

Schuler, S.R., L.M. Bates, and Md.K. Islam. 2002. Paying for reproductive health services in Bangladesh: Intersections between cost, quality and culture. *Health Policy and Planning* 17 (3): 273–280.

Schulz, A.J., and L. Mullings. eds. 2006. Gender, race, class and health: Intersectional approaches. San Francisco: Jossey-Bass.

Segall, M., G. Tipping, H. Lucas, T.V. Dung, N.T. Tam, D.X. Vinh, and D.L. Huong. 2000. *Health Care Seeking by the Poor in Transitional Economies: The Case of Vietnam.* Brighton, Sussex: Institute of Development Studies.

———. 2002. Economic transition should come with a health warning: The case of Vietnam. *Journal of Epidemiology and Community Health* 56 (7): 497–505.

Sen, B. 2003. Drivers of escape and descent: Changing household fortunes in rural Bangladesh. *World Development* 31 (3): 513–534.

Sen, G., A. George, and P. Östlin. 2002a. Engendering health equity: A review of research and policy. In *Engendering International Health: The Challenge of Equity,* edited by G. Sen, A. George, and P. Östlin. Cambridge and London: The MIT Press: 1–34.

Sen, G., A. Iyer, and A. George. 2002b. Class, gender and health equity: Lessons from liberalisation in India. In *Engendering International Health: The Challenge of Equity,* edited by G. Sen, A. George, and P. Östlin. Cambridge and London: The MIT Press: 281–311.

———. 2007. Systematic hierarchies and systemic failures: Gender and health inequities in Koppal District. *Economic and Political Weekly* XLII (8): 682–690.

Sen, G., A. Iyer, and C. Mukherjee. 2009. A methodology to analyse the intersections of social inequalities in health. *Journal of Human Development and Capabilities* 10 (3): 397–415.

Shuey, K.M., and A.E. Willson. 2008. Cumulative disadvantage and black–white disparities in life-course health trajectories. *Research on Aging* 30 (2): 200–225.

Stronks, K., H. van de Mheen, J. van den Bos, and J.P. Mackenbach. 1995. Smaller socioeconomic inequalities in health among women: The role of employment status. *International Journal of Epidemiology* 24 (3): 559–568.

Thurston, R.C., L.D. Kubzansky, I. Kawachi, and L.F. Berkman. 2005. Is the association between socioeconomic position and coronary heart disease stronger in women than in men? *American Journal of Epidemiology* 162 (1): 57–65.

Townsend, P., M. Whitehead, and N. Davidson. 1992. *Inequalities in Health: The Black Report and The Health Divide.* 2nd ed. London: Penguin.

Townsend, T. 2008. Protecting our daughters: Intersection of race, class and gender in African American mothers' socialization of their daughters' heterosexuality. *Sex Roles* 59 (5): 429–442.

Van Doorslaer, E., C. Masseria, and X. Koolman. 2006. Inequalities in access to medical care by income in developed countries. *Canadian Medical Association Journal* 174 (2): 177–183.

Vlassoff, C. 1994. Gender inequalities in health in the third world: Uncharted ground. *Social Science and Medicine* 39 (9): 1249–1259.

Wagstaff, A., and E. Van Doorslaer. 2003. Catastrophe and impoverishment in paying for health care: With applications to Vietnam 1993–1998. *Health Economics* 12 (11): 921–934.

Walsemann, K.M., A.T. Geronimus, and G.C. Gee. 2008. Accumulating disadvantage over the life course: Evidence from a longitudinal study investigating the relationship between educational advantage in youth and health in middle age. *Research on Aging* 30 (2): 169–199.

Walters, V. 1993. Stress, anxiety and depression: Women's accounts of their health problems. *Social Science and Medicine* 36 (4): 393–402.

Walters, S. and M. Suhrcke. 2005. *Socioeconomic inequalities in health and health care access in central and eastern Europe and the CIS: A review of the recent literature,* WHO European Office for Investment for Health and Development, Working paper 2005/1.

Wamala, S.P., J. Merlo, G. Boström, and C. Hogstedt. 2007. Perceived discrimination, socioeconomic disadvantage and refraining from seeking medical treatment in Sweden. *Journal of Epidemiology and Community Health* 61 (5): 409–415.

Weber, L., and D. Parra-Medina. 2003. Intersectionality and women's health: Charting a path to eliminating health disparities. In *Gender Perspectives on Health and Medicine: Key Themes,* edited by M.T. Segal, V. Demos, and J.J. Kronenfeld. Amsterdam: Elsevier Ltd: 181–230.

Whitehead, M., G. Dahlgren, and T. Evans. 2001. Equity and health sector reforms: Can low-income countries escape the medical poverty trap? *The Lancet* 358 (9284): 833–836.

Wilkes, A., Y. Hao, G. Bloom, and G. Xingyuan. 1997. Coping with the costs of severe illness in rural China. *IDS Working Paper 58.* Brighton, Sussex: Institute of Development Studies.

World Bank. 2001. *Kosovo Poverty Assessment. Volume I. Poverty Reduction and Economic Management, Europe and Central Asia Region.* Washington, DC: World Bank.

Xu, K., D.B. Evans, G. Carrin, A.M. Guilar-Rivera, P. Musgrove, and T. Evans. 2007. Protecting households from catastrophic health spending. *Health Affairs* 26 (4): 972–983.

Xu, K., D.B. Evans, K. Kawabata, R. Zeramdini, J. Klavus, and C.J.L. Murray. 2003. Household catastrophic health expenditure: A multicountry analysis. *The Lancet* 362 (9378): 111–117.

4 Gendered Health Outcomes of an 'Endless' War on Terror[1]

Rosalind Petchesky and Melissa Laurie

The camp is the space that is opened when the state of exception begins to become the rule. (Sergio Agamben, *Homo Sacer*, 1998, pp. 168–169)

CONCEPTUAL FRAMEWORK

This chapter sets out from several key premises. First, we agree with the observation of contemporary political theorists that under present conditions of militarized global capitalism and a 'war on terror' that knows no limits of time or space, what Agamben calls "states of exception" have increasingly become a "normal situation"—the everyday condition of life for millions of people across the globe (Agamben, 1998, p. 168; Papastergiadis, 2006; Hyland, 2001).

By "state of exception," Agamben means a juridical situation in which a declaration of emergency powers, a temporary imposition of martial law entailing suspension of ordinary constitutional norms and civil rights (usually in time of war, threat of armed attack or civil unrest), becomes indefinite if not permanent. In this condition, sovereignty itself, increasingly centralized, is defined by the capacity to determine when and where the state of exception exists, and more and more people find themselves reduced to "bare life," stripped of the ordinary rights of citizens or those with "the right to have rights" (Agamben, 2005, pp. 1–7; Papastergiadis 2006).[2]

Second, we adopt Agamben's focus on "the camp" as the quintessential site where the state of exception is manifest in the contemporary global landscape. Agamben's paradigm is the Nazi concentration camps, but the analysis applies just as well to all the proliferating sites of involuntary detention across the globe, from detention points for suspects in the US-led 'war on terror' (Guantánamo, Abu Ghraib, Baghram, and numerous secret sites of 'extraordinary rendition'), to camps for refugees and internally displaced persons (IDPs), to prisons with physical walls as well as those with legal and civil barriers that constitute the limbo in which undocumented migrants and trafficked persons find themselves all over the world. Despite the alleged disintegration of borders commonly associated with globaliza-tion, national borders have hardened and anti-immigrant policies have intensified in the US, UK, EU, and Australia since September 11, 2001, resulting in what Papastergiadis (2006) calls an "invasion complex." There-fore, paradoxically, both mass exclusions and forced migrations have come to typify the current state of global geopolitics.

Furthermore, in an increasingly militarized world, 'the camp' becomes symptomatic not only of a generalized kind of order but also of the merger of order and violence, war and peace, and the penetration of 'armed con-flict zones' into 'normal' life:

> Throughout much of the world, war is increasingly waged on the bod-ies of unarmed civilians [now 60–90% of all conflict casualties]. Where it was once the purview of male soldiers who fought enemy forces on battlefields quite separate from people's homes, contemporary conflict blurs such distinctions, rendering civilian women, men, and children its main casualties. The violence of such conflict cannot be isolated from other expressions of violence. In every militarized society, war zone, and refugee camp, violence against women and men is part of a broader continuum of violence that transcends the simple diplomatic dichotomy of war and peace . . . [and] resists any division between pub-lic and private domains. (Giles and Hyndman, 2004, p. 3)

'The camp' is thus both "a permanent spatial arrangement . . . outside the normal order," one where "law and fact . . . have become indistinguish-able," and a moral and ontological situation. Despite its variations, those who reside in it have in common their exclusion from the circle of persons recognized as citizens or even fully human beings. Yet, paradoxically, these individuals come to typify the current state of geopolitics (Agamben, 1998, pp. 169–171).

Conceptually, states of exception reveal 'bare life' as everyday life stripped down, where it is impossible to separate health from war and human insecu-rity or gender relations from economic and political inequalities. Thus the camp offers an opportunity to apply up close our third underlying premise: that gender equity in health care always and everywhere intersects with a whole series of social, economic, and cultural forces, including levels of armed and physical violence, employment and livelihood conditions, basic infrastructure (water, sanitation, transport), cultural norms and practices regarding gender, race, ethnicity, and religion, and possibilities for politi-cal participation and empowerment. Related to this is an understanding of gender as integral, context-specific, and inclusive of men as well as women and transgender persons. Men of all ages are among the vastly growing number of globalized and militarized bodies thrown into sites of exclu-sion, even though women and children may be the majority in many sites.

Gay men, lesbians, and transgender persons are both denied entry as cross-border migrants and denied full citizenship rights in their natal countries. Clearly the conditions of bare life have different meanings based on gender, sexuality, and race/ethnicity as well as local and cultural circumstances (Indra, 1999; Giles and Hyndman, 2004; Luibhéid, 2002; Luibhéid and Cantú, 2005; Petchesky, 2005; Corrêa et al., 2008).

We argue that foregrounding states of exception as a way of understanding current gender dynamics in the social determinants of health is both conceptually useful and epidemiologically necessary. From an epidemiological perspective, the aggregate of all these sites of exclusion constitutes the real space where untold millions of people live, on the bare margins of national regimes and sometimes under contested international jurisdiction. As such, it represents an enormous concentration of the most vulnerable and at-risk groups as well as a key transfer point for viruses, violence, and damaged, discarded bodies. Yet major health surveys, from the Human Development Reports to UNAIDS reports, and much of the literature on social determinants of health, still take national health systems as their statistical base; the populations residing in camps, whether those physically contained/detained or the huge number of cross-border and virtually stateless migrants, simply are not counted.

Our fourth and final premise is that a human rights approach to gender and health equity issues is *both indispensable and insufficient.* Again, sites of exclusion—'the camps'—reveal this most directly, insofar as their residents are precisely persons who have been cast outside the protections of citizenship and state laws. As Agamben notes, following Hannah Arendt, the situation of refugees embodies a paradox, since one would imagine people forcibly cast out from their homelands to be the 'purest' subjects of human rights. Yet such people are also those most lacking in any reliable forms of protection, respect, accountability, and methods of making claims and seeking enforcement. If they are "so completely deprived of their rights and prerogatives that no act committed against them could appear any longer as a crime," how can they be said simultaneously to be subjects of rights (Agamben, 1998, pp. 126, 171; Papastergiadis, 2006, p. 435)? With regard to health, international recognition of "the right to the highest attainable standard of physical and mental health" as a fundamental human right, and one that is indivisible from all the other economic, social, and cultural as well as civil and political rights is solidly elaborated in a number of international documents (CESCR, 2000; Hunt, 2007). But the verbal pronouncement of this right and its full application to *all* persons regardless of gender, race, or ethnicity, *including "asylum seekers and illegal immigrants" as well as "prisoners or detainees,"* is still a far cry from its practical realization, and nowhere more starkly than in the camps. As one writer puts it:

> 'human rights' clearly remain grounded in 'belonging' to a Nation-State, and consequently are of no use to those who find themselves

Stateless, having left the country they were born in (whether for fear of 'martyrdom' or as a matter of material necessity) and been refused 'naturalization' elsewhere. . . . Consequently, alienation of 'rights' grounded in national citizenship and the urgent need for another, less passive conception of subjectivity and freedom appear destined to become generalized conditions. (Hyland, 2001, p. 3)

Thus, sites of exclusion both mark the limits of human rights as currently understood, and help to illuminate how gender equity in health access and outcomes always, and everywhere, intersects with a whole series of social, economic, and cultural forces.

We have defined sites of political exclusion very broadly and believe it is urgent that public health advocates and practitioners bring this larger array of temporarily or permanently stateless populations into their priority agendas. Nevertheless, for practical reasons this chapter will focus mainly on one particular kind of site—camps containing 'refugees' or 'asylum seekers' (the terms for those who flee across national borders) as well as those harboring IDPs.[3] While forced migration may be the result of a variety of crises, including economic displacement from famines or development projects, and displacement from natural disasters (e.g., floods, hurricanes, tsunamis, earthquakes), because of space limitations, most of the examples of health and gender justice issues we will consider reflect displacement due to armed conflict, violence, and persecution.

Refugee and IDP Camps

There are currently approximately eight 'major wars' (defined by the United Nations as inflicting at least 1,000 deaths on the battlefield a year) under way. Along with these, more than two dozen smaller conflicts in Asia, Africa, the Middle East, and Latin America have been raging for decades and continue still.[4] Besides acting as a green light to all kinds of repressive regimes, the US-led war on terror has "been used to justify new or intensified military offensives," particularly in Aceh, Afghanistan, Chechnya, Georgia, Iraq, Pakistan, Palestine, and Somalia (UNHCR, 2005). In addition, it has made the situation of people forcibly displaced by local violence much more precarious, as they face closed borders, deportations, and the extremes of human insecurity.

According to recent estimates, in 2007 there were some 11–14 million refugees and asylum seekers worldwide, and an additional 26 million IDPs.[5] This number has increased significantly in the last two years reversing a five-year trend (UNHCR, 2007). Women and children constitute between 70% and 80% of all IDPs, and women are roughly half of all refugees and asylum seekers (Buscher and Makinson, 2006; Norwegian Refugee Council, 2008; UNFPA, 2006, p. 57). The gender disparity in IDP situations is directly related to militarized violence, many men and boys having been killed or recruited to join combatant groups.

Weiss and Korn (2006, p. 1) point out the "dramatic reversal" in the ratio of refugees to IDPs in the past twenty-five years, from 1982, when the number of international refugees was ten times greater than that of IDPs, to the present, when the latter have become two and a half times more numerous. This reversal reflects a number of global changes but, particularly, (a) the ascendancy of local, ethnic, and communal conflicts and imperial (US-led) 'policing' operations over international and regional wars; and (b) the recent backlash against the waves of cross-border exiles fleeing economic as well as military crises, with the consequent hardening of national borders to 'aliens.'

Despite the widely hailed open borders of globalization, national sovereignty claims slam the door on cross-border migrants and with a vengeance since September 11, 2001. Although they are most frequently fleeing the worst human rights violations, international asylum seekers not only face ethnic profiling, but also stringently policed borders and impossible visa requirements. In the globalized state of exception—but especially in the US, UK, EU, and Australia—they also meet the threat of indefinite detention as suspected 'terrorists' in jails, camps, or airport transit zones without the possibility of appeal or habeas corpus, contrary to all human rights norms, sometimes at great risk to their health and life.

Border policing and surveillance techniques also take aim at those deemed sexual and gender outlaws as well as the more predictable political, religious, and racialized targets of the 'war on terror.' Contributions to the scholarly anthology *Queer Migrations* document a century and a half of a "federal immigration control regime that sought to ensure a 'proper' sexual and gender order" by excluding Asian women (assumed to be prostitutes), cross-dressers, or anyone of "suspicious" sexual or gender identity, and more recently those infected with HIV/AIDS (Luibhéid and Cantú, 2005; Luibhéid 2002).[6] If anything, September 11th provided an excuse to intensify these more traditional forms of policing borders based on racial, gender, and heteronormative stereotypes. As Loescher puts it, "The war on terrorism has given policymakers and law enforcement agencies a ready pretext to abuse the rights of refugees and other immigrants" (2002, p. 52).

GENDERED HEALTH ISSUES IN FORCED MIGRATION SETTINGS

Militarization and Systemic Violence

Contemporary wars occur in the sites of the most severe social divisions, calling forth multiple forms of crisis all at once. It is, therefore, impossible to draw boundaries between war and peace, or between physical and social violence (including gender, race-ethnic, and class inequalities) (Giles and Hyndman, 2004). Civilian exposure to death and morbidity from armed attacks or land mines, absence of clean water and adequate sanitation, loss of arable land and shelter, severe nutritional deficits, and lack of access to health care, along with drastic human insecurity of every kind, all form part of a single disastrous web. Militarization is integrally linked to systemic violence (Grein et al., 2003; Gyles and Hyndman, 2004; Norwegian Refugee Council, 2006; Petchesky, 2008; Kottegoda et al., 2008; Al-Adili et al., 2008).

When we consider the much higher proportion of women and children in IDP camps relative to refugee camps, the disparity in health conditions and outcomes between them becomes another clear but unnoticed gender issue that arises in situations of armed and ethnic conflict. A 2001 *Lancet* article reports evidence that IDPs suffer "higher rates of morbidity," especially from malnutrition and infectious diseases, than do refugees, as well as greater incidence of "forced isolation, torture or abuse, lack of shelter, and forced separation from family members" (Salama et al., 2001, 4.13). Such differences are not only gendered but also highly political, and need to be understood as such. For example, the international community's failure to address effectively the IDP crisis stems from the old habit of deference to national sovereignty, fear of endangering existing UN programs in countries, and a 'development'-oriented mind-set that finds it difficult to relate to human rights and humanitarian issues (Weiss and Korn, 2006, p. 19). In addition, malnutrition and famine are most always socially constructed, abetted by the politics of internal ethnic conflicts and governments' refusals to allow transport of food and medical supplies (Norwegian Refugee Council, 2006). Even among IDPs, there are differences in treatment and health consequences, and these are often based on race-ethnic exclusions or other political considerations.

In Iraq, evidence-based estimates of 'the human cost of the war' were made in a study by an American and Iraqi team of public health researchers from the Bloomberg School of Public Health at Johns Hopkins University. Based on a population survey drawn from randomly selected clusters of households nationwide, the study estimated, for the period 2002–2006, over 600,000 'excess deaths' (that is, "number of persons dying above what would normally have been expected had the war not occurred") from violent causes, and an additional 53,000 from "non-violent causes," most likely from deterioration of health services and the environment (Burnham et al., 2006, pp. 1, 6). While small in comparison to civilian deaths during the Vietnam War, or in the Congo more recently, these numbers "[dwarf] the median number of 18,000 deaths for all civil wars since 1945" (Sambanis, 2006, 4. 13).

The gendered profile of casualties in today's wars, furthermore, is complex. According to the Hopkins study, the overwhelming preponderance of the estimated 600,000 violent deaths in Iraq has been among males of all ages, the majority ages 15–44, many of them belonging to or targeted by warring insurgent and rival sectarian groups. But other evidence suggests that the majority of those killed by 'coalition forces' (the US and UK primarily) have been civilian women and children. And among children (under 15) in Iraq, violent deaths (and, one supposes, 'excess' deaths from nonviolent causes) have been remarkably gender egalitarian (Burnham et al., 2006, pp. 9, 10).

When we widen the definition of 'human cost' to include more than deaths and morbidities, the impact on women and girls becomes much more visible. The Norwegian Refugee Council (2006, p. 23) estimates "that up to one-third of the internally displaced do not have regular access to clean drinking water and adequate sanitation facilities," and emphasizes their greater vulnerability "to malnutrition and diseases than the non-displaced population." One can only imagine (because we have no empirical studies) what the lack of sanitary facilities and supplies must mean for displaced women and girls. No toilets or paper or sanitary napkins; waiting all day until dark to relieve yourself; wearing dirty rags during menstruation; the related reproductive tract infections, fistulae, pain, festering, and possible infertility; the abjection, rejection, and shame (Mukherjee, 2002). Yet, the prevailing tendency for research and analysis in international public health, still invested in the 'global burden of disease' framework, is to concentrate on conditions of mortality and severe morbidity that threaten productivity, and to ignore the kinds of daily suffering that women—especially the poorest and most vulnerable—have been socialized to endure without stopping their daily tasks of maintaining families, even in the most deprived circumstances of the camps. Reproductive tract infections, lack of contraceptives or sanitary supplies, abdominal and back pain, vaginal discharges, sexual abuse, emotional stress, domestic violence—all become part of everyday life rather than health problems meriting intervention (Petchesky, 2003). In a study of Iraqi women and girls who had fled the war into Jordan, the Women's Commission for Refugee Women and Children found "significant gaps" in delivery of services for prevention of sexual violence, HIV prevention, and emergency obstetric care, among others (Chynoweth, 2008).

Both women and men in conflict-affected sites of displacement must make strategic decisions about just keeping themselves and their children alive. Macklin's (2004) description of the gendered fears of Dinka and Nuer in southern Sudan might represent the agonies of IDPs and refugees in many similar bare-life situations:

> Men worry about being killed by the GoS [Government of Sudan] or its allies, whether as civilians or as combatants in rebel forces. Women worry that they and their children will be abducted and enslaved by government-sponsored militia—if they are not killed outright. They also dread the moment when their boy children will be turned into child soldiers to fight in rebel armies against the GoS. Women fear rape by militia, rape by men who distribute aid in exchange for sex, and rape by husbands who demand that they replace dying children by producing still more children who will grow up to wage the national

struggle—that is, if the women survive their pregnancies and the children survive to adolescence. (2004, p. 82)

Ultimately, the most severe constraint determining lack of access to nutrition and health care among so many IDPs and refugees is the militarization of their environment. Military insecurity and armed conflict interfere with food distribution and often mean the complete breakdown of health services and depletion of aid workers. A study by Spiegel and his associates (2002) of health programs in refugee camps in seven countries found that better health indicators and lower mortality rates correlated not only with more adequate water supplies and higher numbers of health workers per person but also with the camp's location. Camps "situated closer to the border or area of conflict" experienced "increased trauma morbidity" and crude mortality rates ten times higher than those located at least 50 km from the border or conflict zone (Spiegel et al., 2002, p. 1932).[7]

This raises a critical question that is a subject of constant debate and anguish among humanitarian organizations, especially since the Rwandan genocide of the 1990s. What should be the relation of humanitarian efforts to outside military intervention? When if ever should such intervention be called for? Fiona Terry of Médecins sans Frontières (MSF) points out the sobering truth that humanitarian relief in the form of food supplies and medical care is useless "when the civilians it is intended to assist are in greater danger of losing their lives to violence" (Terry, 2001, p. 1432). On the other hand, except in cases of outright genocide, military action by outside powers has more often led to more killings, genocide, and mass expulsions rather than protecting civilians (as in Kosovo and Iraq). Several assessment studies call for greater coherence between military/political and humanitarian agendas (Salama et al., 2004; Waldman and Martone, 1999). But military organizations and humanitarian organizations have very different purposes as well as cultures: "the imposition of peace, like the creation of all political order . . . , inevitably generates its quota of 'victims,' 'excluded' and 'powerless' people who are either doomed to violent death or deprived of water, food, medical care and shelter—precisely the purposes that humanitarian relief is supposed to serve" (Weissman, 2004, p. 208). Moreover, "Military forces are trained and equipped to provide medical care and facilities to a predominately male, adult, healthy population." The medical supplies they do have are insufficient in quantity and "not adapted to the needs of refugees"—certainly not to those of women and girls facing rape, unwanted pregnancy, reproductive tract infections, and obstetric emergencies (Terry, 2001, p. 1431).

Reproductive Health Care

It seems self-evident that women and girls caught in armed conflict situations and refugee and IDP camps are at high risk of rape, unwanted pregnancies, unsafe delivery, and sexually transmitted infections (STIs), including HIV and AIDS. This is all the more likely given that the countries that have generated the greatest number of refugees, asylum seekers, and IDPs are to a large extent those with the highest under-five mortality rates, highest fertility rates, and youngest populations (USCRI, 2008; Spiegel, 2004).[8]

Until quite recently, international agencies and NGOs concerned with the health of refugees and IDPs were focused primarily on malnutrition and communicable diseases. In the past decade, however, they have come to embrace access to reproductive health information and services as a basic human right, thanks to groups like the Women's Commission for Refugee Women and Children and the Reproductive Health Access, Information and Services in Emergencies (RAISE) Initiative (Austin et al., 2008; Girard and Waldman, 2000, p. 167; Hynes et al., 2002; McGinn et al., 2004). Awareness was transformed into explicit policy guidelines in the 1999 Interagency Field Manual governing Reproductive Health in Refugee Situations, which introduced a Minimum Initial Service Package and guidelines related to safe motherhood, sexual and gender-based violence, sexually transmitted infections including HIV and AIDS, and family planning (UNHCR, 1999). The Sphere Project in 2004 built on these guidelines to further define standards and "establish clear guidance for humanitarian responders in all sectors" (Austin et al., 2008, p. 12). These guidelines reflect the coincidence of two world events during the mid-1990s: the humanitarian crises in Bosnia and Rwanda, and the 1994 International Conference on Population and Development (ICPD) in Cairo, whose Programme of Action defined reproductive and sexual health in a broad, integrative way, as part of primary health care and of basic human rights (United Nations, 1994). In a survey of all the international legal norms—conventions, resolutions, guidelines, field manuals, etc.—related to sex and gender in situations of conflict-induced displacement, Audrey Macklin confirms that the framework of protections within the UN system and international law is extensive indeed (Macklin, 2008).

Yet, this formal recognition on paper does not necessarily signify effective implementation on the ground, especially for IDPs. As both Macklin and Austin and colleagues conclude, substantial gaps between theory and practice persist. In a paper commissioned by the London-based Humanitarian Practice Network, McGinn and colleagues (2004) attempted to assess the implementation of the Interagency Field Manual and the 2004 revision of the Sphere guidelines with respect to "reproductive health for conflict-affected people." They found a mixed picture and still a shortage of empirical evidence. Fertility rates and pregnancy outcomes among populations in conflict-ridden zones tend to vary in relation to the stage and level of the conflict, with birthrates going down and incidence of unsafe abortion and maternal mortality ratios (already quite high in the countries affected) going up during the most intense phases. The location of camps,

in relation to both conflict areas and obstetric services, is a critical determinant of maternal risk. A large-scale study by Michelle Hynes and colleagues (2002), reported that "no camp had an operating theatre in which
life-saving surgery such as repair of a ruptured bowel or caesarean section
was possible. Time and distance to referral hospitals can affect maternal
mortality and obstetric intervention rates" (Spiegel et al., 2002, p. 1932;
Hynes et al., 2002). Though reliable data is scarce, some evidence suggests
very high rates of unsafe and self-induced abortions, and abortion complications, in conflict settings in sub-Saharan Africa and Burma (Jok Madut,
1999a). Moreover, services geared specifically to adolescents—for whom
STIs and unsafe abortions remain major health risks—are lacking in most
settings (McGinn et al., 2004). In their review of the existing evidence,
Austin and colleagues find "that advances in service coverage have been
largely concentrated in stable, refugee camp settings," whereas, again, IDPs
are largely neglected (2008, p. 16).

Despite good intentions, many failures in practice stem from the structural and systemic problems of the camps, including 'lack of coordination'
among different responsible agencies, 'serious gaps in services,' and 'a verti-
cal approach to reproductive health services' that is inconsistent with the
ICPD's integrated approach. In addition, "many of the most needed and
simplest reproductive health interventions for refugees, such as emergency
contraception or condom distribution to adolescents, remain mired in
ideological controversies" (Girard and Waldman, 2000, pp. 167, 172). US
government policies, under the Bush administration, have exacerbated reproductive health needs in sites of exclusion by restricting funds for UNFPA,
imposing the 'global gag rule' on any abortion counseling or advocacy, and
prioritizing abstinence over condom use in HIV/AIDS foreign aid programs
(Corrêa et al., 2008; Girard, 2004). This is despite UNFPA reports that
"an estimated 25% of refugee women of reproductive age will be pregnant
at any one time," and that unprotected sex and high-risk pregnancies are
particularly common among teenage girls in camps: "In war-torn southern
Sudan, girls were found to be more likely to die in pregnancy and childbirth
than [to] finish primary school" (UNFPA, 2006, p. 63).

One of the most dramatic examples of the meaning war gives to
health care and human rights is Afghanistan. After five years of US- and
NATO-led military intervention to root out Al Qaeda and end Taliban
rule, the government in Kabul is barely holding on, and Al Qaeda training camps, tribal warlords, and Taliban strongholds are resurgent (Mazzetti and Rohde, 2007). When the Taliban were in power in the 1990s,
prior to the US invasion after September 11th, Afghanistan had one of the
world's highest maternal mortality ratios—reported by WHO as 820 per
100,000 live births, and attributed largely to the draconian restrictions on
women's mobility and health care access under the world's most misogynist
regime (del Valle, 2004, p. 10). Yet two years after the Taliban had been
ousted, documented maternal mortality ratios were even higher at 1,600

per 100,000 and reaching in one province the highest rate recorded any-where at 6,500 per 100,000 live births (Salama et al., 2004). Hernan del Valle (2004), of MSF, questions the tendency to explain this reproductive disaster in terms mainly of cultural and religious factors, pointing instead to the war's total destruction of Afghanistan's infrastructure, roads, hos-pitals, clinics, and human resources—a calamity that affects everyone and not just pregnant women:

> For the vast majority of rural Afghans, health facilities remain inac-cessible, under-staffed, and under-equipped. Roads and transport are rarely available, and pregnant women often have to travel several hours by donkey to seek health care. It is not surprising that almost all of them deliver at home without qualified assistance . . . the issue in Af-ghanistan is arguably not so much one of access to health services for women but rather . . . absolute lack of facilities. (del Valle, 2004, p. 11; Salama et al., 2004)

In the Palestinian territories, besieged on all sides by Israeli Defense Forces, curfews, restrictions on movement, and the need to pass through severely guarded checkpoints to reach functioning health care centers and obstetric services, the reproductive health toll has also been dramatic. In a large-scale representative study of Palestinian women, Rita Giacaman and her associ-ates at Bir Zeit University (2006) report an increasing number of women who have given birth at checkpoints because of being detained there and of neonatal deaths as a consequence. These actual documented cases are only the "tip of the iceberg," since the stresses associated with constrained con-ditions of childbearing for Palestinian women no doubt produce additional maternal and infant mortalities and morbidities and affect both refugee and non-refugee women (Bosmans et al., 2008). Complicating the situation are tensions between biomedical and more traditional models of birthing (administered by TBAs, or *dayats*) (Giacaman et al., 2005). Most Palestin-ian women, reflecting the prevailing biomedical thinking, state a preference for hospital over home births (coinciding with historic Israeli government policy, which viewed hospital births as a means to register and count Pal-estinian population growth). But government maternity services operated under the Palestinian Authority since the Oslo Accords have been unable to meet basic needs or provide a sufficient number of birth attendants due to the continuing emergency, lack of resources, and withdrawal of interna-tional aid—most stringently since the election of a Hamas government in 2006 (Giacaman et al., 2006; Bosmans et al., 2008) and more recently the siege on Gaza residents.

In Iraq as well, physical conditions present an appalling list of everyday threats to life and limb: lack of medicines, sanitation, or adequate nutrition; over two-thirds of the population without potable drinking water; preva-lent diarrhea and pulmonary infections among children and the elderly;

overtaxed and shrinking health care facilities; a countryside riddled with unexploded ordinance, land mines, and depleted uranium; and of course the constant threat of suicide bombs as well as the US's stepped-up aerial war that never, ever avoids killing and maiming civilians (Lasky, 2006). In April 2005 doctors in Baghdad reported a "significant increase in the number of babies born with deformities" attributed to depleted uranium (Lasky, 2006, p. 10). A letter presented to Prime Minister Tony Blair in 2007 and signed by 100 doctors asserts "that conditions in Iraqi hospitals constitute a breach of the Geneva Convention" and are costing the lives of hundreds of sick and injured children left to die because of the lack of medicines, antibiotics, milk, and other basic medical and nutritional supplies (Brown, 2007). Infant mortality and child malnutrition rates have nearly doubled since the invasion. It is suspected that pharmaceuticals are being diverted from Iraqi warehouses into a regional black market, and the shortage of doctors—with some 2,000 murdered and 250 kidnapped between the invasion and the end of 2006—has reached devastating proportions (Chelala, 2007).

Conditions in Iraq make it impossible to get accurate figures on recent maternal mortality, but a UNFPA study in November 2003 found the ratio had nearly tripled since 1990, to 370 in 100,000 (31 times the US ratio) (UNFPA, 2003; Ciezadlo, 2005). While other countries have higher maternal mortality rates, this increase is more than any other country in the world (Save the Children, 2007). A lot is due to harsh UN sanctions during the 1990s, when Saddam Hussein was still in power, but even conservative estimates find a post-invasion increase in infant mortality of 37% (Roberts et al., 2004). Even under Saddam Hussein, women in Iraq prior to the US-led war had full access to prenatal care and trained birth attendants as well as to education and professional employment (Lasky, 2006). In contrast, the UNFPA study found that 40% of pregnant women got no prenatal care and up to 65% gave birth at home, without skilled attendants (UNFPA, 2003). Doctors in the few functioning hospitals are way too overwhelmed with the dying and wounded to bother with women undergoing childbirth, to say nothing of those who have been raped. We can only imagine how the maternal death and morbidity figures must have increased with the escalating violence and civil war the occupation triggered and continues to foment, even as official figures on violence decline.

Three important conclusions are evident from this assessment and case studies. First, in spite of excellent efforts by agencies to provide a high standard of reproductive health services to refugees in camps, most of these services are presently going to people in relatively stable, post-emergency situations, but far less to IDPs, whether in camps or dispersed outside them. Those caught in the most acute and dangerous stages of complex emergencies, and who are thus most at risk, are not getting the services. This underscores the second conclusion: the location of camps in relation to both conflict areas and obstetric services is a critical determinant of maternal risk. Third, even where immediate conflicts have stabilized, the decimated political and economic infrastructure may completely undermine the delivery of vital health care, including for reproductive health.

Finally, it is important to remark that 'poor maternal and pregnancy outcomes' may reflect a variety of factors, and not always women's helplessness. Childbearing becomes a terrain of ethnic struggle in armed conflict and displacement sites. In highly racialized ethno- and nationalist conflicts, such as in Bosnia, rape may be used as a way of 'planting the seed' in the 'enemy' population or, in response, childbearing may become a "demographic weapon" to "replace children or adults lost to war" (Eisenstein, 1996; McGinn et al., 2004, p. 6). However, women do not always respond passively to these demands on their reproductive capacity. Research among the western Dinka shows that women IDPs in Sudan (and likely elsewhere), facing sole responsibility for their children, under constant threat of sexual and military violence, insecurity, and harsh deprivation, cope with their 'reproductive suffering' through a common though clandestine practice of unsafe abortions, even where the practice is not accepted (Jok Madut, 1999a, 1999b; McGinn et al., 2004, pp. 96–97).

HIV/AIDS

If anything has conjoined with fears of terrorism and racism to feed the recent 'invasion complex,' it has been the HIV/AIDS pandemic. Yet, because of the multiple assaults and exclusions they confront, internal and external migrants are more likely to be the victims of transmission than its vectors (Spiegel, 2004; UNFPA, 2006, p. 16). Forced migrants (those fleeing economic as well as political and military crisis) are caught in the double bind that exclusion creates: "Discrimination, already endemic to the migrant and refugee's position, is exacerbated by HIV/AIDS, preventing [migrants] from seeking out appropriate health care and social support" (Williamson, 2004, 12). Besides outright discrimination, government policies simply let displaced populations fall through the cracks in this area of health care and service provision. National HIV/AIDS strategic plans and requests to donors almost never take into account their refugee populations and often ignore their internally displaced citizens as well (Spiegel, 2004). Not only national governments but also international agencies have been slow to recognize HIV/AIDS prevention and treatment as a critical priority for refugees and IDPs. It was only at the end of January 2007 that UNHCR launched a policy to ensure that HIV positive refugees and IDPs across the globe have access to necessary ARV treatment, care, and support in the "earliest possible stages of an emergency response to forced displacement" (IRIN News, 2007).

Forced migrants and civilians caught in armed conflict situations, especially women and youths, are particularly vulnerable to HIV infection (Save the Children, 2002; Spiegel, 2004). In a working paper for the Oxford University Refugee Studies Center, Katherine Williamson (2004) summarizes factors that confirm this general perception. First, female forced migrants "are exposed to exploitation by soldiers, rebels, officials, the military and other refugees [including husbands]." The risk here is not only sexual violence and degradation but also infection, since male combatants in civil conflicts and military personnel generally—including UN peacekeepers—are known to have HIV prevalence rates two to three times higher than those of civilian populations (Williamson, 2004, pp. 2, 13, 15; Spiegel, 2004). Second, the conditions in the camps—overcrowding, poor sanitation, insecurity, unemployment—also contribute to exposure of women and youths to unsafe sex, both unwanted and wanted. Whether in the form of rape, extortion, survival sex for money, food, or safe passage out of the country (documented among women in Sierra Leone), or just turning to sex for diversion or comfort, women and young male and female refugees and IDPs may face elevated risks of infection. "In Guinea, Liberia and Sierra Leone it has been found that refugee children and internally displaced youths are being forced to exchange sex for relief supplies and security by local aid workers, peacekeeping soldiers and refugee leaders in a system so endemic and prolific that many involved have no idea that relief is meant to be free" (Williamson, 2004, pp. 13–15).

As in the case of maternal and reproductive health risks, more evidence-based studies present a mixed picture. The general perception that IDPs have consistently higher HIV infection rates than the general population and that conflict necessarily increases the risks of transmission is not supportable (Norwegian Refugee Council, 2006, p. 25). The relationship between HIV and armed conflict is both 'complex' and 'context-specific,' depending on a range of factors. These include, once again, the phase and level of a conflict; the camp's location, accessibility, and exposure to interactions of people; and the degree to which basic social structures (including health services) have broken down. In addition, "HIV prevalence among the affected community pre-conflict, the HIV prevalence among the surrounding community for those who have been displaced, exposure to violence during conflict and flight and the level of interaction between the two communities" will affect vulnerability (Spiegel, 2004, p. 324; Salama et al., 2004).

Gender, Sexual Violence, and the Complexities of Power

Threading through every aspect of our analysis thus far has been the recurrent theme of violence—sexual, gender-based, military, and existential, in a dense continuum. Since the Vienna Conference on Human Rights and Declaration on Violence against Women in 1993, a global feminist movement has brought sexual and gender-based violence out into the open as a serious human rights issue. More recently, under the statute of the International

Criminal Court, gender-based violence was recognized as a war crime, a crime against humanity, in some circumstances a form of genocide (Bunch and Reilly, 1994; UN/ICC, 1998; Copelon, 2000; Spees, 2003). The UNHCR, the Inter-Agency Standing Committee (IASC), and the Commission on Human Rights have all published safeguards and standards to address gender-based violence in humanitarian crises (Commission on Human Rights, 1998; UNHCR, 2001; IASC, 2004, 2005). Nevertheless, the magnitude of the problem of persistent gender and sexual violence in complex emergencies is still formidable.

Ample qualitative and anecdotal reports make it clear that refugees and displaced persons, especially women and girls, are exposed to relentless risks of abuse by armed combatants, government soldiers, peacekeepers, aid workers, guards, brigands, and, sometimes, their own spouses. Marsh, Purdin, and Navani (2006, p. 135) divide these acts into two categories—"sexual violence perpetrated as a method of warfare" and "opportunistic sexual violence perpetrated within the climate of impunity present in war zones." In a 2005 joint study conducted in Darfur, UNFPA and UNICEF found "that women and girls are subjected to sexual violence on a daily basis" (UNFPA and UNICEF, 2005; Marsh et al., 2006, p. 142). Macklin (2004, p. 90) describes how, once in IDP camps, women find themselves "sexually blackmailed" by military, police, and security personnel for entering and leaving the camp and exposed to sexual rampages after curfew. Similar experiences have been documented among Somali refugee women in northeast Kenya (Hyndman, 2004), Sudanese women and girls as young as ten years old in Chad (UNFPA, 2006, p. 62), as well as in the Eastern DRC, Sierra Leone, Liberia, East Timor, Ivory Coast, Colombia, and Burundi (Marsh et al., 2006, p. 137; Longombe et al., 2008). The health consequences of such sexual violence are bad enough in themselves, but are compounded when rape survivors, especially young unmarried girls and boys, do not seek medical attention because of shame, or avoid medical assistance for births and infants that result from rape.

Patterns of sexual and gender-based violence intersect with both the economic deprivations of exclusion and deeply entrenched traditions of gendered labor. Somali and Ethiopian refugee women in Kenyan camps, Sudanese in eastern Chad, and women and girls in IDP camps in Darfur have all been terrorized by armed groups who rape them when they leave the camps in search of firewood (Hyndman, 2004; UNFPA, 2006, p. 61). As women, they are the ones expected to tend to food-related tasks and collect firewood. Not only is this seen as 'women's work' in normal conditions, but also it is considered less dangerous for women in armed conflict and displacement zones because of "the commonly held belief that men and boys would be killed if they were the ones to leave the security of the camp." This belief leads the family to the decision to send out women and girls, who are seen as risking 'only rape' (Marsh et al., 2006, p. 142; Editorial, 2007, p. 42). Violence in the camps may also result from physically or socially structured insecurities. The physical space of IDP and refugee camps is rarely designed with the security, or the needs for privacy, of women and girls in mind. So the standard humanitarian aid practice of separating potable water from groundwater means that latrines and showers are located at the opposite end of the camp from wells and taps, and women must walk far from their living areas at night to use the toilet or shower, thus risking assault from male residents (de Alwis, 2004; UNFPA, 2006).

One of the most disgraceful aspects of sexual violence aimed at refugees and IDPs is that inflicted by peacekeepers and aid workers, the very persons mandated to provide protection. In 2002, there were shocking reports that UN peacekeepers, as well as UN and NGO relief staff, were systematically bartering food and supplies in exchange for sex from female camp residents, especially adolescent females, but probably also from young boys (UNFPA, 2006, p. 61). This information prompted a General Assembly resolution, calling for an investigation and a 'zero-tolerance' policy on the part of the secretary-general (UNFPA, 2006). Sadly, this is nothing new. The sordid shadow of militarist sexual behavior in armed conflict settings is cast over much of recent history, including evidence of sexual violence against children in Kosovo, and against Iraqi women, men, and girls by soldiers and 'peacekeepers' from the US (Enloe, 2000, 2007; Gyles and Hyndman, 2004; Hersh, 2004; Corrêa et al., 2008).

Nonetheless, it is important not to see the camp as a monolith, but to recognize the ways in which it often reflects survival strategies, including anger and active resistance on the part of residents, especially women. We need to avoid imposing a clichéd victimization rhetoric on women, a rhetoric that reinforces paternalistic attitudes in relief programs and overlooks the active responses of women refugees and IDPs (Turner, 1999; Harrell-Bond, 2002; Miller, 2004; Petchesky, 2005; Papastergiadis, 2006, p. 437). Malathi de Alwis (2004) tells the story of displaced Muslim women in northwestern Sri Lanka who refused to go along with the aid agencies' "grids of intelligibility" and rejected the hazardous "scurrying back and forth between well and toilet" during the night; they simply appropriated the outdoor area near the wells as their toilet. In Darfur, humanitarian workers have introduced women's centers and community-based networks, where women's groups can devise their own strategies for addressing "gender-based violence through community structures." One of the most successful of these strategies has been 'firewood patrols' organized by committees of displaced women leaders. The committee meetings become a kind of forum where women and girls can discuss their concerns; one such meeting in west Darfur "brought together over 400 women and girls to discuss coordination with African Union representatives" (Marsh et al., 2006, p. 142; Patrick, 2007, p. 40).

Indeed, it is clear that gendered relations of power in sites of exclusion are highly complex, context- and culture-specific, and begging for further research. Simon Turner (1999), in a working paper for UNHCR based on fieldwork among Burundian Hutu refugees in Tanzania, shows how structural and social conditions within the camp may work to undermine traditional patriarchal relations, and how deliberate attempts to overturn patriarchal power relations may be fraught with complications. Turner describes how "gender equality was an explicit aim of the relief operation," including active efforts to promote women's and girls' vocational training, women's committees, and their election to positions of camp leadership. However, the lack of privacy and visibility in the camp contributed to the breakdown, not only of gender, but also of generational and intra-male hierarchies, as children and women become aware that 'big men' and fathers no longer control incomes or receive more and better food (1999, pp. 146, 149–150). Yet, Turner found that, despite a pervasive sense of declining male authority, young men had developed a number of economic and political strategies to reassert their 'manhood' and, hence, their power. At the same time, men and boys within camps remain vulnerable to being conscripted into military roles, even when they are still just children and, thus—as intensely as but differently from women and girls—are subject to continual risk of death and brutalization.

All this points to the critical need for humanitarian agencies and NGOs to develop gender-sensitive policies and programs that address the needs and disempowerment of men and boys, as well as those of women and girls, to discard old stereotypes of women as always victims and men as always abusers (Brun, 2000, p. 10). Such programs would have to encompass all aspects of service provision, including reproductive, sexual, and primary health care, sexual and gender-based violence, employment, and decision-making. Like the emergencies themselves, responses must be complex and multidimensional.

CONCLUSIONS—BEYOND THE CAMPS?

Humanitarianism in the State of Exception

Despite great differences in settings and inconsistencies in practices across sites, much of the evidence reviewed earlier tells us that refugees in camps are more likely to receive services of all kinds than are IDPs and displaced persons scattered outside camps or, in some cases, even local residents who are not displaced. Further, a growing body of evidence shows some of the highest, and most prolonged, increases in 'excess mortality' occurring outside camps in provinces, regions, and countries affected by conflict. This is especially true in countries or territories such as Iraq, Afghanistan, and Palestine, where the whole society, in effect, becomes a camp, not of refugees but of IDPs and military prisoners. At the same time, the pattern we observed of flows back and forth between camps, armed conflict zones, and endangered or neglected rural and urban areas suggests that camp boundaries in many complex emergencies cannot easily be immunized against viruses, violence, or marauded food and medical supplies. As health researchers begin to address these problems, by calling for greater 'coverage' beyond the camps, with more coordination with and responsibility of national governments, they are implicitly raising questions about the viability of the camp as a model of 'protection' (Waldman and Martone, 1999; McGinn et al., 2004; Salama et al., 2004).

In our analysis, we have shown that refugee and IDP camps embody a number of striking contradictions. First, while they are supposedly governed by international law and human rights, in reality, the operation of such law and rights in these 'exceptional' spaces is often nonexistent (Slim, 1997; Macklin, 2008). Second, the lines between war-making and nation-building, and between the peacekeeping and humanitarian functions of UN agencies, have blurred (Donini et al., 2004). Traditionally, humanitarian work was supposed to be politically neutral, but in reality humanitarian aid workers and efforts frequently are caught up, and both compromised and endangered, in raging political conflicts. Political neutrality becomes a barrier to reporting and enforcing human rights violations against displaced populations. The third contradiction is the camp's inaccurate conceptualization as an 'emergency' intervention, thus a temporary way station en route to someplace else (whether repatriation or permanent asylum and naturalization). The reality for millions is in sharp contrast to this scenario. According to a recent UNFPA (2006) report, the average stay in refugee camps is 17 years. Moreover, as many critics of the current displacement regime note, the 'emergency mind-set' induces a 'crisis management' approach among camp personnel that treats refugees or IDPs as passive victims, thereby undermining their autonomy or even their humanity (Van Damme, 1995, p. 361; Harrell-Bond, 2002; Hyndman, 2004, p. 203; Pallis, 2005).

This leads to a final key contradiction: refugee and IDP camps are supposed to be just that—refuges, shelters—yet, typically they are places of demoralization, dehumanization, and extreme danger. Many researchers, speaking from direct field observation, critique the ways in which local residents, the media, and policy makers perceive refugees and IDPs as both economically burdensome and morally and physically threatening—as sources of pollution and contamination if not terrorist attacks. "The refugee is malevolent and indolent; prepared to risk everything in order to get in, then happy to retire at the expense of the state" (Papastergiadis, 2006, p. 433; Loescher, 2002; de Alwis, 2004;. As with all forms of racism, these stereotypes have distinct sexual dimensions as well, with women refugees characterized as 'loose' or as bad mothers, and men as emasculated, or sexual predators (de Alwis, 2004). Degrading stereotypes may infect the attitudes of humanitarian workers, "whose interests are served by pathologizing, medicalizing and labeling the refugees as helpless and vulnerable" or, alternatively, as cheaters, schemers, and obstacles to efficiency (Harrell-Bond, 2002, pp. 57–58).

The underlying assumption of UNHCR operations—"that refugees can best be cared for when they are settled in camps" (Van Damme, 1995, p. 361)—constructs an "asymmetrical power relationship" between forced migrants and "those upon whom they are dependent for the means of survival and security" (Harrell-Bond, 2002, p. 55). Harrell-Bond analyzes the structural conditions in refugee camps that foster inhumane, at times even violent, behavior toward refugees on the part of camp administrators. These conditions entail the 'strict control' thought necessary to distribute food and medical aid 'equitably' and in a way that prioritizes account-ability to donors; indeed, any accountability of aid organizations seems directed toward donor governments rather than to aid recipients. Mecha-nisms to enforce such control can often be degrading and objectifying—for example, organizing the camp into a grid, having people line up or herding them into groups for head counts and food or medical distribu-tion, and generally treating refugees of all ages like children. Harrell-Bond (2002, pp. 57–60) calls this "undignified humanitarianism" and suggests that it induces servile, helpless, and dependent behavior, rather than giving people the tools to regain some control over their lives. Rigid bureaucratic rules result in absurdities, such as refusing medical care to elderly or dying refugees whose cases were deemed too costly, or to fall outside the defi-nitions of 'primary health care,' and denying assistance to any refugees except those living full-time in the camps (and hence under agency control) (Harrell-Bond, 2002, pp. 65–66). In general, aid givers "assume the power to decide who is deserving," and this is the crux of the power asymmetry (2002, p. 68).

New Directions

In a suggestive study from the mid-1990s comparing the case of Rwan-dan Tutsi refugees in Goma, Zaire, with that of refugees in Guinea in the same period, Van Damme (1995) argues that in Guinea, where refugees were deliberately not placed in camps but rather settled among the resi-dential population, everyone benefited. The refugees had more autonomy and self-respect, and both refugees and local residents experienced signifi-cantly improved health outcomes. This was because the Guinean govern-ment used the inflow of refugees as an opportunity (rather than a threat) to set up health stations offering free health care to all inhabitants, regardless of nationality. As a result, "the health care system in the refugee-affected region is now by far the best developed in the country, benefiting Guinea and refugees alike." In contrast, the camps in Goma suffered huge chol-era and other epidemics involving 50,000 deaths, and refugees sank into passivity, dependence, and nutrition-related diseases that grew worse the greater the size of the camps (Van Damme, 1995).

Harrell-Bond (2002, p. 80) and Kälin (2006b, p. 9; 2007, p. 6) suggest that the best way to assure accountability and enforcement for IDPs and refugees is "to invest in strengthening local and national institutions," giving local governments "adequate human and financial resources to fulfill their obligations." There is a fallacy in the belief "that it is possible to bring about improvement in isolation from the state that hosts the refugees, its institutions of governance and civil society"—and, one would add, its basic health and transportation infrastructure (Harrell-Bond, 2002, pp. 80–85).

An alternative approach is one that stresses greater coordination across agencies and a multisectoral model of responsibility that would actually broaden and deepen the existing international regime. In this view, given the reality that millions of displaced people do live in camps, and have no safe or welcoming place to go, the urgent need is to promote their human rights. This would be accomplished by vastly improving their health, housing, educational, and economic possibilities; expanding their physical safety, freedom of movement and expression; and giving them—especially disempowered women and girls—a voice in all key areas of decision-making (Marsh et al., 2006, p. 140). This international or multisectoral model recognizes that gender equity and health rights are inseparable from a wide range of other economic, social, and political rights, which no single agency can guarantee by itself (Hunt, 2007; Kälin, 2006a; Macklin, 2008; Petchesky, 2008).

We view the national capacity building and international/multisectoral approaches to enforcing the human rights of excluded and displaced persons as interdependent rather than oppositional. Walter Kälin (2006b, p. 5) has formulated this hybrid perspective thus: "Where governments lack the will or capacity, international actors will need to be more directly involved in protecting the rights of the displaced, but in a way that seeks to reinforce rather than substitute for national [and also local] responsibility." A genuine 'human rights approach' to relief work will require dissolving the artificial boundary between 'political' and 'humanitarian' functions. As such, international organizations and NGOs will have to decide strategically when it is necessary to step out of the cover of neutrality, make demands on states to live up to their human rights obligations (including health and all other economic and social rights), and when to call governments to account when they refuse. That is, demand that refugees and IDPs be given all the basic rights due to citizens. Ultimately, protecting the human rights of those in camps has to mean actively abolishing the states of exception.

Yet, neither model of accountability, nor some kind of hybrid, can be an effective guarantor of human rights for refugees and IDPs without continual pressure and activism from transnational movements and grassroots organizations that authentically advocate for, and give voice to, refugee/IDP subjects themselves. This has special importance for issues of gender equity in sites of exclusion as everywhere else. From the 1990s United Nations conferences to the present, transnational women's movements have sought to secure international recognition and concrete implementation of women's rights to decision-making power, as well as gender-specific guarantees in the realms of health, nutrition, sexuality, freedom from violence, sustainable livelihoods, and education. Simultaneously, movements to defend the rights of migrants and stateless persons, and to challenge restrictive conceptions of 'citizenship,' have gained ground in both national settings and international norms.

Impressive examples exist of practical efforts to enforce recognition and implementation of refugee and displaced women's rights to decision-making power and gender-specific protections and amenities in the realms of health, nutrition, sexuality, freedom from violence, and economic and educational opportunities. Such efforts put a high priority on women's direct participation, enlisting women frontline workers as well as international agency representatives and NGOs "to facilitate a systematic consultative process with women in the day-to-day management of the camps and membership in camp committees." Gururaja (2000) describes the work of UNICEF in Palestinian refugee camps in Lebanon, where (similar to the Tanzanian camps Turner visited) men traditionally controlled the "popular committees" responsible for local camp policy. Through a series of seminars with women's association members as well as consultations with the male heads of committees, UNICEF workers helped the women to select their own representatives and to lobby for their appointment to the committees, training them in organizational, communication, and lobbying skills along the way. The women succeeded in obtaining representation on four popular committees (Gururaja, 2000). This effort is reminiscent of the women's committees and 'firewood patrols' established in Darfur IDP camps and illustrates the ways in which feminist activists on the ground have become critical to the implementation of gender equity principles in camps (Marsh et al., 2006). Likewise, evidence of "community resilience" and survival against odds among displaced Lebanese during the July 2006 war reaffirm the need to see populations besieged by crisis as agents, not just victims (Nuwayhid et al., 2006).

Another recent example is a set of "Guidelines for Gender Sensitive Disaster Management" produced by the Asian Forum on Women in Disasters, a group of NGOs and aid agency representatives that met in Chennai following the 2006 tsunami. Though related to a 'natural' rather than the 'unnatural' disasters we have been discussing, this report thoroughly outlines every conceivable dimension of women's health, security, and nutritional needs in 'camp' situations, including the structural design of camps and "adequate toilet and bathing facilities." It could serve as a useful guide for all agencies and NGOs involved in relief work—a spelling out of the concrete meaning of 'gender equity' in sites of exclusion (APWLD, 2006; Silverstein, 2008). It also reinforces once again the fact that both policies of gender equity and women's empowerment and their practical implementation are the result of women's movement activism and the alliance, and sometimes overlap, between activists and service providers (Petchesky, 2003).

Finally, Turner's (1999) analysis reminds us of the deeply entrenched codes of masculinity and femininity that make realization of such 'best practices' quite difficult in many local contexts. Part of the answer here has to be a much more thoughtful and deliberate effort to engage men and boys in programs to empower (not just protect) women and girls, including reproductive and sexual health, HIV/AIDS, and sexual and gender-based violence programs. However, such 'male involvement' has to be fully sensitive to local cultural and religious norms, knowledgeable about local histories, and not simply imposed in a way that might be perceived as intrusive if not neocolonial (Harris, 1999). Moreover, it needs to be framed in terms of a gender analysis that brings into the open the reality of sexual abuse and violence against men and boys, as well as transgender persons, and understands that too as 'gender-based violence.' Moving beyond the stereotypes of women as victims and men as abusers, like moving beyond the camp, will require a thorough rethinking of gender meanings and how to transform them in some of the most resistant, violent, and resource-deprived conditions on the globe. This work—which is really the work of transnational gender and sexual rights movements—has only just begun.

Policy Recommendations

Given the complex realities described here, we propose the following considerations for policy makers and advocates concerned about the injustices and deprivations of existing camp situations. In the long term, we agree with the integrationists who propose to abolish camps as intrinsically unjust because founded on the violence of forcible uprooting and exclusion. An 'abolitionist' path would favor strategies to integrate displaced populations as quickly and safely as possible back into viable, secure communities, whether their own or new and welcoming ones. This would mean treating refugees and IDPs as full citizens of the societies where they are located and at the same time focusing on providing good quality health services, housing, livelihoods, protection from violence and abuse, and access to education and participation in political decision-making to *all* persons, regardless of their place of origin (Guinea in the mid-1990s is a good model). We believe international agencies and NGOs working in the areas of humanitarian and refugee services, peace-building, health, and gender equality have a moral obligation to bring pressure on governments to welcome and integrate forcibly displaced persons, both from among their own citizens and from elsewhere, and to call upon wealthy countries, donors, and the international community to generate the resources to make this a practical possibility. A human rights and social justice perspective on humanitarian assistance, as well as the principles of health as a human right, ultimately can only mean this.

At the same time we recognize that in the world as it is, a range of man-made and natural disasters may make returning home or being at home temporarily unthinkable. In addition, some states and communities are not healthy or hospitable environments for whole groups of people—hence the mass voluntary as well as forced migrations that now characterize the planet. Extreme violence and insecurity, exacerbated if not caused by racial and ethnic hatreds, may make camps a necessary evil in the short term and place particularly onerous burdens on women, children, and youths. In such situations, we urge the following measures to ensure the safety, dignity, and empowerment of those who reside in camps or their equivalent:

1.   Humanitarian, health, and relief workers and agencies should adopt conscious programs to discourage 'victimization rhetoric,' racist and sexist stereotypes of either dependency and helplessness or cheating and wiliness among the populations they serve, and attitudes that promote such dependency. Instead, in providing services and assistance, they should seek out and build on local networks, traditions, and practices of 'community resilience,' self-help and mutual aid; enlist local leaders and speakers—particularly women—in making decisions and designing relief programs concerning everything from camp layout to food and job distribution to child care and health priorities; and attempt to develop democratic, participatory methods for engaging camp residents' involvement across gender, age, and ethnic divisions. (Firewood patrols and committees in Darfur offer a good model.)

2.   Where such networks and traditions tend to be heavily patriarchal and male-dominated, camp workers should see educational efforts concerning women's equality and empowerment and against sexual and gender-based violence as an integral part of their mandate. Such efforts should fully engage men and youth as well as local women and should address male subordination in age and military hierarchies as well as violence against and subordination of women and girls. At the same time, they should be conducted in ways that take into account and respect local beliefs, traditions, and values, raising questions and promoting open discussion rather than imposing alien values and moral judgments. (See Harris, 1999 and 2003 for an excellent example.)

3.   Gender equity, women's empowerment, and participation in decision-making across lines of gender and age difference are difficult if not impossible in the absence of the most basic enabling conditions. Health rights and other social, economic, and cultural rights are indivisible. Humanitarian and health workers in camps must work to assure the structural determinants that underlie an ability to participate, including decent housing, safe water, sanitation, physical safety, affordable cooking fuel, child care, care for the elderly, educational and sustainable livelihood possibilities, and freedom of movement and expression.

4.   To reside in sites of political exclusion is by definition to lack accountability mechanisms for bringing grievances and gaining redress

for abuses and wrongs—including those perpetrated by caregivers and peacekeepers. A new ethos of rights-based humanitarian service delivery to address this problem is emerging, as reflected in documents like Sphere and the International IDP guidelines. International donors should devote sufficient resources to support and strengthen new models of accountability and empowerment for camp residents and UN bodies should work to assure that local governments respect and enforce these efforts. Wherever possible, on-site accountability and grievance processes—for example, establishing a camp ombudsperson or complaints committees—should be linked to existing international human rights machinery, including the human rights treaty bodies and special rapporteurs as well as national and transnational human rights groups engaged in creating shadow reports. At the same time, efforts should be made to strengthen the capacity of local and national courts and administrations as enforcers of refugee and IDP rights. International, national, and local strategies can reinforce one another.

5.   Where conditions in surrounding locales and communities are relatively stable and functional (i.e., not ridden with extreme armed violence and ethnic hatred), efforts should be made to better integrate displaced populations into these communities. Integrative and multisectoral models for meeting the needs of refugees and IDPs are not mutually exclusive but complementary. On the one hand, health, nutritional, and other services provided to camp residents should be available to populations living near the camps, to break down the isolation of camps and to discourage their use as military staging areas. On the other hand, local clinics, services, schools, and community- and faith-based organizations should open their doors to and interact with camp residents on a voluntary basis. Attempts should be made to transcend the prevailing fragmentation of both services and donor streams into compartmentalized pockets (development, humanitarian assistance, post-conflict relief and reconstruction, health services, gender equity, and women's empowerment). The realities of complex emergencies and of the real lives of people caught in displacement and catastrophe call for a much higher level of cooperation across agencies, sectors, and physical boundaries than currently exists.

Building effective mechanisms for participation in decision-making and nurturing respect and empowerment for women and girls—both among refugees and IDPs and between them and those who are there to provide assistance and care—is a necessary part of a rights-based health program, in camps or anywhere else. Increasing civil (as opposed to hostile) interconnections between camp residents and their neighbors in surrounding areas is a strategy to recognize the human rights and full citizenship of refugees and IDPs and eventually to transform camps from isolated depositories or detention centers into actual communities if not homes—that is, to make camps as unlike camps as possible.

Postscript

This chapter was written before the election of Senator Barack Obama to be president of the United States beginning January 2009. We are hopeful that, with an Obama administration, the 'endless' war on terror will come to an end and a new era in which diplomacy and human rights supersede militarism, globally and locally, will begin.

NOTES

1. This article contains material previously published in Laurie and Petchesky (2008), Petchesky (2008), and Corrêa, Petchesky, and Parker (2008).
2. Agamben is elaborating on Foucault's concept of biopolitics, which Foucault defined as technologies of power applied to regulate entire populations—their mortality, morbidity, numbers, and movement—and associated with modernity. Agamben expands the reach of Foucault's analysis to argue that governance over life itself, the very conditions of life (i.e., survival)—throughout much of ancient and early modern history, a function associated with the "private" domain of the household—has become the primary function of State (or imperial) power. See Agamben (1998, pp. 5, 9; 2005, pp. 1,2; and Foucault, 2003).
3. The 1959 Refugee Convention and its 1967 Protocol define a refugee as:

   > any person who: owing to well-founded fear of being persecuted for reasons of race, religion, nationality, membership of a particular social group or political opinion, is outside the country of his nationality and is unable or, owing to such fear, is unwilling to avail himself of the protection of that country; or who, not having a nationality and being outside the country of his former habitual residence as a result of such events, is unable or, owing to such fear, is unwilling to return to it.

   The UN secretary-general's representative for IDPs, endorsed by UNHCR, defines such persons as those "who have been forced or obliged to flee or to leave their homes or places of habitual residence, in particular as a result of or in order to avoid the effects of armed conflict, situations of generalized violence, violations of human rights or natural or human-made disasters, and who have not crossed an internationally recognized State border" (Commission on Human Rights, 1998).
4. See the Global Security Web site for this data, at http://www.globalsecurity.org/military/world/war/index.html. Last accessed September 25, 2008.
5. Numbers vary depending on the method and who is doing the counting (UNHCR, 2007; USCRI, 2008; Norwegian Refugee Council, 2008; Weiss and Korn, 2006). Spiegel and colleagues (2002) place the estimated number of people "displaced by complex humanitarian emergencies" at 35 million, but they are no doubt combining IDPs and refugees here.
6. On immigration restrictions for people with HIV and AIDS, see Herdt (1997) and Haour-Knipe and Rector (1997).
7. The study was conducted between 1998 and 2000 in a total of 52 camps in Azerbaijan, Ethiopia, Myanmar, Nepal, Tanzania, Thailand, and Uganda.
8. These include Afghanistan, Iraq, Palestine, Sudan, Democratic Republic of Congo, Burundi, Somalia, Liberia, and Colombia.

REFERENCES

Agamben, G. 1998. *Homo Sacer: Sovereign Power and Bare Life.* Trans. D. Heller-Roazen. Stanford, CA: Stanford University Press.

———. *State of Exception.* Trans. K. Attell. Chicago: University of Chicago Press.

Al-Adili, N., M. Shaheen, S. Bergström, and A. Johansson. 2008. Deaths among young, single women in 2000–2001 in the West Bank, Palestinian occupied territories. *Reproductive Health Matters* 16: 112–121.

APWLD. 2006. *Guidelines for Gender Sensitive Disaster Management.* Chiang Mai, Thailand: Asian Pacific Forum on Women, Law and Development. www.apwld.org/asianforum_women_in_disasters.html.

Austin, J., S. Guy, L. Lee-Jones, T. McGinn, and J. Schlecht. 2008. Reproductive health: A right for refugees and internally displaced persons. *Reproductive Health Matters* 16: 10–21.

Bosmans, M., D. Nasser, U. Khammash, P. Claeys, and M. Temmerman. 2008. Palestinian women's sexual and reproductive health rights in a long-standing humanitarian crisis. *Reproductive Health Matters* 16: 103–111.

Brown, C. 2007. The battle to save Iraq's children: Doctors issue plea to Tony Blair to end the scandal of medical shortages in the war zone. *The Independent,* January 19, www.independent.co.uk/news/world/middle-east/the-battle-to-save-iraqs-children-432770.html (accessed October 2, 2008).

Brun, C. 2000. Making young displaced men visible. *Forced Migration Review* 9: 10–12.

Bunch, C., and N. Reilly. 1994. *Demanding Accountability: The Global Campaign and Vienna Tribunal for Women's Human Rights.* New Brunswick, NJ: Centre for Women's Global Leadership.

Burnham, G., S. Doocy, E. Dzeng, R. Lafta, and L. Roberts. 2006. *The Human Cost of the War in Iraq: A Mortality Study, 2002–2006.* Bloomberg School of Public Health, JHU and School of Medicine, Al Mustansiriya University. Baltimore, MD and Baghdad, Iraq

Buscher, D., and C. Makinson. 2006. Protection of IDP women, children and youth. *Forced Migration Review* 24: 15–16.

CESCR. 2000. General Comment No. 14. The right to the highest attainable standard of health. *United Nations Economic and Social Council. Doc. No. E/C.12/2000/4.* Geneva & New York.

Chelala, C. 2007. Iraqi survivors face health-care collapse. *The Japan Times,* February 23.

Chynoweth, S.K. 2008. The need for priority reproductive health services for displaced Iraqi women and girls. *Reproductive Health Matters* 16: 93–102.

Ciezadlo, A. 2005. In Iraq, giving birth is complicated by war. *The Christian Science Monitor* (June 30): 7.

Commission on Human Rights. 1998. Guiding principles on internal displacement. *UN Document E/CN.4/1998/53/Add.2.* Geneva.

Copelon, R. 2000. Gender crimes as war crimes: Integrating crimes against women into international criminal law. *McGill Law Journal* 46 (1): 217–240.

Corrêa, S., R. Petchesky, and R. Parker. 2008. *Sexuality, Health and Human Rights.* London and New York: Routledge.

de Alwis, M. 2004. The 'purity' of displacement and the reterritorialization of longing: Muslim IDPs in northwestern Sri Lanka. In *Sites of Violence: Gender and Conflict Zones,* edited by W. Gyles and J. Hyndman. Berkeley: University of California Press. 213–231.

del Valle, H. 2004. Beyond the *burqa*: Addressing the causes of maternal mortality in Afghanistan. *Forced Migration Review* 29: 10–12.

Donini, A., L. Minear, and P. Walker. 2004. The future of humanitarian action: Mapping the implications of Iraq and other recent crises. *Disasters* 28 (2): 190–204.

Editorial. 2007. Listening to the women of Darfur. *Forced Migration Review* 27: 42–43.

Eisenstein, Z. 1996. *Hatreds: Racialized and Sexualized Conflicts in the 21ˢᵗ Century.* New York: Routledge.

Enloe, C. 2000. *Maneuvers: The International Politics of Militarizing Women's Lives.* Berkeley: University of California Press.

———. 2007. *Globalization and Militarism: Feminists Make the Link.* Lanham, MD, and Plymouth, UK: Rowman and Littlefield.

Foucault, M. 2003. *"Society Must Be Defended": Lectures at the Collège de France, 1975–1976.* New York: Picador.

Giacaman, R., N.M. Abu-Rmeileh, and L. Wick. 2006. The limitations on choice: Palestinian women's childbirth location, dissatisfaction with the place of birth and determinants. *European Journal of Public Health* 17 (1): 86–91.

Giacaman, R., Wick, L., Abdul-Rahm, H., and Wick, L. 2005. The politics of childbirth in the context of conflict: Policies or de facto practices? *Health Policy* 72: 129–139.

Girard, F. 2004. Global implications of US domestic and international policies on sexuality. *IWGSSP Working Papers, No. 1 (June), Centre for Gender, Sexuality and Health, Dept. of Sociomedical Sciences, Mailman School of Public Health.* New York: Columbia University.

Girard, F., and W. Waldman. 2000. Ensuring the reproductive rights of refugees and internally displaced persons: Legal and policy issues. *International Family Planning Perspectives* 26 (4): 167–173.

Grein, T., F. Checchi, J.M. Escriba, A. Tamrat, U. Karunakara, C. Stokes, V. Brown, and D. Legros. 2003. Mortality among displaced former UNITA members and their families in Angola: A retrospective cluster survey. *British Medical Journal* 327: 1–5.

Gururaja, S. 2000. Gender dimensions of displacement. *Forced Migration Review* 9: 13–16.

Giles, W., and J. Hyndman. 2004. Introduction: Gender and conflict in a global context. In *Sites of Violence: Gender and Conflict Zones,* edited by W. Giles and J. Hyndman. Berkeley: University of California Press. 3–23.

Haour-Knipe, M., and R. Rector, eds. 1997. *Crossing Borders: Migration, Ethnicity, and AIDS.* London: Taylor and Francis.

Harrell-Bond, B.E. 2002. Can humanitarian work with refugees be humane? *Human Rights Quarterly* 24 (1): 51–85.

Harris, C. 1999. Reproductive health of refugees: Lessons beyond ICPD. *Paper Prepared for the Conference on Refugees and the Transformation of Society.* The Netherlands. April 21–24.

Harris, C. 2003. Involving Men: The Khatlon Women's Health Project in Tajikistan. In *Global Prescriptions,* edited by R. Petchesky. London: Zed Books.

Hersh, S.M. 2004. *Chain of Command: The Road from 9/11 to Abu Ghraib.* New York: Harper Collins.

Herdt, G. 1997. *Sexual Cultures and Migration in the Era of AIDS.* Oxford: Clarendon Press.

Hunt, P. 2007. Report of the special rapporteur on the right of everyone to the enjoyment of the highest attainable standard of physical and mental health. *United Nations Human Rights Council, 4ᵗʰ Session. Doc. No. A/HRC/4/28.*

Hyland, M. 2001. Refugee subjectivity: 'Bare life' and the geographical division of labour. *Log* 13. www.physicsroom.org.nz/log/archive/13/refugeesubjectivity/.

Hyndman, J. 2004. Refugee camps as conflict zones: The politics of gender. In *Sites of Violence: Gender and Conflict Zones*, edited by W. Gyles and J. Hyndman. Berkeley: University of California Press. 193–212.

Hynes, M., M. Sheik, H.G. Wilson, and P. Spiegel. 2002. Reproductive health indicators and outcomes among refugee and internally displaced persons in postemergency phase camps. *Journal of the American Medical Association* 288 (5): 595–603.

IASC. 2004. *Statement of Commitment on Gender Based Violence in Emergencies*. Geneva: IASC.

———. 2005. *Guidelines for Gender-Based Violence Interventions in Humanitarian Settings: Focusing on Prevention of and Response to Sexual Violence in Emergencies*. Geneva: IASC.

Indra, D.M. 1999. Not a "room of one's own": Engendering forced migration knowledge and practice. In *Engendering Forced Migration: Theory and Practice*, edited by D.M. Indra. New York: Berghahn Books: 1–22.

IRIN News. 2007. UNHCR launches policy to provide refugees with access to antiretroviral treatment. *Integrated Regional Information Networks (IRIN) of the UN Office for the Coordination of Humanitarian Affairs News. January 29.* www.irinnews.org/report.aspx?reportid=66309 (accessed October 2, 2008).

Jok Madut, J. 1999a. Militarism, gender, and reproductive suffering: The case of abortion in western Dinka. *Africa: Journal of the International African Institute* 69 (2): 194–212.

———. 1999b. Militarization and gender violence in south Sudan. *Journal of Asian and African Studies* 34 (4): 427–442.

Kälin, W. 2006a. The future of the guiding principles on internal displacement. *Forced Migration Review* 24: 5–6.

———. 2006b. Specific groups and individuals: Mass exoduses and displaced persons. *Report of the Representative of the Secretary-General on the Human Rights of Internally Displaced Persons. United Nations Economic and Social Council. Doc. No. E/CN.4/2006/71.* Geneva & New York.

———. 2007. Report of the representative of the secretary-general on the human rights of internally displaced persons. *United Nations Human Rights Council, 4th Session. Doc. No. A/HRC/4/38.* Geneva & New York.

Kottegoda, S., K. Samuel, and S. Emmanuel. 2008. Reproductive health concerns in six conflict-affected areas of Sri Lanka. *Reproductive Health Matters* 16: 75–82.

Lasky, M. P. 2006. Iraqi women under siege. *A Report by CODEPINK. Women for Peace and Global Exchange. CODEPINK.* www.codepink4peace.org.

Laurie, M., and R.P. Petchesky. 2008. Gender, health, and human rights in sites of political exclusion. *Global Public Health* 3: 25–41.

Loescher, G. 2002. Blaming the victim: Refugees and global security. *Bulletin of the Atomic Scientists* 58 (2): 46–53.

Longombe, A.O., K.M. Claude, and J. Ruminjo. 2008. Fistula and traumatic genital injury from sexual violence in a conflict setting in eastern Congo: Case studies. *Reproductive Health Matters* 16: 132–141.

Luibhéid, E. 2002. *Entry Denied: Controlling Sexuality at the Border*. Minneapolis: University of Minnesota Press.

Luibhéid, E., and L. Cantú Jr., eds. 2005. *Queer Migrations: Sexuality, U.S. Citizenship, and Border Crossings*. Minneapolis: University of Minnesota Press.

Macklin, A. 2004. Like oil and water, with a match: Militarized commerce, armed conflict, and human security in Sudan. In *Sites of Violence: Gender and Conflict Zones*, edited by W. Gyles and J. Hyndman. Berkeley: University of California. 75–107.

———. 2008. Legal aspects of conflict-induced migration of women. *Reproductive Health Matters* 16: 22–32.

Marsh, M., S. Purdin, and S. Navani. 2006. Addressing sexual violence in humanitarian emergencies. *Global Public Health* 1 (2): 133–146.

Mazzetti, M., and D. Rohde. 2007. Terror officials see Al Qaeda chiefs regaining power. *The New York Times*, February 19.

McGinn, T., S. Casey, S. Purdin, and M. Marsh. 2004. *Reproductive Health for Conflict-Affected People: Policies, Research and Programmes.* London: Humanitarian Practice Network, Overseas Development Institute.

Miller, A. 2004. Sexuality, violence against women, and human rights: Women make demands and ladies get protection. *Health and Human Rights* 7 (2): 16–47.

Mukherjee, V.N. 2002. Gender matters. *Seminar* 511: 67–75.

Norwegian Refugee Council. 2006. *Internal Displacement: Global Overview of Trends and Developments in 2005.* Geneva: Internal Displacement Monitoring Center.

———. 2008. *Internal Displacement: Global Overview of Trends and Developments in 2007.* Geneva: Internal Displacement Monitoring Center.

Nuwayhid, I., C.S. Cortas, and H. Zurayk. 2006. Resilience during war and its implications for public health interventions, education, and training. *Paper Presented at Global Forum for Health Research Annual Meeting, October 29–November 2 (revised).* Cairo.

Pallis, M. 2005. The operation of UNHCR's accountability mechanisms. *International Law and Justice Working Paper 2005/12, Institute for International Law and Justice.* New York: New York University.

Papastergiadis, N. 2006. The invasion complex: The abject other and spaces of violence. *Geography Annual* 88 (4): 429–442.

Patrick, E. 2007. Sexual violence and firewood collection in Darfur. *Forced Migration Review* 27: 40–41.

Petchesky, R. 2003. *Global Prescriptions: Gendering Health and Human Rights.* London: Palgrave; New York: Zed Books.

———. 2005. Rights of the body and perversions of war—ten years past Beijing. *International Social Science Journal* 57 (184): 310–318.

———. 2008. Conflict and crisis settings: Promoting sexual and reproductive rights (editorial). *Reproductive Health Matters* 16: 10–21.

Roberts, L., R. Lafta, R. Garfield, J. Khudhairi, and G. Burnham. 2004. Mortality before and after the 2003 invasion of Iraq: Cluster sample survey. *The Lancet* 364: 1857–1864.

Salama, P., P. Spiegel, and R. Brennan. 2001. No less vulnerable: The internally displaced in humanitarian emergencies. *The Lancet* 357: 1430–1431.

Salama, P., P. Spiegel, L. Talley, and R. Waldman. 2004. Lessons learned from complex emergencies over past decade. *The Lancet* 364: 1801–1813.

Sambanis, N. 2006. It's official: There is now a civil war in Iraq. *The New York Times*, Op-Ed, July 23. 4.13

Save the Children. 2007. *State of the World's Mothers 2007.* London: Save the Children.

Save the Children UK. 2002. *HIV and Conflict: A Double Emergency.* London: Save the Children.

Silverstein, L.M. 2008. Guidelines for gender sensitive disaster management by Asia Pacific Forum on Women, Law and Development: A revolutionary document. *Reproductive Health Matters* 16: 153–158.

Slim, H. 1997. Doing the right thing: Relief agencies, moral dilemmas and moral responsibility in political emergencies and war. *Disasters* 21 (3): 244–257.

Spees, P. 2003. Women's advocacy in the creation of the international criminal court: Changing the landscapes of justice and power. *SIGNS* 28 (Summer): 1233–1254.

Sphere Project. 2004. *Humanitarian Charter and Minimum Standards in Disaster Response*. Geneva: The Sphere Project.

Spiegel, P.B. 2004. HIV/AIDS among conflict-affected and displaced populations: Dispelling myths and taking action. *Disasters* 28 (3): 322–339.

Spiegel, P., M. Sheik, C. Gotway-Crawford, and P. Salama. 2002. Health programmes and policies associated with decreased mortality in displaced people in post-emergency phase camps: A retrospective study. *The Lancet* 360: 1927–1934.

Terry, F. 2001. Military involvement in refugee crises: A positive evolution? *The Lancet* 357: 1431–1432.

Turner, S. 1999. *How Life in a Refugee Camp Affects Gender, Age and Class Relations*. Geneva: UNHCR.

UNFPA. 2003. *IRAQ Reproductive Health Assessment*. New York: United Nations Population Fund.

———. 2006. *State of World Population 2006: A Passage to Hope, Women and International Migration*. New York: United Nations Population Fund.

UNFPA and UNICEF. 2005. *The Effects of Conflict on Health and Well-being of Women and Girls in Darfur: A Situational Analysis*. United Nations Population Fund and United Nations Children's Fund. www.unicef.org/infobycountry/files/sitan_unfpaunicef.pdf. New York.

UNHCR. 1999. *Inter-Agency Field Manual on Reproductive Health in Refugee Situations*. Geneva: UNHCR.

———. 2001. *Prevention and Response to Sexual and Gender-based Violence in Refugee Situations. Inter-agency Lessons Learned Conference Proceedings, March 27–29, 2001—Geneva*. Geneva: UNHCR.

———. 2005. *Global Refugee Trends*. Geneva: UNHCR.

———. 2007. *Global Refugee Trends*. Geneva: UNHCR.

UN/ICC. 1998. Rome statue of the international criminal court. *United Nations General Assembly. Doc. A/CONF.183/9, July 17*. Geneva & New York.

United Nations. 1994. *Programme of Action of the International Conference on Population and Development, Cairo*. Geneva: United Nations.

USCRI. 2008. *World Refugee Survey*. Arlington: USCRI.

Van Damme, W. 1995. Do refugees belong in camps? Experiences from Goma and Guinea. *The Lancet* 346: 360–362.

Waldman, R., and G. Martone. 1999. Public health and complex emergencies: New issues, new conditions. *American Journal of Public Health* 85 (10): 1483–1485.

Weiss, T.G., and D.A. Korn. 2006. *Internal Displacement: Conceptualization and Its Consequences*. London and New York: Routledge.

Weissman, F. 2004. Humanitarian action and military intervention: Temptations and possibilities. *Disasters* 28 (2): 205–215.

Williamson, K. 2004. AIDS, gender and the refugee protection framework. RSC Working Paper No. 19, Refugee Studies Centre. Oxford: University of Oxford.

5 Gender, Health, and Poverty in Latin America

Karina Batthyany and Sonia Corrêa

INTRODUCTION

This chapter analyzes the interface between three sets of policies—poverty alleviation policies, health sector reforms, and sexual and reproductive health policies—in Latin America. The choice of policies reflects the fact that there are critical linkages among them, which affect their collective impact on women's health and gender equity in health. These linkages, as we will show, can be synergistic, but can also act as barriers. Furthermore, there have been significant shifts in each of these policies over the last three decades, creating a rapidly changing and sometimes contradictory policy environment for gender equality and equity in health. As such, the analysis of specific policies in five important countries in the region provides comparative insights that illumine how the structural factors embedded in the policy environment constitute key social determinants of health.

This chapter analyzes the connections and dissonances among the three sets of policies in Argentina, Brazil, Chile, Mexico, and Uruguay. These include the biggest countries in the region, as well as countries where key policy shifts have occurred. However, the selection of countries is, to some extent, arbitrary as it was determined by the availability of literature. Much of the literature accessed by us for this review is in Spanish and Portuguese, and this has been a major plus as we have been able to go deeper than the literature in English would allow.

A SHIFTING POLITICAL AND ECONOMIC LANDSCAPE

Since the late 1970s the political and economic landscape in these five countries has changed substantially. Between the mid-1970s and the late 1980s democracy was restored in Argentina, Brazil, Uruguay, and Chile after periods of military dictatorship. In Mexico, the political transition that began in the late 1980s left behind the one-party system that had existed since the 1920s under the hegemony of the Revolutionary Institutional Party (PRI). In the 1970s and 1980s the regional economy experienced the oil and debt crises and saw the start of structural adjustment programs in Chile following the military overthrow of the Allende government. Ironically, the consolidation of democracy coincided with the expansion of neoliberal state and economic reforms to other countries in the 1990s, and the resulting fiscal stringency impacted significantly on social policies. The whole region was also affected by the paradoxes of globalization that either did not generate growth, or implied greater inequality, informalization of labor, and, in some cases, higher poverty levels (Stiglitz, 2002; López et al., 2006).

By the end of the decade, the impact of the Asian financial crisis of 1997 was acute in all five countries. In its aftermath, left-wing political parties that contested the dominant neoliberal economic models of the 1990s won a series of electoral victories: the Workers Party in Brazil (2002, PT); the Left Front in Uruguay (2004, *Frente Amplio*); in Argentina, sections of the Justice Party (*Partido Justicialista*) who disagreed with the neoliberal policies of the Menem administration. In Mexico, although the end of the PRI rule was followed by two consecutive victories by the conservative National Action Party (PAN), the left-wing Party of the Democratic Revolution (PRD) has retained power since 1994 in the politically important Federal District. In Chile, the Socialist–Christian Democrat coalition that had been in power since 1990 was not dislodged, but issues of inequality and social policy distortions gained greater attention. These new trends coincided with a period of global economic growth in the 2000s, from which all five countries benefited. It is not trivial either that two women were elected as presidents: Michelle Bachelet in Chile (2004) and Cristina Kirchner in Argentina (2007).

This trajectory has meant consolidation of democratic institutions, more effective social policies, and cultural changes in regard to gender. However, patterns of economic, ethnic, racial, and gender inequality have persisted even when poverty indicators have improved (UNDP, 2005, 2006; Social Watch, 2006). Democratization evolved hand in hand with symptoms of social disruption. State violence has not been eliminated, nor have nepotism and corruption been contained. While the influence of the Catholic Church over politicians and states has been long-standing in these countries, in the last 10 to 15 years the religious landscape has been changing, as evangelical churches proliferate, particularly in Brazil (Castilhos, 2008). Religious dogmatism expanded in both electoral politics and influenced over public policies. Since the mid-1990s, opinion polls have detected important gaps between the levels of confidence in democratic institutions and societies' perception about their concrete outcomes (UNDP, 2004; Latinobarómetro, 2000).[2]

This environment—including elements of neoliberal economic policies, challenges to such policies in a more democratic and leftward-leaning polity, the continuing strength of the Catholic Church, the spread of evangelical churches, and the growing global discourse on sexual and reproductive health and rights—provided a contradictory policy space and cultural milieu for women's health and rights. The five countries we examine in this chapter negotiated this complex terrain in different ways and with mixed results, as we show in the next sections. A consideration of the three sets of policies in the countries points to the ways in which policy synergies can be built to support positive social determinants of health, such as women's rights, but also points to the risks and the challenges posed by dilution and narrowing of policies so that they treat women as instruments to meet social goals without adequate attention to their own health or rights. We first discuss health sector reforms that were introduced to the region as part of the neoliberal package of economic reforms. This is followed by an examination of sexual and reproductive health policies that focuses on both the impact of reforms in the health sector and of the changing cultural milieu for gender and women's rights. Finally, we discuss the recent directions in antipoverty policies, and how these intersect with women's health.

HEALTH SECTOR REFORM: TRAJECTORIES AND OUTCOMES

The main motivation behind the first phase of health sector reforms proposed by international financial institutions in the late 1970s was to reduce fiscal deficits, control inflation, and improve national savings. During the 1980s the reduction of public funds for health and the resulting privatization resulted in wide social gaps in health status and access to health care (Standing, 2000). By the 1980s, the universal publicly funded models of earlier decades had eroded. In all five countries, health systems had been based on a tripartite model: workers protected by formal labor contracts were covered by a social security financed health system; those engaged in the informal labor market had access to public health systems managed by Ministries of Health, whose funding depended directly on fiscal resources through budget appropriations; and higher-income groups resorted directly to private providers, or else were covered by private insurance schemes (that started operating in the late 1960s). The inequities of the tripartite model, wherein the large numbers of people in the informal sector or who were dependent on their relationship to someone in the formal sector often had much worse health care, provided a strong rationale for health reforms.

In 1993, the World Bank launched the report "Investing in Health" (World Bank, 1993) in which these failures were recognized and recommendations were made to restore public investments in health to ensure access for the poor, to improve specific health indicators such as infant and child mortality, and to address the growing incidence of HIV/AIDS. The report also prescribed decentralization, participation, and the creation of accountability mechanisms so as to ensure access to and quality of health care.

A second phase of reforms ensued, based on this new approach. However, although public investment in health increased, this did not mean the full revival of the publicly funded universal models of the 1950s and 1960s.

Public investments remained limited to so-called 'basic health packages,' while more complex procedures were covered by user fees, and higher-income groups were supposed to pay for the totality of their health costs. It has been argued that such an approach impairs the implementation of comprehensive health care and compromises the principle of universality, a cornerstone of the right to health (Almeida, 2002; Standing, 1997, 1999).

In Latin America, these health reforms were implemented as components of broad state reform agendas and, in particular, reforms of social security systems (Mesa-Lago, 2005; Alneida, 2001).[3] When the reforms were adopted, they aimed at separating health financing from service provision; decentralizing health management and services; reducing or eliminating the social security financing of health care; improving cost-effectiveness; adopting user fees; reallocating public investment to the poor and to redress regional disparities; and improving health management and promoting technological innovation.

The reforms deeply altered the structure and functioning of health systems. By the 2000s, as shown in Table 5.1, in the five countries under examination the level of health expenditure in relation to GDP is not low, but the proportion of private expenditures is high. Decentralization and coverage have expanded, and health systems became increasingly sophisticated in terms of rules and managing structures. But the weaknesses of the tripartite model have not been fully addressed everywhere. Access to health care is more fragmented, and neither universal access to health services nor standardized quality of care was achieved. In the 2000s, concerns about the disparities in access to health care gained policy legitimacy and efforts began to correct obvious distortions in the emerging system. These trajectories have varied among the five countries examined in this chapter.

Table 5.1 National Health Expenditure As a Percentage of GDP (2005)

Country	Public Expenditure 2000/03	Private Expenditure 2000/02
Argentina	4.7	3.7a
Brazil	3.2	5.3b
Chile	4.4	3.9c
Mexico	2.7d	3.3d
Uruguay	4.7	5.6a

a Health, unspecified
b Medical expenses and personal care
c Medical care and health maintenance
d Estimates based on national studies
Source: Gender, Health and Development in the Americas: Basic Indicators 2005. PAHO/UNFPA/UNIFEM.

Chile

The model adopted in Chile, during the Pinochet regime, implied decentralization and drastic reduction of public expenditure. Social Security Health Institutions (ISAPREs) were created that function as private insurance companies offering health packages determined by the premium paid by beneficiaries (Tajer, 2006). The public health system operates on an equal distribution scheme offering limited health benefits for all (*Fondo Nacional de Salud*, FONASA). Workers (active and retired) contribute 7% of their taxable income to the health system. This contribution can be made either to FONASA or to an ISAPRE. Those who opt for an ISAPRE may pay additional premiums to have access to a wider range of services or better quality of care. FONASA coverage is automatic for those not affiliated to an ISAPRE: dependent relatives of a contributor, the unemployed, pensioners, pregnant women who do not have other health coverage, people with disabilities, and the very poor. In 2000, the majority of the population (66.5%) was covered by the public subsystem (FONASA), 19.8% were affiliated to the ISAPREs, and 9.7% resorted to private providers (PAHO/WHO, 2002). However, public hospitals lacked funds and municipalities faced financial constraints to sustain primary health care. ISAPREs remained totally unregulated and disparities related to income, gender, and age were glaring. When democracy was restored in Chile in 1990, these distortions were acknowledged.

A series of measures were gradually adopted to resolve these biases. An agency was created to regulate the ISAPREs, the public health budget expanded by 50% and the rules for financing primary health care were modified. Between 2004 and 2005, new laws were approved that expanded the basic health package and created a compensation fund to redress age and gender discrimination in access to health care (Tajer, 2006).

Argentina

Until the early 1990s, the operations of the Argentine health system were guided by rules established in the 1930s, when the public social security systems incorporated and expanded the health care network created by immigrant workers' associations (*Obras Sociales*) in the early twentieth century. A major argument of health reformers was, as usual, that those who were not in the formal labor market did not have proper access to health care. While this distortion existed and should have been addressed, as the reform progressed it became clear that its main objective was the reduction of public expenditure and privatization.

Priority was also given to decentralization, and by 2005 roughly 60% of public health funding and provision of health care was already under the direct responsibility of provincial governments (Romero and Macieira, 2006). A universal public basic health insurance package (*Paquete Médico*

Obligatório) was created, which is managed by both national and provincial governments. Interventions of higher complexity are subject to user fees or covered by the modified health insurance schemes resulting from the deregulation of *Obras Sociales*. While in the past a worker and his/her family were 'attached' to a specific health insurance and provider, people now can choose among the various health insurance schemes. But no proper standards for service delivery were defined to guide the contracts signed between health insurance schemes and clients, and no formal procedure was established to assess costs or user satisfaction. According to Belmartino (Belmartino et al., 2002):

> The implementation of 'free choice' of health insurance was delayed and when finally it happened it was not accompanied by sufficient information that would allow persons to make a conscious option in respect to potential benefits and risks implied in their choice. (p. 13)

Although the reduction of public funding and state regulation in Argentina was not as drastic as in Chile, growing privatization was reflected in health expenditures., In 2000, public investment in health was reduced to 2.4% of GDP, while private expenditure accounted for 6.1% of GDP. As new policy directions were adopted by Argentine governments after the 2001–2002 crisis and the political discrediting of neoliberalism, there was some reverse swinging of the pendulum and public investment in health increased to 4.7% in 2000–2003 (Table 5.1).

Mexico

In Mexico, after many years of debate, a health reform law was approved in 2003 (Frenk et al., 2006). The reform aimed at ensuring access to health care for those sectors excluded from the formal labor market, the so-called 'general population' that could not access the networks funded by the Mexican Institute of Social Security (IMSS), which was responsible for pensions and health services of private employees, and the National Social Security Institute of Public Workers (INSTE).

A System for the Social Protection of Health (SPSS) was established to manage a basic health package (*Seguro Popular de Salud*) offering free access to a predefined and limited set of health care interventions. The SPSS package also comprises a mechanism of prepaid premiums through which the scope of services can be expanded. The premium is calculated on the basis of a progressive means-tested sliding scale to ensure that public subsidies are inversely proportional to family income levels. Health interventions not covered by the package are paid either directly through user fees or financed through these additional subsidies (provided by both federal and state governments). The poorest 20% of families are exempt from contributions. Cost-effectiveness parameters based on DALYs were adopted to guide the priorities of public investments, and novel structures were created to improve management and operational activities.[4]

The reform kept intact the constitutional principle of health as a right and is credited with having overcome some of the barriers created by poverty and labor market status to access to health care. However, the structure of the health system has not been substantially altered, as the SPSS basic package coexists with IMSS and INSTE publicly funded services whose level of funding has not decreased. In 2002 these two subsystems consumed more 60% of public funds invested in health (Sánchez, 2004). The national health budget decreased by 12% between 1995 and 2001. In the years 2000 to 2003, Mexico spent the lowest percentage of GDP for public investment in health (a mere 2.7% of GDP) among the five countries (Table 5.1). Private expenditures (3.3%) correspond to household and employers expenditures in private health insurance schemes and out-of-pocket fees. The latter spending is higher in Mexico than in other countries with similar levels of economic development (Knaul et al., 2005).

Brazil[5]

The Brazilian health reform was triggered by the critiques of two distortions of the health system of the 1970s: disparities in access to and quality of care between the social security (formal labor force) and the Ministry of Health networks (informal labor force); and a bias towards hospital-centered care resulting from the expansion of the social security–linked health network through the contracting of private providers. A broad health reform movement emerged to fight these distortions and became a key actor in the democratizing process, achieving major victories in the 1988 constitutional reform. The reformed constitution recognized the right to health and defined the principles of the Unified Health System (*Sistema Único de Saúde*, SUS) as a publicly funded, universal, decentralized, and comprehensive system, with built-in participatory and accountability mechanisms at all levels. The 1991 National Health Law defined the rules for merging the social security and Ministry of Health networks, and to guide decentralization and create the SUS management structure involving federal, state, and municipal administrations.[6]

In terms of decentralization, federal funds (roughly 65% of the national health budget) are transferred to municipalities that can become mainly responsible for management and provision of health services whenever local health funds and health councils are established, while the role of state health departments is mainly of planning and supervision. From 1994 on, a strategy was designed to improve primary health care: the Family Health Program (*Programa de Saúde da Família*, PSF) operating through basic health units with a small team of medical doctors, nurses, and community health workers. New rules were also defined for the payment of hospital-based, clinical, and primary care procedures (Médici, 1999).[7]

SUS coexists, however, with a supplementary private health system comprised of insurance schemes that are paid for by employers and individuals, and that cover 30% of the population. In 1998, a new public agency (*Agência Nacional de Saúde Suplementar*, ANS) was established to regulate this wide and powerful system.

In 1996, in order to resolve the financial constraints of the system, a new source of health funding was created—the Financial Transactions Tax (CPMF)—that remained in place until 2007. That same year a new financing modality was created to support basic health care (*Piso de Assistência Básica*, PAB). It transfers nonearmarked (per capita) amounts to municipalities to sustain clinics and primary care costs. In 1999, a new constitutional provision was adopted (PEC 20–1999) establishing that 20.6% of health financing must be provided by state governments and 16.4% by municipalities, and that the national health budget must increase in tandem with GDP growth.

Though the Brazilian reform contrasts with the models adopted in Chile, Argentina, and Mexico, problems remain in terms of access to services and quality of care. SUS is a gigantic machine delivering services to millions of people across an extremely diverse and unequal country. Though decentralization favored accountability and the expansion of basic health care, considerable unevenness exists at municipal levels in terms of technical capabilities and human resources; and local health systems are more prone to corruption and clientelism.

The partition of financial responsibilities between federal, state, and municipal levels has not been yet fully implemented. Hospital expenditures, especially in the case of complex procedures (like heart surgery, kidney dialysis, transplants, etc.), consume the bulk of public resources. As national policy guidelines translate poorly at local levels, access and quality tend to be compromised. The coexistence of the SUS and the private system is a perennial source of tension. Whenever an SUS 'crisis' becomes visible, space is opened for the private sector to expand its reach.

Uruguay[8]

Differently from other countries the Uruguayan health system has not been subject to a full reform. However, since the mid-1980s piecemeal measures were adopted that modified the structure established in the 1930s. In 1987, the State Health Services Administration (ASSE) was created to enhance decentralization. In the mid-1990s, World Bank funded state reform programs, included privatization proposals, and suggested the creation of a basic health package. Though these ideas gained much legitimacy during the economic crisis, critiques were raised in relation to the basic package as a health model designed 'only for the poor.' As no policy consensus was reached, the modification of the health system was silent, slow, and partial.

The system includes the public health network that covers 40.83% of the population (low-income recipients) with special emphasis on primary health care. It is managed by the Ministry of Public Health (*Ministerio de Salud Pública*, MSP), which both regulates and provides services. The other key component of the system is the Social Security Bank (*Banco de Previsión Social*, BPS) through which the formal labor force has access to health insurance and care through the so-called 'Collective Medical Care Institutions' (*Instituciones de Asistencia Médica Coletiva*, IAMCs; also established by European migrants in the early twentieth century). The IAMCs are private nonprofit organizations providing prepaid full-coverage health insurance to roughly 50% of the Uruguayan population (2000). Though they enjoy much autonomy, ceilings on premiums are defined by the state. BPS health insurance is financed by employee and employer contributions (90%) and national fiscal funds (10%) and the bank also manages a general hospital and six mother and child care centers in Montevideo.

Municipal health services constitute the third pillar of the public system, providing clinical and primary care to the 'general population.' It is funded by local tax resources, complemented by international grants and the national health budget. The Montevideo municipal health network offers the widest coverage, through 18 polyclinics, mobile clinics, and health centers. The private sector includes the IAMCs, but also other insurance schemes that provide partial coverage, specialized hospitals (that are private but also receive public funds), and hospices, clinics, and homes for the elderly (usually charging user fees).

Though reform measures have not been as clear-cut as in the other countries, the system has become more decentralized; since the 1980s mechanisms of social participation have proliferated, and primary health has expanded. A study carried out by the National Medical Union found that during the economic crisis 264 people lost their IAMC coverage each day and had to resort to the public health system. But in 2004, no systematic studies were available to fully assess how this piecemeal reform affected equity, efficiency, access to services, and quality of care. A full health reform began to be discussed in 2007.

*   *   *

To sum up, health reforms in the five countries have had different trajectories since the 1970s. The neoliberal reforms have themselves had two phases of discourse and implementation—the first was linked to the harsh structural adjustment reforms of the 1980s, and essentially reduced public health expenditures, speeded up privatization, and resulted in huge inequities and reduction in access wherever it was implemented. The second phase of health reform ideology, as propounded by the World Bank in its 1993 World Development Report, was more subtle and based its proposals on a critique of the tripartite systems which had evolved in the earlier part of the century under the influence of unionization (fuelled by import substitution industrialization and expansion of the public sector).

While the critique of the tripartite system was undoubtedly valid, there were different trajectories possible for reforms. The problem was the great inequalities between the health care available to those in the formal sector versus those in the informal labor force. One way to correct this inequality was by *expanding* the kind of care available under the social security–linked system to those in the informal sector. This is what was attempted in Brazil, using innovative public funding to support expanding a solidaristic and rights-based system to all. The reverse approach was the one proposed by the World Bank. It attempted to reduce inequality by *shrinking* the social security–based system and creating a new system based on a minimal package that would be publicly funded, with privatization and user fees to take care of the rest. It was implemented in different measure and with different degrees of effectiveness in Chile, Argentina, and Mexico. The harshest changes were under the 'pure' neoliberal reforms implemented by the Pinochet regime in Chile. Argentina's reform was in between, while Mexico provided some protection for the bottom quintile in the population. While this approach probably increased access for those at the very bottom, it was highly self-limiting, depended on privatization and user fees for anything outside the basic package, had its own inefficiencies, and did little to prevent health care costs from fueling poverty.

The irony is that, except for the tax on financial transactions used for a time in Brazil, the top tier of the old tripartite system was left to care for itself through private providers (as it always had) without much demand on it to contribute to the public health care system on grounds of solidarity, equity, or efficiency.

GENDER EFFECTS OF HEALTH REFORMS

Gender inequity and discrimination in access and service provision were not, by and large, consistently addressed by the health reform agendas. This contrasts with women's role in health, as they represent 80% of the health services labor force, perform 90% of community health work, and are fully responsible for household health needs. Research also indicates that women have a greater *objective* need for health services as their reproductive functions generate specific needs related to contraception, pregnancy, birth, and postnatal care. Male–female differentials in the demand for health care also reflects distinct patterns of socialization that impact on perceptions of symptoms. Though male mortality is higher, female morbidity and disability rates are higher, and, due to greater longevity, women are more prone to suffering chronic illnesses associated with age (Anderson, 2000; Chacham et al., 2003; Health Canada, 2003; Sen and Östlin, 2002.

Historically, in all countries of the sample, the majority of the labor force engaged in the formal sector had access to health care through social security–based solidarity funds. In all countries, except Brazil the reform logic made access to health care more dependent on income. This is important because, as noted by Pollack (2002), gender inequities in health can be explained either by the characteristics of the health system or by social and economic determinants, such as women's participation in the labor market, female wages, and household decisions regarding health investments. Though the available literature does not allow for a detailed analysis of the gender effects of health reform in each country, it is possible to broadly examine the implications of the shift from publicly funded solidarity systems to insurance schemes dependent on income, decentralization, and basic health packages.

From Publicly Funded Solidarity Systems to Income-Dependent Health Insurance Schemes

As described previously, one key impact of health reform processes was the transfer or transformation of solidarity funds into risk-based insurance schemes. Even when such schemes are publicly funded and subject to effective regulation, the scope of coverage they offer is dependent on the potential individual health risks assessed according to sex, age, and number of dependents. Before the reforms, public health systems in Argentina, Chile, and Mexico did not always offer good quality health care and had serious regional imbalances. However, among those who were covered, they tended to be more equitable in terms of access and coverage and did not present major gender-related distortions deriving from labor market participation or income differentials. Inequities were mostly related to the scarcity of comprehensive services, paternalistic attitudes of practitioners, and excessive medicalization of women's health.

While these preexisting distortions have not been consistently tackled, the new health insurance modalities, the dissociation between financing and provision of services, and self-regulation imposed on both public and private health providers have created new distortions. Today users can access only a certain level of services guaranteed by the publicly funded packages. Health care is no longer offered to respond to health needs but determined by managing and financial criteria of insurance schemes. One clear gendered implication of the shift is that women in the reproductive age-group pay higher premiums because of deliveries and other obstetric risks. Also, since women live longer, they also may be compelled to spend more in a phase of life when their income is probably lower. Women's ability to pay higher premiums or additional costs is impaired because they are mainly engaged in informal activities and have lower salaries than men (roughly 70%) (Gomez, 2002a, 2002b).

While the assumption made by health economists is that households are homogeneous and equitable and will invest in health if needed or as a way to prevent major health costs in the future, feminist analysis has shown that this is not exactly the case (Kabeer, 1994; Gomez, 2002a).

In all the countries being examined, a significant percentage of house-holds are headed by women and, even in other households, since solidarity within the household is not a given, nothing ensures that income will be invested in girls' and women's health as needed. Tajer (2006) analyzed gender-based intra-household inequities in a study of Argentine women affected by heart conditions who were treated in the public hospital. She concluded that when these women were in the hospital they had access to medication, but when they became outpatients, very often treatment collapsed because they tended to lose out in household negotiations and could not afford out-of-pocket expenses. Also as shown by Tajer (2006) and Mesa-Lago (2005), in some cases private insurance companies openly avoid providing insurance for women because they are considered to have higher potential health risks.

The gendered impact of income-dependent health schemes is evidently more acute in cases where privatization has been more drastic (Chile) or where the proportion of out-of-pocket expenditures is higher (Mexico). Women's ability to pay for private health insurances also requires further research in Brazil, where the inefficiencies of the SUS compel low-income individuals and families to contract limited private health insurance for hospital-based care and diagnosis. Evidence available from other contexts has shown the detrimental impact of user fees and other modalities of pri-vate access on women because they resort more frequently to health ser-vices for their own needs, but also for their children and other dependent relatives' health problems (UNRISD, 2005).

Decentralization

When health systems were highly centralized, women with reduced mobility were negatively affected because secondary and tertiary units were distant from where they lived. Though decentralization tends to improve access to services, other aspects must be taken into account. For instance, at local levels, the mind-set of health providers is more likely to adapt to dominant cultural norms that restrict the access of women and girls to health care. Also, while decentralization made municipalities responsible for basic or primary health, the responsibility for more complex services has in many cases remained in the hands of national or state/provincial governments and this affects the functioning of referral systems.

Basic Health Packages

Basic health packages adopted in Chile, Mexico, and Argentina have been also proposed and discussed in Brazil and Uruguay as a strategy to real-locate public funds to the poorer sectors. One way of examining the gen-dered effects of such packages is to assess its impact in terms of horizontal fairness. If universal access to a certain package exists, it can be said that horizontal equity has improved. As mentioned before, the previous tripartite models were not equitable. But in countries where social security–funded health systems covered a higher percentage of the population, such as Argentina and Chile, the shift towards basic packages compromised gender equity because of the income limitations and other barriers analyzed earlier (Gomez, 2002b).

Although basic health packages have, in most cases, defined women as their main beneficiaries, they tend to concentrate on traditional maternal and child care, leaving aside other health needs such as cervical and breast cancer, HIV/AIDS and STI screening and treatment, contraception, occupational health, mental health, and chronic diseases. By and large basic packages revived the maternal and child paradigm of the 1970s, and are at odds with the policy paradigm shift of the International Conference on Population and Development (Cairo, 1994) and the Fourth World Conference on Women (Beijing, 1995). According to Almeida and colleagues (2004):

> The mother and child basic health packages do not fulfill minimal requirements to be considered a consistent social insurance scheme . . . A basic package of medical interventions can be an efficient tool in countries experiencing great deficits in terms of health care coverage (such as Bolivia and some Argentine provinces). However the lack of connections between the basic package and wider health system at large, in particular effective referral to more complex level of care, make them (only) a valid short term policy intervention. But they do not constitute an effective long term strategy of social insurance. Basic packages must necessarily be combined with structural mechanisms that imply additional efforts in terms of both health and macroeconomic policies. (p. 69)

Gender Distortions in the Chilean Reform[9]

The Chilean experience strikingly illustrates some of the distortions listed earlier. In Chile only 39% of women are in the workforce, the average female wage is 30% lower than men's wages, and 45% of working women are in the informal sector. In 2000, the FONASA basic package covered 65% of the population, and its beneficiaries were 57% male and 43% female. While this proportion is not too unbalanced, when the status of the affiliates is taken into account the picture is different. In 2004, 28% of female beneficiaries of the basic package were dependents of another affiliate.

In the case of ISAPREs (the private insurance plans covering 19.8% of the population) only 35% of the insured are women. This is explained by ISAPREs' logic: the contract is individual, and the cost of the premium is defined by, among other factors, the paying capacity of beneficiaries. As women have lower salaries, they are usually not accepted, and even when they are able to sign a contract they have access to limited insurance schemes. In 2001, premiums for women of reproductive age were between 2.4 and 3.1 times higher than men's premiums for the same age-group. Although these higher premium costs are partly explained by the fact that maternity leave was initially paid for by ISAPREs, even plans that exclude medical care for delivery had higher premiums for women than for men of similar ages.

The creation of a public subsidy for maternity leave, irrespective of the chosen insurance system and income level, was the first step to correct these long-standing distortions. But the subsidy itself is highly regressive, as it is paid in proportion to salaries. In consequence, half of the ISAPREs affiliates who have higher incomes receive 80% of the total state investment in maternity leave. As mentioned before, in 1995 a new law altered some aspects of the health model, but it did not address the other gendered distortions. Finally in 2004, after Bachelet's election, an expanded basic health package was adopted that is now provided by FONASA and ISAPRE networks, irrespective of the sex of the beneficiary and cannot be linked to higher premiums. In 2005, a compensation fund was created to reduce gender- and age-based discrimination in both FONASA and ISAPRE insurance schemes. The state has also set limits to the annual increase in premium costs.

The Chilean experience sharply illustrates the negative potential of this type of health reform for gender equity and women's health. But, even though less acute, similar problems have shown up in the other countries as well. Ironically, the same period of the 1990s saw significant advances at the global level in the discourse on and commitments to sexual and reproductive health and rights (SRHR) at both the Cairo (1994) and Beijing (1995) conferences, although the political weight of the Catholic Church and its lay arm, Opus Dei, continue to act as a counterpoint in the region. To examine the effect of these contradictory tendencies, we turn next to look more closely at SRHR policies, their interplay with health sector reforms, and the impacts in the five countries.

SEXUAL AND REPRODUCTIVE HEALTH POLICIES

As sexual and reproductive autonomy is a key dimension of gender equity, it is also necessary to verify if health sector reforms have favored sound sexual and reproductive health policies. This is also relevant because in the five countries, since the 1970s, feminists and other actors have struggled to transform health systems to respond to women's needs and to respect their rights. While in Mexico and Brazil these struggles mainly focused on the distortions of population control, in Uruguay and Argentina, they challenged pro-natalist assumptions. As a result, in Brazil and Uruguay, novel and early women's health policies were crafted: the PAISM (in Brazil, 1984) and the PAIM (in Montevideo, 1992). In Chile, efforts were made to improve maternal health and access to contraception and provide safe abortion, despite stringent legal restrictions (Faúndes and Barzelatto, 2004). Everywhere, from the mid-1980s on this policy area would be impacted by the HIV/AIDS epidemic.

During the 1990s, the relative political stability and the impacts of Cairo and Beijing favored greater visibility and legitimacy for sexual and reproductive health demands. But fiscal restrictions and, in most cases, health reform created constraints for the advancement of sound sexual and reproductive health. Quite often international commitments made by governments did not fully translate into national policies, and electoral and administrative changeovers implied erratic policy progress. In the 2000s, though the sexual and reproductive policy agendas were not abandoned, leftward political shifts have not meant major steps forward, among other reasons because the influence of moral conservatism and dogmatic religious views has increased.[10]

Argentina

In 1974, a governmental decree was issued prohibiting the supply of contraceptives, and this was later ratified during the military regime (1977). As democratization evolved, a public debate on women's reproductive self-determination started. Between 1986 and 1998 two bills were presented to the house of representatives and the senate to create a national family planning program. They were immediately attacked by conservative sectors. In 1989, despite stringent fiscal constraints, a family planning program began to be implemented in the metropolitan area of Buenos Aires. In 1990, Carlos Menem was elected president, even as a new family planning law was drafted. But it was never voted on because a strong alliance was established between the Menem administration and the Catholic Church.[11]

In 1995, a new bill was presented to congress and approved by the house to guide a national sexual and reproductive health framework. Though the senate did not ratify the law, a lively public debate ensued, leading to the adoption of progressive legislative initiatives at provincial and municipal levels. Concurrently, the Argentine government started to implement a national program of HIV/AIDS prevention and treatment. Finally, in 2001, at the end of the Duhalde administration when the political and economic crisis was at its height, Law No. 25.673 that defines the National Program on Sexual Health and Responsible Procreation was finally approved.[12] Dominguez and colleagues (2004) interpret the shift as a result of the greater visibility of unwanted pregnancies and maternal mortality rates among poor women, particularly teenagers. By late 2004, roughly 13 million contraceptives had been distributed by the public health system to 1.5

Table 5.2 Women's Health and Reproductive Health: Selected Indicators

Country	Total fertility rate	Percent of women who gave birth by age-group		Births within 24 months after last delivery (percent) 1996/2003	Estimated death rates (per 100,000 women) due to		Prevalence of anemia (percentage of women)		maternal mortality ratio (per 100,000 live births) 1997/2003
		Age 15 to 19 2004	Age 35 to 49 2004		malignant neoplasm (uterus) 1997/2002	malignant neoplasm (breast) 1997/2002	Pregnant 1990/2000	Nonpregnant 1985/1997	
Argentina	2.4	6	2	-	14	30	24	18	46.1
Brazil	2.2	7	2	29	11	13	42	20	45.8
Chile	2.3	4	2	-	13	15	20	8	16.7
Mexico	2.4	6	3	-	11	8	26	14	63.9
Uruguay	2.3	7	2	-	16	39	-	-	a

a: The ratio is not calculated if the relative standard error is higher than 23%.
Source: Gender, Health and Development in the Americas: Basic Indicators 2005. PAHO/UNFPA/UNIFEM.

million users through 5,076 hospitals and clinics that also offered STI prevention, and in April 2005, the government announced that the program
would be expanded.[13]

Even so, according to Dominguez and colleagues (2004), no consistent
linkages were built with the national HIV/AIDS and the adolescent health
program (*Programa de Atención a Menores en Riesgo*, PROAME). The
effectiveness and quality of services varied widely across provincial and
municipal levels. Furthermore, the guidelines of the sexual and reproductive program were not properly incorporated by the newly deregulated
social security health schemes (*Obras Sociales*), to which the majority of
women resort. Until 2004, poverty and economic deprivation resulting
from the economic crisis had not totally receded, women's access to sexual
and reproductive health care was restricted by user fees or higher premiums, and no consistent links had been built between poverty alleviation
programs and the sexual and reproductive health program.[14]

However, it is also important to underline the fact that these two decades
of struggles also raised the visibility of abortion. When efforts were made
to ensure access to the procedure in the only case permitted by the penal
code (the rape of mentally disabled women), the Catholic Church and other
conservative sectors systematically interposed juridical contestations. In
2005, the church hierarchy directly attacked the minister of health as a
proponent of abortion. In the same year a national feminist campaign for
legal abortion took off and by 2007 had resulted in a draft legal provision
and triggered mobilization across the country.

Brazil

The Brazilian women's health policy launched in 1984 (*Programa de
Assistência Integral à Saúde da Mulher*, PAISM) encompassed prenatal,
birth, and postnatal care, cervical cancer and STI prevention, adolescent and menopausal care, and contraceptive assistance. The policy was
crafted in tandem with the health reform process, and the struggle for
women's health and reproductive autonomy also impacted on the Constitutional Reform (1988). A definition in regard to family planning was
adopted and, despite a strong Catholic Church lobby, the text did not
include the defense of the right to life from the moment of conception. In
1988, a National HIV/AIDS program was created that is globally recognized as a policy model for prevention and treatment, and much synergy
between these two policy areas would develop in the years to follow (Corrêa, 2006b; Parker, 1997).

Until the mid-1990s, though PAISM implementation was impaired by
political instability and health financing concerns, positive experiences
developed at local levels, as in the case of the first service established in São
Paulo (1989) to provide abortions in the two cases permitted by law (rape
and women's life risk). Brazilian feminists intensively mobilized for Cairo

and Beijing, and the Brazilian government played a key role in these negotiations. In 1996, a new law was approved to regulate access to contraception in the SUS (*Lei do Planejamento Familiar*, 1997). A year later as the
PAISM was revitalized, a new strategy was defined to: improve prenatal,
childbirth, and postnatal care to meet the maternal mortality targets and
reduce the proportion of cesarean sections; ensure the provision of male
and female sterilization and reversible methods according to the family
planning law; improve postabortion care; expand the prevention and treatment of cervical and breast cancer; prevent and treat STIs and HIV/AIDS
infections among women; and a Ministry of Health protocol was approved
to guide abortion services and expand services to respond to gender-based
and sexual violence. The implementation of these guidelines required systematic negotiations with SUS management structures at all levels.

The 2002 general elections resulting in the PT victory did not imply major
policy discontinuity. In early 2004, the National Women's Health Policy
defined gender equality, women's human rights, and comprehensive care as
its guiding principles. New targets were set for maternal mortality reduction and a compact was signed by the federal, state, and municipal health
managers to achieve these goals. The distribution of reversible contraceptive methods was restructured and access to vasectomies was prioritized.
In 2005, the 1998 abortion protocol was reviewed to include postabortion care, and in 2007, a new plan to tackle the feminization of HIV/AIDS
was also made public (Pinto, 2008; Corrêa, 2006b). These efforts have
resulted in the expansion and improvement of prenatal care, epidemiological surveillance of maternal mortality (including the creation of maternal
mortality committees), and services responding to gender-based violence
(including abortion provision in the case of rape).

But even when public distribution of reversible methods improved,
problems persisted in terms of logistics. The response to HIV transmission among women remained limited until 2007.[15] The results of campaigns
implemented to improve cervical and breast cancer screening and prevention
were far from ideal. Most importantly, much remains to be done in regard
to the quality of obstetric and postabortion care and maternal mortality.

Even though policy performance has been uneven, data collected in 2006
by the National Survey on Demography and Health (*Pesquisa Nacional em
Demografia e Saúde*, PNDS) indicates that these continuing investments
are positively reflected in key indicators: 61% of pregnant women had
seven or more prenatal consultations (in contrast to 48% in 1996); 81%
of women in unions use a contraceptive method (67% in 1996), and this
expansion has mainly occurred among lower-income women; the bias in
contraceptive mix towards female sterilization (40% in 1996) is more balanced: female sterilization, 29%; pills, 25%; condoms, 12% (4% in 1996);
injectables, 4%,[16] and vasectomies 5%. In relation to obstetric care the
results are poorer, as no reduction was detected in relation to C-sections,
and even though 98% of women deliver in hospitals, the quality of care is

not satisfactory. Though roughly 65% of maternal deaths occur in hospitals, according to Lago [17]:

> A perverse combination exists between archaic gender relations and disrespect to women in health services. Even today maternal health care and, in particular, obstetric care is seen and implemented in the worst conditions, because it is a procedure that pays less. Maternal deaths are still perceived by society and the health establishment as an inevitable event.

This mixed picture must be placed against the background of structural factors that hamper the overall performance of SUS: the scale of the system, the enormous challenges in logistics, and the effects of decentralization, since sexual and reproductive health services are highly dependent on local technical capacity and the surrounding cultural and social conditions.

This long trajectory also included a steady struggle for safe and legal abortion that, in 2004, culminated in two parallel initiatives. The Supreme Court was called upon to judge a request to permit abortion in the case of anencephaly, and the National Conference on Women's Public Policies issued a recommendation to revise the existing abortion legislation. A Tripartite Commission, involving the executive and legislative branches and civil society representatives was created to propose a law reform. When it concluded its work in 2005, a political corruption crisis had erupted and the interest and commitment of the executive branch waned. When the provision was tabled it was heavily attacked by conservative sectors, and the momentum died down in early 2006. In 2007, right before the Pope's visit, the health minister declared that abortion was a grave public health problem and appealed for a wide public discussion. Though this inaugurated a new advocacy cycle for legalizing abortion, a stalemate ensued because antiabortion forces kept gaining strength. In 2008, a clinic in the state of Mato Grosso was anonymously denounced to be performing abortions and was invaded by the police who collected all medical records in the files. Subsequently, around 10,000 women were formally accused for having aborted, and a few of them have already been condemned to community services. This was followed by a Supreme Court debate on abortion in the case of anencephaly that is still pending a final decision (Castilhos, 2008). In March 2009 another abortion-related episode captured the attention of the international media, when the archbishop of Recife excommunicated the doctors who performed a legal abortion on a nine-year-old girl who had been raped by her stepfather. There was open public outrage at the position taken by the church, and both President Lula and the Minister of Health supported the doctors.

Chile

Until the dictatorship, Chile probably had the most progressive and effective reproductive health policy in South America. Under Pinochet even when the MCH and family planning programs were not completely dismantled, access to and quality of health care was negatively affected by health reform. Also the moral conservatism of the regime was totally at odds with women's self-determination: sexual education was suspended, and at a late moment of the dictatorship therapeutic abortion was abolished by the Supreme Court. In the early 1990s, 55 in every 100 pregnancies were terminated, which implies that women had difficulties in accessing contraception and that the prohibition of abortion did not imply its elimination as a means of fertility control.

The Socialist-Christian Democrat coalition in power since 1990 implemented broad and effective gender equality policies. But sexual and reproductive health, sexuality, and abortion remained subject to major controversies, as the Catholic Church's influence on political institutions did not diminish. The struggle for SRHR has therefore been unrelenting. Though divorce was approved in Chile in 2004, the Supreme Court in May 2008 suspended the distribution of emergency contraception included in a new Ministry of Health guideline. An assessment made by the Gender Equity in Health Observatory in 2005 concluded that, despite domestic and international commitments, no substantive progress has been observed in the areas of sexuality education, adolescent health, or HIV/AIDS surveillance, prevention, and treatment for women (Observatório de Equidad de Género en Salud, 2005). Of note is the fact that the sexual and reproductive rights law presented in 2000 had not yet been approved. [18]

However, maternal health policies have evolved positively. Lago (2006) notes that in Chile maternal mortality rates have been declining since the 1950s, when the National Health System was created and began effectively engaging midwives. This created favorable conditions for the investments made after 1990 to have positive results, as maternal death ratios decreased from 40 to 19 per 100,000 live births. This outcome contrasts sharply with the absence of comprehensive sexual and reproductive health care and the gender-based distortions of health reform previously analyzed.

Mexico

In Mexico, a family planning program based on fertility control and contraceptive prevalence as a target was established in 1974, which would be systematically criticized by feminists and other actors. In the 1990s, due to the mobilization of women's organizations for both Cairo and Beijing, Mexico was also a main player in these conferences. In 1994, an ICPD follow-up commission was established, involving state agencies, academics, and feminist NGOs. Policy guidelines then adopted prioritized: the expansion and improvement of prenatal, obstetric, and postnatal care; maternal mortality; correcting the distortions of the family planning program through the implementation of informed consent; expansion of services to rural areas, poorer urban sectors, and the indigenous population; improvement of postabortion care; training of health professionals; expansion of cervical cancer screening and HIV/AIDS prevention; and development of protocols to guide health response to gender-based violence. In society, the struggle for safe and legal abortion was also reactivated.

But these policy efforts coincided with the approval and gradual implementation of health reform that, as previously seen, weakened the rights-based dimension of health policy by reducing the scope of universal care to the basic insurance package. After the PAN victory in 2000, though the previously adopted sexual and reproductive health remained formally in place, the political climate changed drastically. The main reproductive health policy of the Fox administration was the "Fair Start in Life" (*Programa Arranque Parejo a la Vida*) that prioritized maternal and infant mortality through a rather conventional approach (Sánchez, 2004).[19] This shift is not, however, followed consistently across the country as state administrations today have much more autonomy in policy design and implementation. The most striking example is the Federal District, which has been governed by the PRD since 1994.

Legal abortion has been part of the feminist agenda since the 1970s and gained much visibility after Cairo and Beijing. In 1999, the debate was fuelled by the case of Paulina, a teenager raped in Baja, California, who could not access abortion even when the state penal code allowed it.[20] In the 2000s strong feminist advocacy for reforms of abortion laws began in the Federal District, since, during the 2000 electoral campaign, presidential candidate Vicente Fox had declared that if elected he would promote the "right to life from the moment of conception." Rosario Robles, then governor of the Federal District, drafted a bill to expand access to abortion in the cases of health risks and grave fetal abnormality. Though the bill passed, antiabortionists appealed to the Supreme Court, and the state law was upheld until late 2002. Finally, in a political context of polarization between the recently elected PAN federal administration and the PRD that governs Mexico City, in April 2007 a provision for legalizing abortion was approved by the Federal District Assembly. Antiabortion forces once again contested the law at Supreme Court level, but in August 2008 the Court issued a decision that affirmed its constitutionality. Since 2007, roughly 10,000 abortion procedures have been performed under the law.

Uruguay

The evolution of reproductive health policies must be traced back to the 1950s, when a coherent mother and child program expanded prenatal care services and ensured hospital-based deliveries across the country. From the 1960s on, contraceptive prevalence also increased, both through market outlets and national family planning NGOs. By the late 1980s, indicators in these two areas were fairly good by Latin American standards, but comprehensive women's health policy was not in place, female sterilization was not permitted, and resistance prevailed with respect to abortion. In the early 1990s the Left Front was elected in Montevideo and a comprehensive women's health program (PAIM) began to be implemented within the municipal health network.

Cairo and Beijing gave a further boost to a broader SRHR perspective. With UNFPA support the PAIM in Montevideo and the Maternity and Paternity Program (*Programa Maternidad-Paternidad Elegida*), under the responsibility of the Ministry of Health, expanded. In 2000, a national Comprehensive Women's Health Program (*Programa de Salud Integral de la Mujer*, SIM) was launched under the responsibility of ASSE, the main implementing agency of the Ministry of Health. In 2004, a National Commission on Sexual and Reproductive Health was created.

Abracinskas and López (2004) assessed this trajectory, concluding that health policies had moved beyond maternal health to provide access to contraceptive methods, STI/HIV prevention, screening, and treatment, and the start of adolescent health interventions. But they also remarked that private providers and the IAMCs did not always include contraceptive provision in their packages and that the national policy framework did not pay enough attention to inequalities and discrimination based on gender, race, ethnicity, and sexual orientation. The report also observes that though in official documents sexual and reproductive health was linked with poverty concerns, this did not easily translate to program implementation.

In 2004, the victory of the Left Front would imply new policy directions. A report published in 2006 by the National Commission for the Beijing Follow-up analyzed the shifts observed since 2004 as a slow but steady advance in terms of sexual and reproductive health policies including: the creation of a National Program on Women's Health and Gender in the Ministry of Health that expanded the previous framework to incorporate gender-based violence and masculinity. However the report also calls attention to the fact that the program, though national in design, only covered the Montevideo metropolitan area and that its various protocols had not been effectively disseminated across the public health system and other relevant public and private health care institutions (Comisión Nacional de Seguimiento, 2006).

Abortion debates constitute another main feature of the Uruguayan trajectory as efforts to legalize abortion can also be retraced back to the 1980s. These efforts gained increased political relevance in the 2000s when data was released on the increased rates of abortion-related deaths. This triggered a new wave of mobilization, and in 2002 the house approved the Sexual and Reproductive Law Provision that included access to abortion on demand until the 12th week of pregnancy. Even when a public opinion poll concluded that 63% of Uruguayans approved law, in May 2004 the bill was defeated in the senate. In 2005, the recently elected president Tabaré Vásquez declared that if the bill were retabled, he would veto it. In October 2007, the bill was finally retabled and approved by the senate and is still pending approval by the house. Since the threat of the presidential veto remains in place, an unrelenting debate has evolved since 2005, within the Left Front and in society at large, which has led to abortion being addressed not just as a key women's rights and health issue, but also as a political topic that challenges the very principles of democracy.

*   *   *

The preceding discussion points to two key elements that have affected women's access to sexual and reproductive health services and policies. Health reforms have clearly intersected with the evolution of SRHR policies. Interestingly, in Brazil, which followed the most progressive health reforms, there was significant realization of synergies between the SUS on the health reform side and the PAISM on the women's health side, even though gaps and bottlenecks remain. Where health reforms have been more neoliberal, as in Chile, they have been significantly at odds with women's SRHR. This has been the pattern in other countries as well, although there have been many ups and downs as economic and political crises and changes have played out.

The other major element is the ongoing battle between women's organizations and their supporters versus the Catholic Church, not only on abortion but even on the availability of contraception, as in Argentina. This struggle has been going on almost independently of health reforms at the legislative level; however, the limits placed by health reforms on access have hampered and distorted SRHR program advances even when women's advocates are able to gain victories in their struggles with the church.

In addition, health reforms and SRHR policies have been intersected since the 1990s by antipoverty programs that have been spreading rapidly in the region. In the context of rapidly rising health costs, and given the limited nature of basic health packages and the expansion of user fees, poverty alleviation programs constitute a third important policy input to the social determinants of health in the region. In the next section, we examine these links and their gender implications in brief without going into detailed country-level analysis.

POVERTY ALLEVIATION PROGRAMS

Since the mid-1990s poverty alleviation policies have been implemented in Latin America, including income transfer programs, which provide a minimum allowance to poor households. In our sample of countries, one of the earliest programs was implemented in Mexico under the name of *Progresa* (in 1997), later renamed *Oportunidades*. In Brazil in 1996, the School Grant Program (*Programa Bolsa Escola*) started in specific municipalities and by 2001 was expanded, though not yet to the whole country. In 1996 a specific income transfer program was also created to eradicate child labor (*Program de Erradicação do Trabalho Infantil*, PETI). In 2003, the Zero Hunger Program *(Fome Zero)* established a food subsidy and the previously existing programs were consolidated in the Family Grant (*Bolsa Família*) that presently covers all households whose income is below the nationally defined poverty threshold. In 2000, Argentina adopted the Heads of Household Program (*Programa Jefas y Jefes de Hogar*); in 2002, Chile initiated the Solidarity Program (*Chile Solidario*); and in Uruguay, a similar initiative, the National Plan of Social Emergency Assistance (*Plan Nacional de Atención a la Emergencia Social*), started in 2005.[21]

The stated goals of these programs are to alleviate poverty in the short run, and enable the households to invest in education and health of future generations. The income transfers to households increase their consumption levels and have positive economic impacts, particularly in small towns and rural areas. However, in all cases, income transfer is conditioned on children's attendance at school and, in some cases, it is also required that young children and pregnant women access health services for specific interventions. In Argentina, where the program was adopted during the economic crisis, it required that beneficiaries work in public construction and community activities.

The programs target the poor or extremely poor sectors and are described as policies based on the right to social inclusion. Managers also claim that they differ from previous policies for the poor because a contract is made between the state and beneficiaries. Everywhere the programs have been encouraged and/or financially supported by multilateral financial institutions, which play a strong supporting role in their design, operation, and evaluation. Input from national economies is moderate, not exceeding 0.35% of GDP. Women are usually the recipients of the transfers, either because this is stipulated in the programs' criteria or simply because this is what happens in practice.

Gender Implications of Poverty Alleviation Programs

Since the late 1970s, a vast amount of research is available about the impacts of poverty on women and the gender dimensions of poverty (Corrêa, 2006a). At that time, some studies identified higher levels of poverty among female-headed households, triggering what become known as the "feminization of poverty" agenda (Buvinic et al., 1978; Merrick and Schmink, 1983). Subsequently, as research revealed that women tended to invest more in the well-being of households whenever they had resources to do so (Bruce and Dwyer, 1988, among others), development institutions began to adopt the 'efficiency' approach to women and poverty (Young, 1991; Arriagada and Torres, 1998). In contrast, other feminist perspectives emphasized the structural roots of poverty and power differentials between women and men (Kabeer, 1998; Sen and Grown, 1986). In the 1990s, gender frameworks were recognized as better tools to address development and poverty trends and policies (Baden and Milward, 1997; Chant, 1997; Fraser, 1997; Kabeer, 1994; Moser, 1995; Young, 1991; UNDP, 1995). Arriagada and Torres (1998) remind us that gender frameworks led development agencies to shift to new approaches based on the "equity" and "empowerment and citizenship" policy frameworks.[22]

This literature provides parameters to analyze how gender inequality, class differentials, and poverty patterns intersect, and to examine how poverty alleviation programs are being implemented. All these studies concluded that female poverty cannot be assessed with the same conceptual tools used to analyze male poverty (Ocampo, 2000; Hopenhayn and Ottone, 2000; Serrano, 2005). Some of them examined factors that hinder the assessment of gender disparities in poverty, such as scarcity of consistent data, the difficulties in capturing differentials of income distribution within households, and in measuring the impact of income on women's autonomy. Research also suggests that while the focus on female-headed households and female informal labor may contribute to measure inequality of income, it does not allow for a generalized assumption about feminization of poverty (Baden and Milward, 1997).

In relation to poverty alleviation programs, various authors consider that the choice of women as their beneficiaries is more in line with the 'efficiency approach' than with the newer gender frameworks. Though policy makers consider these programs as women's empowerment initiatives, the transfer of income is not aimed at women themselves, but at the household's well-being. As the main recipients women become 'household poverty managers' or intermediaries between the state and households. Instead of tackling and transforming the gender division of labor to ensure higher levels of gender equity, the programs make instrumental use of the existing sexual division of labor to optimize the social impacts of women's roles as mothers and caregivers (Klein, 2005).

Programs under way are credited with having expanded school enrolment under the assumption that poverty and wage inequalities are easily overcome when educational levels increase. However, in all countries being examined, while women's educational levels are higher than men's, they still earn on average 30% less: 67% less in Argentina, 55.2% less in Brazil, 66% less in Chile, 55.4% less in Mexico, and 59% less in Uruguay (CEPAL, 2008). This implies that higher levels of education do not automatically translate into higher income. It is also not clear how the increase in education in children immediately impacts on women's personal lack of income and autonomy. It is worth noting that the increases in basic education enrolment are not accompanied by the expansion of day care centers. The study undertaken by Lavinas and colleagues (2008) in Recife found that just 10% of women beneficiaries of the *Bolsa Família* have children in public day care centers. In addition, no consistent strategies have yet been designed to help these women move beyond the condition of recipients and escape economic exclusion and discrimination. Lastly, as highlighted by Daeren (2004), poverty alleviation strategies and opportunities are not being created for those women that are not mothers of young children or caught in extreme poverty. A caveat less discussed is that, as women become intermediaries between households and the state, connections may be lost with surrounding social dynamics that are key to enhancing sociability and citizenship.[23]

The Health–Poverty Link through a Gender Lens

When the links between gender, health, and poverty are examined, other gaps become apparent. In Brazil, health reform evolved in tandem with rather consistent sexual and reproductive policies, and from the mid-1990s on expansion of basic health care programs also converged with the establishment of income transfer programs. The Family Grant includes nutrition interventions for pregnant and nursing women and children under five and access to conventional maternal and child care. In many municipalities, the identification of the target population is made by Family Health Program teams. The Ministry of Social Development reports that health conditionality is being fulfilled by 90% of recipients. However, the research coordinated by Lavinas and colleagues (2008) shows that in Recife, where the Family Health Program is quite effective, all women enrolled in the Family Grant had access to prenatal care through SUS, but not all of them could get contraceptive methods through public outlets, and one-third had not planned their last pregnancy.

In Argentina and Uruguay, even though the crises of 2000 to 2002 opened the space for sexual and reproductive health policies, they are not consistently articulated through income transfer programs. In Chile, the antipoverty program started in early 1990s was converted into an income transfer program in 2000 and a rather successful strategy for maternal mortality reduction was implemented. Yet, the poor still lacked access to comprehensive sexual and reproductive health services because of the narrow focus of poverty programs, and also because the health reform model was fraught with gender biases. In Mexico, the adoption of gender equality and sexual and reproductive health policies coincided with the beginning of health reform and poverty alleviation strategies, and initial efforts were made to link the Cairo and Beijing agendas, the health reform process, and poverty programs. But, under the Fox administration, the federal reproductive health policy retreated to a conventional mother and child approach, a shift that can be explained by the conservative political climate, but is not unrelated to the logic behind the health reform.

In most cases, therefore, the narrow focus of both the basic health care packages and poverty alleviation tend to sideline other key dimensions of sexual and reproductive health such as cervical and breast cancer, STI and HIV/AIDS screening and treatment, access to contraception and postabortion care, and health responses to gender-based violence (or even access to abortion in those cases when the procedures are legal). Other interventions required to tackle the effects of poverty on women's health, such as chronic diseases, in particular high blood pressure, nonreproductive cancers, and mental and occupational health, are also not on the policy radar screen (Aquino et al., 1999). Last but not least, poor women's roles as 'poverty managers' often implies additional burdens that also may have detrimental health effects or impede their search for health care (Aguirre and Batty-hány, 2005).

CONCLUSIONS

When health reform, sexual and reproductive health, and poverty reduction policies in these five countries are examined through a gendered lens the results are paradoxical. On the one hand, health services, in particular of primary health care, have expanded, sexual and reproductive health frameworks have been legitimized despite strong conservative resistance, and income transfer programs have directly transferred cash to poor women. On the other hand, no consistent dialogues have developed, except in the case of Brazil, between actors involved in health reform processes and those engaged in the design and implementation of sexual and reproductive policies, let alone income transfer programs. Conceptual clarity is still lacking in terms of integrating gender equity perspectives in both health reform and income transfer policy frameworks.

Even today a large proportion of women are not engaged in the labor market and among those who are, roughly 50% are engaged in informal activities and are not covered by labor regulations and social protection. Unemployment rates also tend to be higher among women, and even those who are covered by labor rights receive lower salaries. Women's labor is affected by discontinuities related to pregnancy and childrearing. All these factors imply that women have less ability to pay private health insurance premiums or out-of-pocket expenses and are more directly affected by the limited scope or bad quality of public health systems.

Though it is not possible to affirm that poverty rates measured by income are higher among women overall, an important segment of women who are single heads of households experience a greater incidence of poverty. Married women or women in unions may be more protected from extreme poverty but may also lack autonomy either to earn personal income or to freely dispose of their money. Women's health is directly affected by poverty: pregnancy and labor risks, postnatal care complications, STIs, HIV, and cervical cancer rates, nutrition deficiencies, higher rates of chronic, occupational, and mental health impairments. Gender inequalities are also a cause of ill-health, as demonstrated by the effects of gender and sexual violence.

Women also tend to be dependents of their husbands and partners in health insurance schemes and can lose these protections in the event of widowhood, abandonment, or separation. In some countries, insurance schemes and basic packages only provide maternity coverage and, in some cases, the insurance rules discriminate against women of reproductive age because of costs of medical care related to childbirth, certain pathologies, and greater longevity. Moreover the sex-based differentials in the use of services occurs during the reproductive years, which is exactly when non-solidarity insurance plans discriminate most against women. The immediate consequence is that costs for the social function of reproduction fall principally on women and may be aggravated in the case of women who are heads of households and who do not have a partner to share health costs. The adoption of user fees to cover complex health interventions affects all women because their income is lower, and particularly excludes low-income and poor women from access to these procedures.

In poverty alleviation programs the choice of women as beneficiaries may have some immediate positive impacts in terms of raising them above extreme poverty and allowing them to expand household consumption. However, these programs as designed today do not included measures to alter the sex-based division of labor and the gender biases they imply. Rather they make instrumental use of women's socially constructed roles as mothers and caregivers to transform them into poverty managers at the household level. However, the health effects and other implications of increasing women's workload and responsibilities have not been seriously taken into consideration in these programs.

The connections between income transfer programs and education are positive, but have not been accompanied by the expansion of day care centers and do not include systematic mechanisms to enable these women to engage in paid work and increase their income. The links with health interventions have been weak, and most do not guarantee access to comprehensive sexual and reproductive health or to services that respond to other health needs. This tendency is inconsistent with the policy recommendations on gender equality, women's empowerment, women's reproductive and sexual autonomy, and women's human rights more generally, as agreed in the UN conferences of the 1990s and supported by all five countries examined in this chapter.

But while our analysis of policy experiences in the five countries presents a picture of a half-empty–half-full glass in terms of women's health and gender equity, it also offers some clear pointers. It is clear that the cultural struggles over the legitimacy of the women's rights and gender equality agenda and especially of SRHR will continue to be engaged for some time between religious and other conservatives and women's organizations and their allies. However, the more neoliberal and limited the health reform agenda, and the more instrumental and limited the scope and methodology of antipoverty strategies, the less space they offer for advances in women's health and rights. The five countries examined in this chapter offer striking contrasts in this regard, with Brazil and Chile at the two extremes, and with the others going through significant economic, political, and policy ups and downs in between, proving thereby that policies do matter in determining the trajectories, risks, and opportunities for women's health and rights.

NOTES

1. We thank Gita Sen enormously for her insightful editorial suggestions, which greatly improved the clarity of our analysis. We also acknowledge the timely contributions of Keri Bennet, Charlotta Zacharias, and Jonathan Garcia to the English translation and revisions of the many versions of this chapter, and its editing. Keri Bennet is a student at the Law School of the University of Toronto and was an intern with the DAWN Sexual and Reproductive Health Program, at ABIA—*Associação Brasileira Interdisciplinar de AIDS*—in 2007. Charlotta Zacharias is a medical doctor and has a master's degree in International Health from the Karolinska Institutet in Stockholm, Sweden. Jonathan Garcia is a doctoral student in the Department of Sociomedical Sciences of the Mailman School of Public Health at the University of Columbia and a research associate at ABIA.
2. Data collected by the Latinobarómetro informs us that since 1997, on average, support for democracy in the region has ranged between 50 to 60% (54% in 1999–2000). But much variation is found across countries. Taking the example of the five countries of our sample as an illustration, the support for democracy in 2000 and 2007 was as follows: Argentina, 58 and 63% respectively; Brazil, 35 and 43 respectively; Chile, 45 and 46 respectively; Mexico 40 and 48 respectively; Uruguay 73 and 75 respectively. Though the number of people supporting democratic institutions is on the rise, the gap between confidence in the system and satisfaction with its outcomes remains quite striking: in Argentina 33% of those polled said they were satisfied with what democratic institutions deliver, in Brazil this figure was 30%, in Chile 36%, in Mexico 31%, and even in Uruguay where support for democracy has remained high and steady since 1997, those who were satisfied with democratic outcomes (66%) were less numerous than those who support the system.
3. In seven countries (Argentina, Bolivia, Colombia, Chile, El Salvador, Peru, Dominican Republic), health reforms followed the structural reform of pensions. In four cases health reform preceded pension reforms: Brazil, Costa Rica, Mexico, and Nicaragua. In Guatemala, Honduras, Panama, and Paraguay, health reforms have taken place, but no structural pension reforms have occurred. In Uruguay pension reform has been under way for some time, but the health system was not structurally altered.
4. The basic health care package component was funded by a loan of US$310 million from the World Bank and a contribution of US$133.4 million from the Mexican government National Health Council, which is a participatory mechanism at federal level; the Decentralization and Institutional Coordination Advisory Board and the Decentralization Support Units (*Unidades de Apoyo a la Descentralización*, UAD).
5. The content of this section is based on Corrêa, Piola, and Arilha (1999).
6. In 1996 and 2001 operational and financial norms guiding SUS decentralization and other structural guidelines were adopted (*Normas Operacionais Básicas*, NOBs).
7. In 2006 the PSF was implemented in 5,106 municipalities and provided basic health care to roughly 85 million persons (46% of the population).
8. The content of this section is mainly based on Abracinskas and López (2004) and López (2004).
9. This section is mainly based on the 2005 Gender Equity in Health Observatory (Observatorio de Equidad de Género en Salud, 2005).
10. In reference to Argentina, Brazil, Mexico, and Uruguay, the information and analysis offered in this section is mainly based on Corrêa, 2006b. The study mainly covered the 2002 to 2004 period but in some cases included

information on the post-2004 period. The analysis of Chilean policies is based on the report produced by the Observatório de Equidad de Género en Salud.

11. As a result of this alliance the Argentine government was an opponent of SRHR throughout 1990s UN conferences, especially at Cairo (1994) and Beijing (1995).

12. This policy shift was also reflected in Argentine foreign policy, as from there on the government would systematically support the Cairo and Beijing agendas in international negotiations and was particularly active in the regional Cairo Plus Ten Reviews from 2003 to 2004 in Latin America.

13. By 2004, 14 provincial and municipal legislative bodies had approved specific sexual and reproductive health provisions: Buenos Aires (City), Cordoba, Chaco, Chabot, La Pampas, Rio Negro, Juju, Santa Fé, Tierra del Forego, and La Rioja. In 2005, the Minister of Health announced that 10 million condoms, 450,000 IUDs, 1.6 million injectables, and 5.8 million oral contraceptives had been distributed (an increase of 36% from what was distributed in 2004), and that a mass media campaign would start in order to promote access to and use of these methods.

14. The first version of this chapter was finalized in 2007, before the election of Cristina Kirchner (in October). It has not been possible to consistently update information on sexual and reproductive policies. However, Alejandra Domigues, in a private conversation in June 2008, informed the authors of some worrying signs. As soon as she was elected as president, Kirchner declared that she was against abortion and the minister of health who was one driving force behind the sexual and reproductive health program that remained. In addition, problems in the logistics of contraceptive import and provision were detected in early 2008.

15. Though this has been a positive step, according to Pinto (2008), the new plan has conceptual and strategic gaps and distortions. This was recognized by the Ministry of Health, which promoted regional consultations to correct these problems.

16. The increase in condom use is also related to successful strategies for HIV/AIDS prevention.

17. Analysis presented by Tania Lago at the plenary session on "Sexual and Reproductive Rights in the World and in Brazil" at the 2008 Bi-Annual Meeting of the Brazilian Association for Population Studies (ABEP), in Caxambu. Dr. Lago is the current coordinator of the Women's Health Program at the São Paulo State Department of Health.

18. The bill known as "Framework for Sexual and Reproductive Rights" was discarded a month after it was presented. Then in October 2004, a Constitutional Reform provision was drafted to ensure that all persons, in particular women, have the right to choose the most appropriate contraception method approved by existing health legislation. This is still pending approval.

19. The election of Calderon in 2006 has further distanced federal policies from the comprehensive sexual and reproductive agenda of the mid-1990s, as it led to the nomination of a very conservative health secretary and shifts in the general orientation of CONAPO, as well.

20. Paulina Ramírez Hyacinth was 13 years old, and became pregnant when raped by a drug addict in Mexicali. The judge authorized the abortion but the director of Mexicali General Hospital refused to perform the procedure, and the pregnancy was taken to term. Feminist organizations publicized the case widely and started a lawsuit against the hospital director. As the decision from the Mexican court was not favorable, the case was taken to the Inter-American Commission on Human Rights, and in 2006, in a landmark

settlement, the Mexican government agreed to pay a financial compensation to Paulina and issue a decree regulating guidelines for access to abortion for rape victims.

21. Other similar programs include those in Nicaragua: Social Protection Network (*Red de Protección Social*) initiated in 2000; Colombia: Families in Action (*Familias en Acción*), initiated in 2001; Bolivia: Emergency Employment Plan (*Plan de Empleo de Emergencia*), initiated in 2001; Ecuador: Human Development Bonus (*Bono de Desarrollo Humano*), initiated in 2003. In Bolivia, more recently, after the partial state takeover of gas production, a specific income transfer program was established for ageing people.

22. Arriagada and Torres (1998) list as agencies adopting this approach in the early 1990s: the World Bank, the Inter-American Development Bank, the Food and Agricultural Organization, UNICEF, and UNFPA. Later in the decade the Economic Commission for Latin America (ECLAC), the International Labor Organization, and UNESCO have adopted the 'equity framework,' and later still ECLAC itself would move towards a new 'empowerment and citizenship' framework that is also emphasized by the United Nations Development Program (UNDP) and the United Nation Research Institute for Social Development (UNRISD).

23. In addition, it must be noted that income transfer programs will have positive impact in terms of health and education if and when these other two policies are efficient and offer quality education and health care. The long-term impact of income transfers can be compromised by the absence or inefficiencies of structural social policies.

REFERENCES

Abracinskas, L., and A. López. 2004. *Mortalidad Materna, Aborto y Salud en Uruguay en un escenario cambiante*. Montevideo: Mujer y Salud en Uruguay (MYSU).

Aguirre, R., and K. Batthyány. 2005. *Usos del tiempo y Trabajo no Remunerado. Encuesta, Montevideo 2003*. Montevideo: UNIFEM–UDELAR.

Almeida, C. 2001. Reformas del Estado y reforma de sistemas de salud. *Cuadernos Médico Sociales* 79: 27–58.

———. 2002. Reforma de Sistemas de Servicios de Salud y Equidad en América Latina y el Caribe: Algunas Lecciones de los Años 80 y 90. *Caderno de Saúde Pública* 18 (4): 45.

Almeida, C., C.L. Boada, A.C. Gonzáles, M.E. Labra, E.S. Oliveira, R.A. Pêgo, A. Tapia, F.L. Théodore. 2004. *Reformas del Sector Salud y Salud Sexual y Reproductiva en América Latina y el Caribe: Tendencias e Interrelaciones— Una Revisión*. Mexico City: UNFPA/EAT.

Anderson, J. 2000. Participación y reforma de la salud: nuevas expectativas, viejas formas. In *Saúde, Eqüidade e Gênero: um Desafio para as Políticas Públicas*, edited by A.M. Costa, E. Merchán-Hamann, and D. Tajer. Brazil: Editora Universidade de Brasilia.

Aquino, E., T. Araújo, and L. Marinho. 1999. Padrões e Tendências da Saúde Reprodutiva no Brasil: Bases para uma Análise Epidemiológica. In *Questões da Saúde Reprodutiva*, edited by K. Giffin and S. Hawker Costa. Rio de Janeiro: Fiocruz. 187–204.

Arriagada, I., and C. Torres. 1998. Género y Pobreza: Nuevas Dimensiones. *Edición de las Mujeres* 26.

Baden, E., and S. Milward. 1997. *Gender Inequality and Poverty: Trends, Linkages, Analysis and Policy Implications.* Brighton: Institute of Development Studies of the Sussex University. http://www.ntd.co.uk/idsbookshop/details. asp?id=196 (accessed October 2008).

Belmartino, S., C. Bloch, and E. Báscolo. 2002. La Atención Médica en Argentina. Historia, Crisis y Nuevo Diseño Institucional. *Paper Presented at the IV Seminario Salud y Política Pública, Cedes, Buenos Aires, Argentina, July.* Buenos Aires. http://www.cedes.org/informacion/ci/publicaciones/serie_sem.html

Bruce, J., and D. Dwyer. 1988. *A Home Divided: Women and Income in the Third World.* Stanford: Stanford University Press.

Buvinic, M., N.H. Youssef, and B. Von Elm. 1978. Women headed households: The ignored factor in development planning. *Paper Presented at the AID/WID meeting, International Center for Planning.* Washington. International Center for the Research on Money.

Castilhos, W. 2008. *Working Paper No. 5—The Pope's visit to Brazil: Context and Effects.* Rio de Janeiro: Sexuality Policy Watch. http://www.sxpolitics.org/mambo452/index.php?option=com_docman&task=cat_view&gid=7&Itemid=2.

CEPAL. 2008. *Indicadores de Beijing.* Santiago: División de Asuntos de Género. http://www.eclac.cl/mujer/proyectos/perfiles/comparados/trabajo17.htm (accessed October 2008).

Chacham, S., A.Valongueiro Alves, and S. Valongueiro Alves. 2003. *On Gender Equity and Public Health. Achieving the Millennium Development Goals.* Mimeo. Paper comissioned by the PAHO Gender Unit. Unpublished.

Chant, S. 1997. Women-headed households: Poorest of the poor? Perspectives from Mexico, Costa Rica and the Philippines. *IDS Bulletin* 28 (3): 26–48.

Comisión Nacional de Seguimiento. 2006. "Uruguay y las políticas en salud sexual y Reprodutiva. Montevideo.

Corrêa, S. 2006a. Feminização da pobreza: Percursos, revisões, recorrências. *Paper Presented at the International Seminar on Development, Inequality, Poverty and Exclusion, Rio de Janeiro, Brazil, September, 2006.* Rio de Janeiro: School of Economics of the Federal University of Rio de Janeiro. http://www.minds.org.br/arquivos/generopobreza_Sonia%20Correa.pdf (accessed October 15, 2008).

———. 2006b. *Interlining Policy, Politics and Women's Rights and Reproductive Rights—A Study of Health Sector Reform, Maternal Mortality and Abortion in Selected Countries of the South.* DAWN. http://www.repem.org.uy/files/globalinterlinking.pdf (accessed October 12, 2008).

Corrêa, S., S. Piola, and M. Arilha. 1999. *Cairo in Action: The Brazil Case.* Washington, DC: Population Reference Bureau.

Daeren, L. 2004. ¿Mujeres pobres: prestadoras de servicios o sujetos de derechos? Los programas de superación de la pobreza en América Latina desde una mirada de género. *Document Presented at the Reunión de Expertos sobre Políticas y Programas de Superación de la Pobreza desde la Perspectiva de la Gobernabilidad Democrática y el Género.* Ecuador: CEPAL, Unidad Mujer.

Domínguez, A., A.Soldevila, L. Vázquez, M. Rosemberg, Z. Palma, S. Checa, M. Bianco, M.A. Gutiérrez, A. Marino, M. Laski, M. Alanis, and V.J.S. Ambachs. 2004. *Salud y Aborto en Argentina: De las propuestas a los hechos.* Córdoba, Argentina: Se.A.P.

Faúndes, A., and J. Barzelatto. 2004. *O drama do aborto: em busca de um consenso.* São Paulo: Ed. Komedi.

Fraser, N. 1997. *Iustitia Interrupta—Reflexiones críticas desde la posición postsocialista.* Bogotá: Universidad de los Andes and Siglo Hombre Eds.

Frenk, J., E. González-Pier, O. Gómez-Dantés, M.A. Lezana, F.M. Knaul, et al. 2006. Comprehensive reform to improve health system performance in Mexico. Series health system reform in Mexico, no. 1. *The Lancet* 368: 1524–1534.

Gomez, E.G. 2002a. Equity, gender, and health: Challenges for action. *Pan American Journal of Public Health* 11 (5–6): 454–461. May.

———. 2002b. Gender, equity, and access to health services: An empirical approximation. *Pan American Journal of Public Health* 11 (5–6): 327–334.

Health Canada. 2003. *Exploring the Concepts of Gender and Health. Women's Health Bureau.* Ottawa: Health Canada. http://www.hc-sc.gc.ca/hl-vs/pubs/women-femmes/explor-eng.php.

Hopenhayn, M., and E. Ottone. 2000. *El gran eslabón: educación y desarrollo en el umbral del siglo XXI.* Buenos Aires: Fondo de Cultura Económica.

Kabeer, N. 1994. *Reversed Realities: Gender Hierarchies in Development Thought.* London: Ed. Verso.

———. 1998. Tácticas y compromisos: Nexos entre Género y Pobreza. In *Género y Pobreza: Nuevas Dimensiones*, edited by Irma Arriagada and Carmen Torres. Santiago: ISIS. 26–41.

Klein, C. 2005. A produção da maternidade no Programa Bolsa Escola. *Revista Estudos Feministas* 13 (1).

Knaul, F.M., H. Arreola-Ornelas, O. Mendez. 2005. Financial protection in health: Mexico, 1992 to 2004. *Salud Publica de Mexico* 47 (6): 430–439.

Lago, T. 2006. Impactos sobre a saúde das mulheres de diferentes políticas de saúde: o caso da Morte Materna na América Latina. *Paper Presented at the Congress of Brazilian Association of Collective Health (ABRASCO), August.* Rio de Janeiro: ABRASCO.

Latinobarómetro. 2000. Informe de prensa—Encuesta 1999–2000. *Informes de Prensa.* http://www.latinobarometro.org/ (accessed October 12, 2008).

Lavinas, L., J.E.D. Alves, S.M. Cavenaghi, M. Nicoli, R. Loureiro, and C. Simoes. 2008. *Impactos do Bolsa Família e do BPC/Loas na reconfiguração dos arranjos familiares, nas assimetrias de gênero e na individuação das mulheres.* Executive Summary. São Paulo: CCR-PROSARE (unpublished).

López, A. 2004. *Génesis y desarrollo de una nueva política de salud reproductiva. El caso de Uruguay.* Montevideo: Mujer y Salud en Uruguay (MYSU).

López, C., A. Espino, R. Todaroo, and N. Sanchís. 2006. *Latin America, a Pending Debate—Contributions in Economics and Politics from a Gender Perspective.* Montevideo: REPEM.

Médici, A.C. 1999. Uma década de SUS (1988–1999): progressos e desafios. In *Saúde sexual e reprodutiva no Brasil*, edited by L. Galvão and J. Díaz. São Paulo: Hucitec/Population Council. 104–150.

Merrick, T., and M. Schmink. 1983. Household headed by women and urban poverty in Brazil. In *Women and Poverty in the Third World*, edited by M. Buvinic, M. Lycette, and W. McGreevey. Baltimore: Johns Hopkins University Press. 127–145.

Mesa-Lago, C. 2005. *Las reformas de la salud en América Latina y el Caribe: su impacto en los principios de la seguridad social. Serie CEPAL Documentos de Proyectos, no. 63.* Santiago: United Nations/CEPAL.

Moser, C. 1995. *Planificación de Género y Desarrollo: Teoria, Práctica y Capacitación.* Lima: Flora Tristán Ediciones.

Observatorio de Equidad de Género en Salud. 2005. Observatorio de Equidad de Género en Salud—Informe 2005. *Observatorio de Equidad de Género en Salud Publicaciones.* http://www.observatoriogenerosalud.cl/pubs.php (accessed October 2008).

Ocampo, J.A. 2000. *Equidad, desarrollo y Ciudadanía*. Santa Fé de Bogotá: CEPAL and Ediciones Alfaomega.

PAHO/UNFPA/UNIFEM. 2005. *Gender, Health and Development in the Americas. Basic Indicators 2005*. Washington, DC: PAHO/UNFPA/UNIFEM.

PAHO/WHO. 2002. *Discriminación de las mujeres en el Sistema de Instituciones de Salud Previsional. Regulación y perspectiva de Género en la Reforma. Serie Género, equidad y reforma de la salud en Chile, cuaderno 1*. Santiago: Pan American Health Organization/World Health Organization.

Parker, R. 1997. *Políticas, Instituições e Aids*. Rio de Janeiro: Zahar Editores and ABIA.

Pinto, M. E. 2008. Mulheres, AIDS e estratégias de prevenção: para quem? *Monography Presented as Conclusion Paper in the Programa de Especialização Latu-Sensu em Políticas Públicas promovido pelo Instituto de Economia da Universidade Federal do Rio de Janeiro*. Rio de Janeiro: Universidade Federal.

Pollack, M. 2002. *Equidad de género en el sistema de salud chileno. Serie Financiamiento del Desarrollo 123, CEPAL*. Santiago: United Nations/CEPAL.

Romero, M., and Maceira, D. 2006. *Iniciativa por los derechos sexuales y reproductivos en las reformas del sector salud: América Latina. Nuevo Documentos CEDES 2006/20*. Buenos Aires: Centro de Estudios de Estado y Sociedad. http://www.cedes.org/informacion/ci/publicaciones/estudios_c.html (accessed July 2007).

Sánchez, V.C. 2004. *Reforma de Salud: Alcances y retrocesos de la mortalidad materna y al aborto en México*. Guadalajara: Dawn-Repem y Campo.

Sen, G., and C. Grown. 1986. *Development, Crisis and Alternative Visions: Third World Women's Perspectives*. New York: Monthly Review Press.

Sen, G., and P. Östlin. 2002. *Engendering International Health: The Challenge of Equity*. Ed. G. Sen, A. George, and P. Östlin. Cambridge: MIT Press.

Serrano, C. 2005. *Claves de la Política Social para la pobreza. Serie Mujer y desarrollo. CEPAL: Santiago.

Social Watch. 2006. *Social Watch Report 2006: Impossible Architecture*. Montevideo: Social Watch. http://www.socialwatch.org/en/informeImpreso/informe2006.htm (accessed October 2008).

Standing, H. 1997. Gender and equity in health sector reform programmes: A review. *Health Policy and Planning* 12 (1): 1–18.

———. 1999. *Frameworks for Understanding Gender Inequalities and Health Sector Reform*. Cambridge, MA: Harvard Center for Population and Development Studies, Working Paper Series no 99.06.

———. 2000. *Impactos de género de las reformas de salud. Actual estado de las políticas y la implementación. Revista Mujer Salud*. Santiago: Red de Salud de las Mujeres Latinoamericanas y del Caribe.

Stiglitz, J.E. 2002. *Globalization and its Discontents*. Delhi: Penguin Books India.

Tajer, D. 2006. *Globalización, Reformas y el Derecho a la Salud: El caso de América Latina. Revista Mujer Salud* 2. Santiago: Red de Salud de las Mujeres Latinoamericanas y del Caribe.

UNDP. 1995. *Human Development Report 1995*. New York: United Nations Development Program. http://hdr.undp.org/en/reports/global/hdr1995/ (accessed October 2008).

———. 2004. *Human Development Report 2004*. New York: United Nations Development Program. http://hdr.undp.org/en/reports/global/hdr2004/ (accessed October 2008).

———. 2005. *Human Development Report 2005*. New York: United Nations Development Program. http://hdr.undp.org/en/reports/global/hdr2005/ (accessed October 2008).

————. 2006. *Human Development Report 2006*. New York: United Nations Development Program. http://hdr.undp.org/en/reports/global/hdr2006/ (accessed October 2008).

UNRISD. 2005. *Gender Equality: Striving for Justice in an Unequal World*. Geneva: United Nations Research Institute for Social Development.

World Bank. 1993. *World Development Report 1993: Investing in Health*. New York: Oxford University Press.

Young, K. 1991. Reflexiones sobre como enfrentar las necesidades de las mujeres. In Una nueva lectura: Género en el desarrollo. Lima: Entre Mujeres; Flora Tristán Ediciones. 15–59.

6 Gender Norms and Empowerment
'What Works' to Increase Equity for Women and Girls

Helen Keleher

INTRODUCTION

This chapter is about 'what works' in programs that seek to change gendered norms at the level of households and communities that lead to increased equity for women and girls, with a focus on low- to middle-income countries. There are clear rationales for doing so. One is the body of work developed by the Commission on the Social Determinants of Health (CSDH) (WHO, 2005, 2008) for which gender equity was a key priority for action. This volume as well as the final report of the CSDH (CSDH, 2008) attests to the priority placed on increasing equity for women and girls by the CSDH.

Prior to the CSDH was the Fourth World Conference on Women in Beijing (UN, 1995) and the resulting Beijing Platform for Action, which provides a purposeful agenda for empowerment of women and girls in a rights framework. The Beijing Platform for Action emphasizes that the human rights of women and fundamental freedoms of the girl child are "an inalienable, integral and indivisible part of universal human rights" (UN, 1995). Then the Convention on the Elimination of All Forms of Discrimination against Women (CEDAW UN) upheld and affirmed the Beijing Platform for Action, which set an agenda to improve the status and lives of women and girls.

More recently, the Millennium Development Goals (MDGs) (UN, 2005) reaffirmed goals to strengthen gender equity and empowerment of women. Specific MDG targets have been developed in relation to issues about education for women and girls, in particular, equal primary school access and keeping girls at school; women's job opportunities, drawing attention to the poverty trap of insecure low-paid employment; and levels of women's involvement in political decision-making.

These issues are addressed in this chapter as well as key issues of violence against women and programs designed to change the attitudes and behaviors of men and boys toward women and girls. In the lives of women and girls these issues are interdependent social and economic determinants that are critical to their well-being and quality of life. Programs to address these issues work at different levels and with different intent in terms of their desired outcomes. Some programs work directly with women and girls for the purposes of empowerment. Such programs do not necessarily change gendered norms but by strengthening empowerment among women and girls, changes to norms can follow. Effective interventions also work at more one than one level—individual, family, community, and/or policy-maker levels—to more directly seek to change underlying values, norms, and attitudes about women and girls and to challenge stereotypical and traditional male and female roles that are detrimental to the health and well-being of women and girls. Different types of programs will be qualitatively different in what they are seeking to change.

Public health interventions are complex but are easier to understand if they can be understood through frameworks that explain the purpose and outcome measures of various types of interventions. Therefore, in this chapter, the evidence about 'what works' will be discussed in relation to both types of public health interventions and frameworks that assist us to understand the kind of change intended, at what levels the interventions were targeted, and the outcomes intended to guide the programs and their evaluations. Effectiveness in changing norms is highlighted throughout the chapter together with boxes that draw attention to research that has informed actions and interventions.

KEY CONCEPTS

While gender refers to female and male issues, the focus of this chapter is on female gender issues. As discussed earlier, the rationale for this focus is drawn from the Beijing Platform for Action's goals, which were about improving the status and lives of women and girls, CEDAW, the MDGs, and the work emanating from the CSDH and its reports. Since the Fourth World Conference on Women in Beijing in 1995, there has been considerable progress towards overcoming inequitable gendered norms; however, the effects of that progress have not been experienced evenly. The CSDH reports highlight the inequities faced by women and girls in low- to middle-income countries.

Gender Norms

Gender norms are powerful, pervasive values and attitudes about gender-based social roles and behaviors that are deeply embedded in social structures. Gender norms are about power relations, and manifest at various levels including within households and families, communities, neighborhoods, and wider society. Norms ensure the maintenance of particular social orders by punishing or sanctioning deviance from those norms to produce outcomes that are frequently inequitable, and dynamics that are often risky for women and girls. Risks include violence against women and girls, discrimination, denial of education, illiteracy from lack of education, poverty, restrictions on women's physical mobility resulting, for example, in economic and social injustice, honor killings, sexual assault and rape, female feticide, subordination and exploitation, and political disenfranchisement. Norms are perpetuated by social traditions that govern and constrain behaviors of both women and men and by social institutions that produce and reproduce laws and codes of normative conduct that maintain serious gender inequities. All countries, to some degree, experience tensions between emerging roles for women in society and expressions of their social, economic, and political rights, with traditional kinship concepts of women's roles. Such tensions are magnified in low- and middle-income countries regarded as being in development.

Gender Equity

Gender inequity is widely and deeply entrenched in individual and community attitudes and behaviors, societal norms, institutions, and market economies, with their impact apparent in disproportionate inequities among poor women (World Bank, 2005; Grown et al., 2005b). Inequities created by gendered norms affect both women and men, and create the necessity for gender analysis. Dominant forms of masculinity operationalize gendered power relations to produce inequities for women. They sustain power relations and male risk-taking behaviors that impact on women, including street and sexual violence, unsafe sexual practices and misogyny, denial of women's rights (Karlsson and Karkara, 2004), and support for men to have multiple partners or to maintain control over the behavior of their female partners (Pulerwitz et al., 2006). Although male high-risk behaviors also impact on male vulnerability to morbidity and mortality, they are not a focus of this chapter.

Empowerment

Empowerment is a complex but viable strategy if its processes are understood and put into practice. Participatory processes are an essential foundation of empowerment to build capacity to challenge and change norms and institutions to redress power imbalances, and norms must be redefined in order to effect change (Wallerstein, 2006). Operationally, empowerment is both process and outcome and encompasses economic empowerment, human and social empowerment, and political and cultural empowerment (Luttrell and Quiroz, 2007). Wallerstein (2006) found, in an extensive review of the literature, that empowerment of women can be a pathway to changing gendered norms and overcoming inequities if they are designed and implemented at multiple levels to effect change. Conditions for these change processes to be effective include: that projects and interventions are women-specific; that they begin with women's concerns within the social context of their lives; and there is transfer of power to women.

The change process of empowerment begins with the strengthening of individual (self) and collective efficacy, which is a precondition for strong group bonding and the formation of sustainable groups at the levels of community. This foundation leads to increased participation of women in social action. Intersectoral organizing and coalition building are used effectively by women. When women take on leadership at local and political levels and develop critical mass, changes to policy has been demonstrated (Wallerstein, 2006). Women's empowerment is therefore best measured at various levels rather than single measures of empowerment disembodied from their context, which can be misleading. The development of contextually relevant indicators assists with determining outcome measures, but it is necessary that those indicators are based on careful analysis of local power structures in order to highlight which factors are the most significant in creating powerlessness in the first place (Wallerstein, 2006). For example, at the level of households and community, women's empowerment can be measured by the degree of landownership by women, their autonomy and degree of authority in decision-making, mobility for both women and girls (for schooling particularly), and levels of domestic violence. At the national level women's empowerment and gender equity can be measured by the percentage of women in political office and management positions as well as women's share of earned income (Wallerstein, 2006).

METHODS

The methods for the review conducted for the Women and Gender Equity Knowledge Network are reported elsewhere (Keleher and Franklin, 2008). In brief, the search process was set up to answer the question: 'What is the effectiveness of household and community-level strategies and interventions in changing gender norms?' Beginning with an extensive list of search terms, the search was brought down to a manageable number of keywords to frame the search strategy for relevant study populations: women and girls; men and boys; household and community; intervention; gender norms. The inclusion criteria were that to be included in the review, impact evaluation data had been reported, and the report was written in English. Reviews and major reports were given preference over smaller studies and those that did not report outcome measures.

The literature on these keywords is enormous with a predominance of descriptive research methodologies and very few randomized controlled trial studies. It was impossible to conduct quality ratings on individual articles because so many of the papers found were in the form of reviews by UN agencies and NGOs that summarize whole suites of funded programs, country studies, and their outcomes, but do not provide information about actual evaluation design or measures. Overall, the literature reporting evaluations was limited with fewer than expected reports about measurement of changes in gender equity and women's empowerment.

Narrative (table) summaries and key themes were developed around the available data about the scale of issues, intervention types, levels of action, populations of interest, and key outcomes from evaluations. There were key themes that emerged:

- changing gendered norms in relation to education of women and girls
- changing gendered norms in relation to violence against women
- changing gendered norms about female genital cutting
- the challenges of educating men and boys about gender equity
- changing gendered norms in relation to economic empowerment of women

PUBLIC HEALTH INTERVENTIONS

Public health interventions are necessarily complex because for effectiveness, they work across sectors and settings and at multiple levels. A useful framework for understanding different types of public health programs was developed by Rychetnik and Frommer (2002). Interventions can be universal (available to all people), targeted (e.g., individuals, families, communities) or indicated (specified for a particular group or individuals), and, in addition, interventions are also usefully understood across an upstream–downstream continuum in a framework of programmatic interventions. Figure 6.1, Framework for health-promoting actions and capacity building, illustrates this continuum:

Figure 6.1   Framework for health promoting actions and capacity building.

Downstream (individual) focus ⟵⟶ *Upstream (population) focus*			
Communication strategies	Social marketing	Community development	Infrastructure, institutional & systems change
Health information	Health education	Engagement	Organisational change
Behaviour-change campaigns	Develop personal skills and individual capacity	Community action	Workforce development
	Social support	Advocacy	Policy
		Community/institutional support	Legislation
			Organisational development
			Resources

Source: Keleher (2007)

- Downstream interventions are those focused on change or support for individuals and include primary prevention.
- Midstream interventions are those that focus on psychosocial levels and behaviors. Midstream interventions including social marketing and the provision of health information to individuals, communities, and populations more broadly. Community action interventions, which often encompass awareness raising, are also directed at social change, so they are sometimes considered to be more upstream than midstream.
- Upstream interventions take a population focus, and are also intended as umbrella protections, or change mechanisms, to support efforts to promote justice, human rights, and social change. Upstream interventions encompass institutional practices and organizational change to influence social (including gender) norms that create and reinforce social and health inequalities. Developing healthy or just public policy is an upstream intervention that will also require reinforcement through social marketing for awareness raising.

Interventions are more effective when they are integrated and multilevel; therefore, program approaches often use a combination of interventions that work by mutual reinforcement. For example, universal, selected, or targeted interventions may be developed across the continuum from downstream to upstream, although indicated interventions are more likely to be situated towards the downstream.

CHANGING GENDERED NORMS IN RELATION TO EDUCATION OF WOMEN AND GIRLS

Education is a core social determinant of health, one that is infused with gendered norms about the value of education for girls and women, their social status, and traditional attitudes to female roles in households and communities. There are indisputable social, economic, and human rights rationales for increased efforts that strive towards gender parity in education although educational interventions are not sufficient to achieve gender equity. Education is perhaps the most critical mechanism for women's empowerment but it is only over time that the effects of women's empowerment are reflected in outcomes that can be regarded as achievement of gender equity.

Of the 860 million people around the world who are affected by illiteracy, two-thirds are women who experience poorer health, larger families, and few opportunities for any form of economic productivity. Girls' education is affected by: negative perceptions that devalue their capabilities; values about female roles in public and private spheres; beliefs about relative costs to communities of educating females; expectations that males will be

The proportion of children in developing countries who have completed primary education rose from 79 per cent in 1999 to 85 per cent in 2006 although in Sub-Saharan Africa, only 71% of children are enrolled in primary school. But for every 100 boys, only 45 girls are enrolled in school (UNICEF 2008: http://www.irinnews.org/Report.aspx?ReportId=80097).

54 per cent of children of the appropriate age in developing countries attend secondary school. In Oceania, almost two thirds of children of secondary school age are out of school. In sub-Saharan Africa, only a quarter of children of secondary school age are in secondary school. In Mali only 36%) of girls are enrolled in school, in Guinea (41%), Central African Republic (42%), Chad (45%) and Benin (57%), the numbers of higher. But in Nigeria, only 33 percent of the country's girls are enrolled in school. The number is even lower in Congo Kinshasa (32%) and Burkina Faso (28%). These eight countries also showed big differences in gender parity in school enrolment. While the number of girls and boys enrolled in Congo Kinshasa and Nigeria was almost equal, the gender gap reached 24 percent in Chad and 25 percent in Benin. (UNICEF 2005: '25 by 2005', UNICEF's global initiative to accelerate progress on getting more girls into school in 25 countries by the year 2005).

Papua New Guinea (PNG) has the highest gender disparity in education in the East Asia and Pacific region. For every 100 boys in primary school, there are 80 girls; at secondary level there are 65 girls for every 100 boys in school. As a result, the literacy rate for girls is 50.9% compared to 61.2% for boys (UNICEF 2008: http://www.unicef.com.au/mediaCentre-Detail.asp?ReleaseID=799).

Box 6.1   Education of women and girls.

the primary income earners; heavy domestic schedules that place inequitable burdens on females; and distance from schools (Abane, 2004; UNICEF, 2004). Children with low levels of schooling assume the work burdens of adults prematurely, are deprived of opportunities for learning outside the family, and eventually take up gender-stereotyped roles (Lloyd and Grant, 2004). Millions of girls, estimated at one out of every seven, 'disappear' into early marriages before their fifteenth birthday where they are isolated with restricted mobility, limited control over resources, and little power in their new households (Population Council, 2008). Others disappear into hazardous labor or combat roles (UNICEF, 2006).

The continuing need to work towards gender parity in education is reiterated by the MDGs (UN, 2005, 2008). While significant progress has been made in the education of girls, gender parity is much more than school enrolment numbers, which are not a sufficiently robust indicator to measure achievement of gender equity. Indicators that measure girls' actual levels of education, the relevance of the education they receive for their cultural and community context, and the identification of structural barriers, such as school fees, a curriculum perceived as inappropriate for girls, lack of alternatives, lack of gender sensitivity, inflexibility of classroom programs, and lack of safety (UNICEF, 2004), are all critical to measuring gender parity in education. And whilst the broadening of access to education is not yet uniform or universal, more upstream actions are needed to provide change mechanisms and umbrella protections to achieve gender equity. These actions are needed to improve the quality of education, the conditions that allow girls to stay in school, and gender-sensitive professional training, not just of teachers but also at the level of school governance and administration (Smith et al., 2003).

A five-country longitudinal study of programs for women's education that combined literacy, health, and employment skills recommended that beyond individual indicators of empowerment, gender equity be measured against a 56-point index of social and economic development. Key indicators consist of literacy, education, family and reproductive health, income-earning activity, household decision-making, community participation, and legal rights (Burchfield et al., 2002). Other important indicators of gender equity that reflect social and economic development include employment statistics; income data; women's representation in decision-making institutions, particularly in parliaments; and the sexual and reproductive health of women, including social structures and norms that support rights and provide freedoms for women to take control of their fertility (UNICEF, 2005b).

The powerful connections between low-literacy, poverty, and poor health outcomes have been recognized for decades. The year 1990 was declared by the United Nations to be International Literacy Year with female illiteracy its focus (UN Chronicle, 1990), but how much has been achieved since then?

Certainly programs have sought to change gendered norms about education through targeting communities or regions with low total enrolments, and targeting specific populations of marginalized adolescents and poor working women with low levels of literacy. Change is being directed universally at populations of primary and secondary girls with efforts to increase the quality and quantity of education of girls (UN, 2008, p. 13).

Analysis for the Global Monitoring Report (GMR) 2008 (Smith et al., 2007) shows that gender disparities in primary school enrolments have improved between 1999 and 2005 for most countries but many lag behind, particularly in fragile states. Greatest progress towards gender parity is found in South and West Asia, followed by sub-Saharan Africa, but progress is slowed in Arab states. Impoverished rural and urban slum dwellers experience greater gender disparities.

UNESCO (2003) has developed cross-cutting, targeted, multilevel approaches to poverty reduction via teaching both skills for life and work as well as gender rights awareness for suppressed marginalized adolescent girls. Operating in Bangladesh, India, Nepal, and Pakistan, the projects are founded on education and training with a strong rights framework. They have found that when girls are regarded not as a burden but as untapped potential for social and economic transformation, they are enabled to take greater control over their own lives, to shape their own livelihood, and to contribute to the development efforts of their communities.

Girls' education has significant economic benefits. Psacharapoulos and Patrinos (2002) estimate that every year of schooling lost represents a 10% to 20% reduction in girls' future incomes. By contrast, countries can expect per capita annual growth in GDP of between one to three percentage points higher when more equal levels of education are achieved. Economic returns from primary education are slightly higher for girls than boys (Psacharopoulos and Patrinos, 2002; Herz and Sperling, 2004). In a 72-country analysis, as well as country studies in Uganda, Kenya, and Zambia, reductions in HIV/AIDS infection rates are found to be related to literacy and girls' education. In a 63-country study, gains in women's education contributed more than any other intervention to reduce malnutrition between 1970 and 1995, due to more productive farming (Smith and Haddad, 2000; Herz and Sperling, 2004). In other words, girls' education leads to increased income for individuals and for nations as a whole, with compounding economic and social benefits.

Widely replicated studies across comparative databases have shown that an extra year of girls' education can reduce infant mortality by 5% to 10%, especially in low-income countries; and in Africa, children of mothers who receive five years of primary education are 40% more likely to live beyond age five (Herz and Sperling, 2004). Multi-country data show that educated mothers are 50% more likely to immunize their children than uneducated mothers (Gage et al., 1997), and cross-country studies have shown that the education of women promotes the education of children (UNFPA, 2002; Herz and Sperling, 2004).

Education is the key to the fertility transition that contributes to gender equity. A Brazilian study found that illiterate women average six children each, compared to 2.5 children per literate woman (UNESCO, 2000). A 65-country analysis found that doubling the proportion of women with a secondary education would reduce average fertility rates from 5.3 to 3.9 children per woman (Herz and Sperling, 2004).

Primary education seems insufficient to provide women with the knowledge and skills they need to improve and sustain their own health or economic independence. At least some secondary education influences capacity for resistance and opposition to violence and genital cutting (Global Campaign for Education, 2005), while more female secondary education is influential on later age at marriage, fertility control and smaller families, improved material care for children, reduced vulnerability to HIV/AIDS (Grown et al., 2005b), empowerment, democracy, income growth, and economic productivity (Herz and Sperling, 2004).

Investing in the education of girls and women is good economic policy, but education must be empowering for girls by including curricula on: women's rights, gendered norms about access to employment, finances, education, health care, and equity issues. Setting targets for parity in levels of education is meaningless unless countries also develop indicators for quality educational curricula that promote gender equity and the rights of girls. Both universal and targeted programs should be supported to ensure that they reach marginalized and suppressed younger and older girls and women in hard to reach communities.

CHANGING GENDERED NORMS IN RELATION TO ECONOMIC EMPOWERMENT OF WOMEN AND GIRLS

Programs which foster women's economic empowerment are likely to contribute to progress as they can provide incentives to change the patterns of traditional behavior to which a woman is bound as a dependent member of the household, or where women are losing traditional access to economic gain and its associated power.

> Gainful employment empowers women in various spheres of their lives, influencing sexual and reproductive health choices, education and healthy behavior. (UNFPA, 2007b)

Economic empowerment of women is understood as "economic change/ material gain plus increased bargaining power and/or structural change which enables women to secure economic gains on an on-going and sustained basis" (Sudarshan, 2003, p. 384). Another definition is "the expansion of assets and capabilities of poor people to participate in, negotiate with, influence, control, and hold accountable, institutions that affect their lives" (Narayan, 2005, p. 5). Economic and social empowerment are entwined so both must be addressed to increase gender equity. Programs to change gender norms within male-dominated cultural traditions tackle female education, advance their legal rights and participation in decision-making, and allow women to take some control over their lives. Advances in the measurement and monitoring of empowerment (Charmes and Wieringa, 2003; Narayan, 2005) have emphasized the importance of multilevel interventions that tackle multiple complex issues, but many programs are demonstrating success in creating pathways from empowerment to gender equity.

Major barriers to women's ability to participate in economic activity are heavy burdens of domestic and agricultural work, illiteracy, widespread female malnutrition from childhood, which results from complex gender norms about inferior status accorded to women and girls, and low levels of female education. There is a lack of sex-disaggregated nutrition data about malnutrition in many regions, but particularly in sub-Saharan Africa and

South Asia, and women's lower status is regarded as the strongest contributor to the costs of child malnutrition (Smith et al., 2003).

Violence against women increases the risk to child survival, child health, and malnutrition in mothers and children, which is strongly connected to women's status (Sethvraman et al., 2006; Asling-Monemi, 2008). These data indicate the need for multilevel actions to address gender equity to achieve outcomes on all these issues.

There is good evidence that working upstream on empowerment is successful through support for women's organizations. The Self-Employed Women's Association (SEWA) of India is a trade union reaching vast numbers of poor self-employed women. SEWA's approach is multilevel, from the micro levels of skill building to institutional and legal reform and capacity building, to enable local organizations to increase their effectiveness and sustainability (SEWA, 2005). SEWA's achievements have been remarkable, utilizing social protections and innovative services with rapid growth of 25% to 35% percent per year (Grown et al., 2005a).

Another mechanism for empowerment is micro-credit/microfinancing schemes for low-cost, accessible credit. Such schemes are built on assumptions about the empowerment of women through their establishment of small businesses and the resulting capacity of women to contribute to household income and family welfare. However, careful analysis of the gender relations involved and the dynamics of local economies is essential to understand the barriers to women in their local contexts as they attempt to conduct business in male-dominated structures, networks, and communities. Women trying to enter markets face many hazards and constraints, including increased violence, limits on their physical mobility, increasing responsibilities to provide a steady flow of cash and food for the household without changes occurring to inequitable intra-household relations, and difficulties with extracting repayment when selling on credit (Johnson, 2005). High turnover of group membership is a frequent result. Through a series of case studies, Johnson (2005) demonstrates the value of the ways in which micro-credit schemes can be tailored to overcome obstacles, particularly a lack of power among women, and be designed to transform gender relations. She argues (2005, p. 244) that "achievement of a 'double bottom line' of both financial and social performance of [micro-credit] schemes is . . . both a necessity and a reality."

Countering macroeconomic reforms through antipoverty programs can also impact on women's empowerment although they do not of themselves change gendered norms or increase gender equity. The Mexican nationwide PROGRESA program involves the disbursement of cash transfers to women with incentives designed to improve health, nutrition, and education. The program has had significant impacts on women's empowerment and status, access to appropriate health services, and school enrolment among poor families. Careful evaluation is necessary to understand unintended consequences such as disruptions to community social relations and social division (Adato et al., 2000).

Although seemingly gender neutral, macroeconomic reforms have significantly disproportionate impacts on women and girls, particularly women-led households whose livelihoods depended on access to now privatized resources (Mukhopadhyay and Sudarshan, 2003; Van Hue, 2006). Multi-country studies demonstrate the poor quality of employment that has been generated for women:

> although this new employment may have brought women into the global market, it is on terms unequal with men and in conditions of work that have not, so far, created any change in their situation within the home or outside it. Those who have found work are able to contribute to improving the economic situation of the household and reduce the intensity of poverty, but they have not been 'empowered.' (Sudarshan, 2003: 384)

Lack of legal protections and exploitative labor markets have created poverty traps for millions of women. Women with low status have weaker control over household resources, heavier demands on their time, less access to information and health services, poorer mental health, and lower self-esteem.

CHANGING GENDERED NORMS ABOUT FGM/C

Female genital mutilation/cutting (FGM/C) is a manifestation of gender inequality (WHO, 2008). WHO estimates that between 100 and 140 million girls and women in some 28 countries are living with the consequences of some form of female genital cutting,[1] with 91.5 million of those living in Africa where an estimated three million girls each year are at risk of undergoing FGM/C (WHO, 2008; Baumgarten et al., 2004). The health consequences for girls and women are severe. A WHO multi-country study in which more than 28,000 women participated documents the significantly increased risks for adverse events for both women and their infants during childbirth (WHO, 2006).

There is high prevalence also in western and southern Asia and the Middle East, and among some ethnic groups in Central and South America (WHO, 2008). FGM/C is a deeply entrenched social practice through which girls and their families acquire social status or shame and exclusion if there is failure to perform FGM/C. FGM/C practices are based on gendered inequalities driven by norms about women's social status, patriarchal family structures, honor, religious beliefs, and social control over women. Certainly, strong gender disparities within society lead to violations of women's rights, but FGM/C appears to be part of a dense social and cultural fabric, integral to rites of initiation of girls to purify them and inculcate culturally acceptable behaviors in them (Lisy, 2007). It is a tradition that can be dissolved but efforts to do so may counter tremendous resistance (Gruenbaum, 2001).

Upstream interventions, particularly legislation and the use of human rights instruments, are increasingly used to support the eradication of FGM/C practices. International and regional human rights treaties and consensus documents that give strong support for the elimination of FGM/C are listed in Box 2.

While pressure can be brought to bear on countries through conventions, treaties, and legislation, these represent only one approach. Indeed, they can lead to unintended consequences for some women and further entrench adherence to the practice among communities where poverty, economic uncertainty, and social isolation threaten those who challenge norms about FGM/C (Martinez, 2005). There is evidence that FGM/C practices may respond more readily to social change in gender norms than to legislation and policing. In another strategy, medical licensing authorities and professional associations are working with the UN to condemn FGM/C and oppose the involvement by medical professionals in performing FGM/C.

Although there are few evaluated programs, many lessons have been learned, including that programs must empower women if they are to achieve change. Effectiveness is dependent on programs that work at multilevel and multiple sectors in sustained processes that are community led and based on understandings about long-term commitment to change (WHO, 2008):

> Concerted action from many sides and at different levels is needed, from local to global and involving sectors such as education, finance, justice, and women's affairs as well as the health sector; and many different kinds of actors must be engaged, from community groups and nongovernmental organizations including health professional groups and human rights groups to governments and international agencies. (p. 19)

In many communities, changes to attitudes and community-held norms have occurred not through acts of protest or suppression, but through strategies such as intergenerational dialogue (Lisy and Finke, 2005) and multipronged education approaches (Gruenbaum, 2001; UNICEF, 2005a; WHO, 2008). The Senegal project (spearheaded by the NGO Tostan) has been so successful it is now an endorsed regional model by UNICEF. Its success involves public declaration of intent to abandon the practice; slow but steady human rights education programs that encourage villagers to make up their own minds about FGM/C, literacy education, alternative employment for cutters, reproductive health and rights education classes that lift the taboo on talking about health problems associated with FGM/C, and

International Treaties

- Convention against Torture and Other Cruel, Inhuman or Degrading Treatment or Punishment
- Covenant on Civil and Political Rights
- Covenant on Economic, Social and Cultural Rights
- Convention on the Elimination of all Forms of Discrimination against Women (CEDAW)
- Convention on the Rights of the Child
- Convention relating to the Status of Refugees and its Protocol relating to the Status of Refugees

Regional Treaties

- African Charter on Human and Peoples' Rights (the Banjul Charter) and its Protocol on the Rights of Women in Africa
- African Charter on the Rights and Welfare of the Child
- European Convention for the Protection of Human Rights and Fundamental Freedoms

Consensus Documents

- Beijing Declaration and Platform for Action of the Fourth World Conference on Women
- General Assembly Declaration on the Elimination of Violence against Women
- Programme of Action of the International Conference on Population and Development (ICPD)
- UNESCO Universal Declaration on Cultural Diversity
- United Nations Economic and Social Council (ECOSOC), Commission on the Status of Women. Resolution on Ending Female Genital Mutilation. E/CN.6/2007/L.3/Rev.1.

Box 6.2 International and regional sources of human rights that give strong support for the protection of the rights of women and girls to abandon female genital mutilation. Source: WHO 2008, 14

community-decided alternative rites of passage (Mackie, 2000). The model is being adopted in Guinea, Burkina Faso, Mali, and Somalia.

Nonetheless, Gruenbaum (2001) argues that human and economic development are necessary for creating propitious conditions for the abandonment of FGM/C, which may be a relatively low priority where communities lack basic health care and education. Interventions to protect women from

FGM/C have shown that simply affirming a stand against FGM/C is inadequate without close empirical scrutiny of the local, national, and international politics that surround FGM/C and efforts to stop its practices. Other tactics, such as providing alternative employment for the circumcisers or introducing alternative rites of passage, require a comprehensive and multilevel approach to education, social mobilization, and diffusion strategies to spread ideas and change attitudes (Mackie, 2000).

CHANGING GENDERED NORMS IN RELATION TO VIOLENCE AGAINST WOMEN AND GIRLS

Violence against women (VAW), described variously as intimate partner (or domestic) violence (IPV), female genital cutting, sexual violence, and gender-based violence (GBV), are forms of discrimination committed on the basis of sex (UNGASS, 1993). VAW is a clear violation of women's human rights including the rights to life, liberty, and security of person, equality, equal protection under the law, and freedom from all forms of discrimination.

VAW is a direct cost to development, both obstructing women's participation in and contradicting the goals of development (Burton et al., 2000). Women are dependent on their immediate social environment, their vulnerability related to "impossible choices for women between security of shelter, economic dependence or continued abuse" (Bhatla et al., 2006, p. 4). Educational disadvantage and poverty render women and girls more susceptible to elevated risks of abuse (McCloskey et al., 2005). However, where violence continues to be tolerated in both school and family life, VAW will be difficult to overcome.

Evidence about outcomes of program interventions to prevent violence against women is seriously lacking (Jewkes, 2002; Wathen and MacMillan, 2003). There is emerging evidence about protective mechanisms for women against domestic and sexual violence, one of which is education. Women with more education are more highly valued because of employability and have more capacity to leave a relationship if it becomes abusive.

In a multisite study in India and Sri Lanka, women's ownership of property was found to "extend their capabilities, expand their negotiating power, and enhance their ability to address vulnerability" (Bhatla et al., 2006, p. 11). Multifaceted responses are increasingly understood to be the most effective in changing social norms about men's control of, and access to, women's bodies. Embedding of rights frameworks that offer legal protections for women are becoming more widespread, as is recognition of the need for capacity building of staff in health, education, and justice sectors to communicate that violence against women and girls is a serious offense and to become actively involved in prevention work (Jewkes, 2002; WHO, 2002, 2005).

This was the first population study on the association between violence and health outcomes study covering 15 sites and 10 countries:
Bangladesh, Brazil, Ethiopia, Japan, Peru, Namibia, Samoa, Serbia
and Montenegro, Thailand and the United Republic of Tanzania.
Using a standardized and rigorous methodology, the study produced
robust data to enable comparison between survey sites in each country as well as between countries.

The lifetime experience of physical partner violence was13–61%
(in most sites between 23–49%) of ever married women between
15–49 years of age. The lifetime experience of sexual violence was
between 6–59%. Lifetime experience of one or more emotionally
abusive acts was reported among 20–75% of respondents and controlling behaviour by intimate partners among 20–90% of women of
reproductive age. Further, 1–28% of women reported physical abuse
during at least one pregnancy (Asling-Monemi 2008).

- In every setting except Japan, more than a quarter of women in
  the study had been physically or sexually assaulted at least once
  since the age of 15 years.
- At least half of all women in Bangladesh, Ethiopia province,
  Peru, Samoa, and the United Republic of Tanzania said that
  they had been physically or sexually assaulted since 15 years
  of age.
- In most sites women with a higher educational level reported a
  lower lifetime prevalence of partner violence than women who
  had not attended school or had primary education only.
- Women in non-conflict settings are at greatest risk of violence
  from their husband or intimate partner, father or other male
  family members rather than from strangers or others known to
  them. In some sites, teachers were identified as perpetrators of
  violence against women.

A major finding of the study is that the status of women in their own
communities and broader society is a key factor in the prevalence of
violence against them. The findings of the study confirm that tackling
violence against women requires multilevel responses that begin with
addressing women's status and seek to change gendered norms across
all societies.

Box 6.3   Prevalence of violence against women and girls: The WHO Multi-country
Study on Women's Health and Domestic Violence Against Women. Source: Garcia-
Moreno et al 2005

Thresholds for tolerating violence against women vary among and within countries. The development of a measurement scale for countries to assess the degree of tolerance and the degree to which gendered violence has become normalized would inform program interventions. The scale should include the attention paid to issues of gender in both policy proposals and debates on violence within countries.

CHANGING GENDERED NORMS AMONG MEN AND BOYS

In every country, norms of superiority and masculine honor are widespread. Masculine norms are reinforced by the large-scale militarization of many countries, which has devastating impacts on women through economic upheavals, cultural dispossession, violence, deaths of family members, poverty, and hunger due to loss of lands or lack of employment (Becker, 2003). Gender inequity is deeply affected by dominant male behaviors that manifest in violence against women, forced or unsafe sex, sexual assault and rape, inequitable gender relations, and gender stereotypes, all of which impact heavily on women and girls.

There is wide agreement that men need to be part of the solutions to overcoming gender inequalities (Sternberg and Hubley, 2005; Doniach and Peacock, 2006), and many lessons have been learned from program development in the last 10 years. Programs have been developed to find ways to get men involved who might not otherwise be involved in addressing gender equity, and many programs are designed to give men small steps to becoming involved. Programs have targeted both men and adolescent boys to interrupt the internalizing of norms about traditional masculine roles. However, major challenges remain in the translation of programs with men and boys into greater gender equity for women and girls.

Program interventions to change men's attitudes towards women are typically designed around group work in a variety of community-based settings. Programs aim to effect change in knowledge, attitudes, and behavior through strategies that move from the individual to more upstream (see Figure 6.1):

- workshops that encourage men to take action in their own communities
- the media to promote changes in social norms
- collaboration between nongovernmental organizations and grass-roots community-based organizations to strengthen their ability to implement programs
- advocacy for increased government commitment to promoting positive male involvement (International Women's Health Coalition, 2003; Peacock and Levack, 2004; Sternberg and Hubley, 2005; Barker et al., 2007)

Small-scale impact evaluations are beginning to measure behavior change among men. The Gender Equitable Men Scale (GEM Scale), developed by the Instituto Promundo with support from the Population Council, is being used to measure the effects of group education and community programs on gender-equitable behaviors and attitudes associated with the reduction of risk to HIV/AIDS (Pulerwitz et al., 2006; Pulerwitz and Barker, 2008).

Program interventions have achieved some change in terms of changing males' understanding about gender stereotypes, but most program interventions are short term, and few have been evaluated systematically (Barker et al., 2007). Measures of change are focused on men's knowledge, attitudes, and behaviors with regard to sexual and reproductive health, such as family planning and contraceptive use, safe sex, gender roles and relations, challenging men to examine masculinities, sexualities, power, and their manifestation in attitudes and behaviors that put women at risk.

Combinations of intervention methods are proving more effective in achieving sustained behavior change at least in the months that follow the intervention. Program H in Brazil and India, using quasi-experimental evaluation design, found evidence of behavior and attitude change in young men who participated in group education activities. Stepping Stones in South Africa, evaluated rigorously, has found reduced rates of violence against women (reported by women) in emerging evaluation data (Barker et al., 2007).

However, evaluations have not yet been developed to measure how men's involvement in gender equity programs impact on women (White et al., 2003; UNICEF, 2004). There has been substantial rhetoric about men's involvement but little evidence that programs are empowering for women or changing gendered norms, or that men were enabled to resist gendered social norms over time (Sternberg and Hubley, 2005; Verma et al., 2006). Critiques argue that men and boys program interventions are narrowly cast in their approach, theoretically thin, relying on descriptive data and lacking in measures of effects on men or impacts on women (Sternberg and Hubley, 2005), although recent evaluations are working towards more rigorous testing (Pulerwitz and Barker, 2008). Both program interventions and evaluations are targeted in terms of men's pathological behavior, with little acknowledgment of the cultural stereotypes of masculinity that emphasize physical strength, sexual prowess, and male dominance in sexual encounters, and machismo (Verma et al., 2006). In some countries, men often gained more benefits from interventions than women, so even though the interventions were designed to overcome gendered inequalities they can inadvertently increase the gender gap (Jacob et al., 2006). Indeed, Sternberg and Hubley (2005, p. 394) ask if "new, caring, sharing models of masculinity are being formed or are men learning more sophisticated ways to assert their dominance over women?"

While there are indications that men do want to be involved and that many men respond positively to well-designed programs delivered over time, behavioral education programs of themselves do not transform communities and societies in terms of social justice and rights. Yet, there is little evidence that men and boys program interventions take or advocate for a social justice or human rights framework. Questions must be asked about the capacity of programs for social change if they operate in a policy and legislative vacuum. Policy, legislation, political and social justice leadership to ensure a publicly accountable criterion of justice with regard to gender equality are critical (Unterhalter, 2005).

CONCLUSIONS

Public health approaches to gender equity are more than a requirement for programs to be gender aware or gender sensitive. They must also be targeted to indicators of gender equity, many of which are identified in this chapter.

The effectiveness of programmatic interventions to change gender norms at the level of household and community requires multilevel (downstream-midstream-upstream) programs (WHO, 2005) designed to influence the underlying determinants of the problem, and require the protective umbrella of policy and legislative actions that recognize and reinforce the rights of women and girls. Downstream strategies that work with targeted individuals are important but insufficient to raise women's social status. Social change occurs when downstream and midstream programs are conducted in the context of broader systemic (upstream) and intersectoral efforts to increase gender equity.

Indeed, perhaps one of the strongest indicators of gender equity is the number of women in parliaments. Ensuring a critical mass of women in parliaments raises the bar on issues such as violence against women and girls, education, and women's employment, with insistence that these are not just women's issues but core issues for the health of all people and the economies of all countries.

Multilevel program evaluations are needed to effect change, measured against indicators that assess the sensitivity of investments, policies, services, and program delivery to gender equity and transformative social change, and the economic and human rights of women and girls. Without gender-sensitive and rights-sensitive country-level protocols and indicators to guide policies, programs, and service delivery, interventions operate in a vacuum.

All areas addressed in this review demonstrate that the status of women and girls and their opportunities are dependent on protective upstream legislation, whether to increase access to education, to reduce all types of violence, or to protect women and girls from discrimination and exploitation in labor markets. Strategies for increasing the levels of education of girls or raising their access to health services will have little or no effect on lessening the gender gap between men and women, whether rich or poor, if they are not embedded in human rights frameworks that affirm, guide, and monitor violations of equal and universal rights. That there are continuing barriers to and denial of education to girls should be regarded as a global emergency. The integration of gender analysis and economic policy is necessary for a positive effect on women and girls. Closing the gender gap requires nothing less than transformation of social and economic relations as well as gender norms.

ACKNOWLEDGMENTS

I wish to acknowledge the contributions of Lucinda Franklin to the background paper on this topic for the WGEKN.

NOTE

1. The practice of female circumcision is classified into Types (see WHO, 2008) and is variously referred to as infibulation and female genital mutilation, among other practices that are more recently referred to as female genital cutting (FGM/C).

REFERENCES

Abane, H. 2004. The girls do not learn hard enough so they cannot do certain types of work. Experiences from an NGO-sponsored gender sensitization workshop in a Southern Ghanaian community. *Community Development Journal* 39 (1): 49–61.

Adato, M., B. de la Briere, D. Mindek, and A. Quisumbing. 2000. *The Impact of Progresa on Women's Status and Intrahousehold Relations. Final Report.* Washington, DC: International Food Policy Research Institute.

Asling-Monemi, K. 2008. The impact of violence against women on child growth, morbidity and survival. Studies in Bangladesh and Nicaragua. Acta Universitatis Upsaliensis. *Digital Comprehensive Summaries of Uppsala Dissertations from the Faculty of Medicine* 366: 1–88.

Baumgarten, I., E. Finke, J. Manguet, and A. von Roenne. 2004. Intergenerational dialogue on gender roles and female genital mutilation in Guinea. *Sexual Health Exchange* 3 (4): 8–15.

Becker, H. 2003. The least sexist society? Perspectives on gender, change and violence among southern African San. *Journal of Southern African Studies* 29 (1): 5–23.

Bhatla, N., N. Duvvury, and S. Chakraborty. 2006. *Property Ownership and Inheritance Rights of Women for Social Protection—The South Asia Experience, Synthesis Report of Three Studies.* Washington, DC: International Centre for Research on Women.

Burchfield, S., H. Hua, D. Baral, and V. Rocha. 2002. A longitudinal study of the effect of integrated literacy and basic education programs on the participation of women in social and economic development in Nepal. *Girls' and Women's*

Education, Policy Research Activity (GWE-PRA) with funding from USAID World Education, Inc. Cambridge: Harvard Graduate School of Education, Education Development Center, Inc.

Burton, B., N. Varia, and N. Duvvury. 2000. Justice, change and human rights: International research and responses to domestic violence. *ICRW/PROWID Project Synthesis Paper.* Washington DC International Centre for Research on Women (CICRW).

Charmes, J., and S. Wieringa. 2003. Measuring women's empowerment: An assessment of the gender-related development index and the gender empowerment measure. *Journal of Human Development* 4 (3): 419–435.

Doniach, A., and D. Peacock. 2006. Masculinities in motion. In *Men of the Global South,* edited by A. Jones. London: Zed Books. 410–414.

Gage, A.J., A.E. Sommerfelt, and A.L. Piani. 1997. Household structure and childhood immunization in Niger and Nigeria. *Demography* 34 (2): 295–309.

Garcia-Moreno, C., A.F.M.H. Jansen, M. Ellsberg, L. Heisse, and C. Watts. 2005. *WHO Multi-Country Study on Women's Health and Domestic Violence Against Women. Initial Results on Prevalence, Health Outcomes and Women's Responses.* Geneva: World Health Organization.

Global Campaign for Education. 2005. Girls can't wait: Why girls' education matters and how to make it happen now. *Reproductive Health Matters* 13 (25): 19–25.

Grown, C., G. Gupta, and A. Kes. 2005a. *Achieving Gender Equality and Empowering Women, UN Millennium Project.* Los Angeles: Stylus Publishing.

Grown, C., G. Gupta, and R. Pande. 2005b. Taking action to improve women's health through gender equality and women's empowerment. *The Lancet* 365: 541–543.

Gruenbaum, E. 2001. *The Female Circumcision Controversy: An Anthropological Perspective.* Philadelphia: University of Pennsylvania Press.

Herz, B., and G.B. Sperling. 2004. *What Works in Girls' Education: Evidence and Policies From The Developing World.* New York: Council on Foreign Relations. http://www.cfr.org/content/publications/attachments/Girls_Education_summary.pdf.

International Women's Health Coalition. 2003. *My Father Didn't Think This Way: Nigerian Boys Contemplate Gender Equality.* New York: Population Council.

Jewkes, R. 2002 Preventing sexual violence: A rights-based approach. *The Lancet* 360: 1092–1093.

Johnson, S. 2005. Gender relations, empowerment and microcredit: Moving on from a lost decade. *The European Journal of Development Research* 17 (2): 224–248.

Karlsson, L., and R. Karkara. 2004. Working with men and boys to promote gender equality and to end violence and boys and girls. *Report of a Workshop Kathmandu 2004. Save the Children Sweden-Denmark, Regional Programme for South and Central Asia.* Kathmandu: Save the Children.

Lisy, K. 2007. *Promotion of Initiatives to End Female Genital Mutilation. Africa Department, Deutsche Gesellschaft für Technische Zusammenarbeit (GTZ).* Eschborn: GTZ.

Lisy, K., and E. Finke. 2005. *Participatory Impact Monitoring through Action Research: Lessons from the Generation Dialogue and Training for Uncircumcised Girls in Guinea.* Eschborn: GTZ.

Lloyd, C., and M. Grant. 2004. *Growing Up in Pakistan: The Separate Experiences of Males and Females.* New York: Population Council Policy Research Division Working Papers No. 188.

Luttrell, C., and S. Quiroz. 2007. *Understanding and Operationalising Empowerment.* London: Overseas Development Institute, Poverty-Wellbeing net.

Mackie, G. 2000. Female genital cutting: The beginning of the end. In *Female Circumcision in Africa: Culture, Controversy, and Change,* edited by B. Shell-Duncan and Y. Hernlund. Boulder, CO: Lynne Rienner Publishers, Inc: 253–282.

Martinez, S. 2005. Searching for a middle path: Rights, capabilities, and political culture in the study of female genital cutting. *Ahfad (Omdurman, Sudan)* 22 (1): 31–44.

McCloskey, L.A., C. Williams, and U. Larsen. 2005. Gender inequality and intimate partner violence among women in Moshi, Tanzania. *International Family Planning Perspectives* 31 (3): 124–130.

Mukhopadhyay, S., and M. Sudarshan Ratna. 2003. *Tracking Gender Equity Under Economic Reforms: Continuity and Change in South Asia*. Canada: International Development Research Centre (IDRC).

Narayan, D. 2005. *Measuring Empowerment: Cross-Disciplinary Perspectives*. Washington, DC: World Bank.

Peacock, D., and A. Levack. 2004. The men as partners program in South Africa: Reaching men to end gender-based violence and promote sexual and reproductive health. *International Journal of Men's Health* 3 (3): 173–188.

Population Council. 2008. Transitions to adulthood: Child marriage. New York. http://www.popcouncil.org/ta/mar.html.

Psacharapoulos, G., and H. Patrinos. 2002. *Returns to Investment in Education: A Further Update. Policy Research Working Paper 2881*. Washington, DC: World Bank.

Pulerwitz, J., and G. Barker. 2008. Measuring attitudes towards gender norms among young men in Brazil. *Men and Masculinities* 10 (3): 322–338.

Pulerwitz, J., G. Barker, M. Segundo, and M. Nascimento. 2006. *Promoting More Gender-Equitable Norms and Behaviors among Young Men as an HIV/AIDS Prevention Strategy. Horizons Final Report*. Washington, DC: Population Council.

Rychetnik, L., and M. Frommer. 2002. *A Schema for Evaluating Evidence on Public Health Interventions, Version 4*. Melbourne: National Public Health Partnership. http://www.nphp.gov.au/publications/phpractice/schemaV4.pdf.

Sethuraman, K., R. Lansdown, and K. Sullivan. 2006. Women's empowerment and domestic violence: The role of sociocultural determinants in maternal and child undernutrition in tribal and rural communities in South India. *Food and Nutrition Bulletin* 27 (2): 128–143.

Smith, L., and L. Haddad. 2000. *Explaining Child Malnutrition in Developing Countries: A Cross-Country Analysis. Research Report No.111*. Washington, DC: International Food Policy Research Institute.

Smith, L., U. Ramakrishnan, A. Ndiaye, L. Haddad, and R. Martorell. 2003. *The Importance of Women's Status for Child Nutrition in Developing Countries. Research Report 131*. Washington, DC: International Food Policy Research Institute.

Smith, R., M. Wilkinson, and F. Huebler. 2007. *Notes from 2008 EFA Global Monitoring Report: A Review of the Main Gender and Inclusion Issues*. New York: UNIGEI.

Sudarshan, R.M. 2003. Towards integration? Gender and economic policy. In *Tracking Gender Equity under Economic Reforms: Continuity and Change in South Asia*, edited by S. Mukhopadhyay and R.M. Sudarshan. Canada: International Development Research Centre (IDRC): 364–385.

UN Chronicle. 1990. Closing the gender gap. *UN Chronicle* (March): 56–57.

UN. 2005. *The Millennium Development Goals Report*. Geneva: UN Millennium Project.

———. 2008. *The Millennium Development Goals Report*. Geneva: UN Millennium Project.

UNESCO. 2000. *Women and Girls: Education, Not Discrimination*. New York: UNESCO.

————. 2003. *Education for All: Global Monitoring Report 2003/4*. Paris: UNESCO.

UNFPA. 2002. *State of World Population Report*. New York: UNFPA.

————. 2007b. *Women's Economic Empowerment: Meeting the Needs of Impoverished Women*. New York: UNFPA.

UNICEF. 2004. Strategies for girls' education. In *A solution to almost every problem*. New York: UNICEF.

————. 2005a. *Changing a Harmful Social Convention: Female Genital Mutilation/Cutting*. Florence: UNICEF Innocenti Research Centre.

————. 2005b. *Progress for Children: A Report Card on Gender Parity and Primary Education. Number 2, April*. New York: UNICEF.

————. 2006. *The State of the World's Children*. New York: UNICEF.

Unterhalter, E. 2005. Mobilization, meanings and measures: Reflections on girls' education. *Development* 48 (1): 110–114.

Van Hue, Le Thi. 2006. Gender, doi moi and mangrove management in northern Vietnam. *Gender, Technology and Development* 10 (1): 37–59.

Verma, R., J. Pulerwitz, V. Mahendra, S. Khandekar, G. Barker, P. Fulpagare, and S.K. Singh. 2006. Challenging and changing gender attitudes among young men in Mumbai, India. *Reproductive Health Matters* 14 (28): 135–143.

Wathen, C.N., and H. MacMillan. 2003. Interventions for violence against women: Scientific review. *JAMA* 289 (5): 589–600.

White, V., M. Green, and E. Murphy. 2003. *Men and Reproductive Health Programs: Influencing Gender Norms*. Washington, DC: The Synergy Project.

WHO. 2002. *World Report on Violence and Health*. Geneva: World Health Organization.

————. 2005. *WHO Multi-Country Study on Women's Health and Domestic Violence against Women: Summary Report of Initial Results on Prevalence, Health Outcomes and Women's Responses*. Geneva: World Health Organization.

————. 2006. *Study Group on Female Genital Mutilation and Obstetric Outcome*. Geneva: World Health Organization.

————. 2008. *Eliminating Female Genital Mutilation: An Interagency Statement UNAIDS, UNDP, UNECA, UNESCO, UNFPA, UNHCHR, UNHCR, UNICEF, UNIFEM, WHO*. Geneva: World Health Organization.

7 Challenging Gender in Patient–Provider Interactions

Veloshnee Govender and Loveday Penn-Kekana

INTRODUCTION

Quality of health services is an important factor in terms of health care access. Access encompasses a range of dimensions spanning availability (e.g., geographic distribution of health facilities, etc.), accessibility (transport, etc.), affordability (user fees, etc.), and acceptability (referring to the social and cultural distance between health care systems and their users) (Hausmann-Muela et al., 2003). This aspect of analysis recognizes that even if patients do reach health services, and do get to see a health care provider, they will not necessarily be able to access good quality care because of problems with the provider–patient relationship. This dimension of access signifies an important shift away from narrowly defining quality of services in terms of technical and clinical competence towards a broader definition that acknowledges the importance of the quality of interpersonal communication between providers and patients as an importance barrier to access. In this chapter, we define the patient–provider interaction as one that occurs between a patient and a health service provider. Although we recognize the important role that non-biomedical healers play in meeting the health needs of large sectors of the population, we will not be dealing with interactions between them and patients in this chapter.

Across both high- and low-income countries, the patient–provider interface has often been described by patients as discriminatory, marginalizing, abusive, and mirroring the social stratifications of society at large. This, together with a lack of privacy and confidentiality, poor communication between providers and patients, failure to communicate medical and health-related information fully (including side effects), a paternalistic approach that fails to give patients information to enable them to make informed consent, on the part of the provider, we would argue in this chapter, are all important markers of poor quality and as important as whether the 'correct drug' was given, and in cases where the interaction is problematic make it almost impossible to prescribe the 'correct drug.' This experience of discrimination and poor quality care is even more marked for poorer, lower-class, lower caste women and men and is also often mediated by other ethnicity, religion, and language groups.

> Clients often experience providers as powerful individuals, who by social background and training are far removed from their own daily realities and concerns. Clients and providers bring very different expectations to their encounters, and these differences in perspective and power profoundly affect the nature of the interaction. (Simmons and Elias, 1994, p. 4)

While the gender of the patient is important in defining access, we would argue that the *gap* between the provider and patient with respect to gender, class, caste, ethnicity, and other social stratifications (i.e., the social distance) might be even more important in shaping the interaction.

While there have been important regional and country efforts to provide more client-centered care, the particular role of gender as an underlying social determinant in shaping the interaction between clients and providers, while often acknowledged, is still poorly understood and has only received attention in recent years. Gender here is understood to refer to the nature and distribution of roles and power between men and women both within and outside the health system. We recognize that as a socially constructed concept gender is inherently dynamic with the meaning of what it is to be a man and a woman varying across cultures and historical moments. There is, however, in much of the literature we reviewed—and consequently in this review of the literature—some degree of slippage between concepts of gender and sex, as well as relatively ahistorical and decontextualized descriptions of gender roles.

There is a growing literature in health systems research that argues that many of the problems around provider practice in public health systems have been that the health reform and policy implementation agendas in many countries have focused purely on the hardware issues of health systems (i.e., the infrastructure, the technology, the economics) and not focused enough on the 'software' of health systems (i.e., the human and social aspects). Many attempts to reform health systems, and to implement policy are based on what Gregory (1999, p. 65) calls an "economistic reductionism and technocratic structuralism" that fails to take account of the everyday organizational reality of what goes on inside hospitals and of the fact that health care workers are not simply robots who implement policy unthinkingly nor are they angels who only have the best interests of the patients at heart but are living thinking reflexive human beings who live in and reflect the social norms of the societies in which they live and work (Blaauw et al., 2006). People's experiences in using the health system are shaped profoundly by the nature of the relationship with the health care worker and the health care workers attitudes and behavior are shaped partly by the social context in which she/he lives and works.

In this chapter, the question will be addressed in three main sections. In the first section we are interested in mapping the context of how gender shapes provider–client interaction, and the impact of these interactions in four areas:

1. differential patterns of care for men and women for the same health problem
2. differential patterns of care by male and female health workers
3. the gendered division of labor
4. patterns of abuse of patients

The second section of the chapter will provide a detailed breakdown of the nature of provider–patient interactions and how gender impacts on these interactions from the perspective of patients and providers. The chapter will conclude with reviewing gender-specific policies and program interventions *within* the health system for improving the interpersonal dimension of health and hence quality of care. The chapter will not examine those policies and program interventions that aim to bring about changes in the wider sociopolitical context and lie *outside* the health system.

SOURCES FOR THIS REVIEW

Evidence demonstrating impact of gender on patient–provider interactions was relatively hard to come by and synthesis. Apart from some studies documenting different treatment received by men and women, most of the studies described are descriptive, or evaluations of relatively small-scare interventions. This is partly due to lack of funding of gender studies and interventions that tackle gender issues, but also reflects that gender is a socially constructed concept that is inherently dynamic with meaning varying across cultures and historical moments. It is therefore hard to imagine how a multicentered randomized control trial of interventions would work. Other challenges in carrying out the review were that work looking at gender and health is cross-disciplinary and wide-ranging, making comprehensive reviews problematic and time-consuming. The fact that the focus of this chapter was also evidence from low- and middle-income country settings also limited the amount of evidence that we could access.

This chapter is based on a comprehensive literature review of peer-reviewed studies and the grey literature. Initial searches for research studies, reviews, and meta-analyses were carried out on Medline Ovid and PubMed involving combinations of keywords (see Appendix 1). The next step was to narrow down the articles to those that addressed specifically the terms of reference for this review. The articles were then further expanded with additional searches based on bibliographic information from identified articles. Grey literature was identified through general Web searches on Google,

Google Scholar, and from more focused reviews of relevant Web sites. The Web sites reviewed included international agencies and foundations (health, development, and family planning) and governmental agencies: Centre for Health and Gender Equity (CHANGE), Guttmacher Institute, Engender-Health, Centre for Reproductive Rights, Family Health International, The International Planned Parenthood Federation/Western Hemisphere Region (IPPF/WHR), Population Council, Pan American Health Organization (PAHO), IDRC, Maximizing Health and Quality, The Interagency Gender Working Group (IGWG), and WHO. In addition, we also obtained references from colleagues in the WGEKN and more broadly those working in the area of gender and health.

Despite limits and difficulties, we would argue that it is possible to learn from existing experience in order to act. Whereas on a few issues there is clear evidence of the kind conventionally accepted by public health practitioners as 'rigorous,' i.e., that men and women receive different treatment for similar conditions, on other issues action should be taken based on a combination of values and an assessment of how available evidence can be made useful in different contexts. Importantly, we feel that it is imperative to take action in the face of gender inequity, even where there is only limited evidence on appropriate, specific interventions.

In conclusion, this chapter agrees with the conclusion of the health system knowledge network final report, which argued the examples given in the review enable policy makers to adapt interventions to local circumstances. When applying lessons from other settings it is always important to establish monitoring and evaluation processes that allow adjustment in response to the experience of implementation in a particular setting.

Overall we were surprised that although there was a vast literature that stated that gender was an important factor that shaped the quality of care that patients received, very few of the articles looked in detail at the patient–provider interaction and described or theorized the way that gender did impact on this interaction.

REVIEW OF THE EVIDENCE

Mapping the Context

Differential Patterns of Care for Men and Women for the Same Health Problem

A recent review of the gender-based differences in care for men and women presenting with eczema and psoriasis in an outpatient clinic in Sweden reported that men received more intensive treatment (ultraviolet, prescriptions, etc.) than the women (Osika et al., 2005). This example is yet another in a long line of studies that have attempted to understand why and how gender contributes to differences in care for similar illnesses and conditions. To explore this more fully, in this section we will review evidence for two conditions, namely tuberculosis (TB) and depression, which illustrate these differences.

Tuberculosis

TB is commonly described as a 'disease of poverty,' for preying on the poorest and most vulnerable in society. Although the majority of the world's poor are women, two-thirds of all notified TB cases are men (WHO, 2000). In the past, this discrepancy between men and women was ascribed to sex-based immunological differences and men having more social contacts and in so doing, increasing their risk to contagious diseases. In recent years, the wisdom of this has been questioned. Data from Vietnam and Bangladesh suggest that underdiagnosis and undernotification of female TB cases as well as gender-related differences in access to TB services might be the underlying reason (Dolin, 1998; Begum et al., 2001; Thorson et al., 2004).

Studies in India (Raikes, 1992; Rajeswari et al., 2002; Sudha et al., 2003) and Vietnam (Johansson et al., 2000) have shown that when women accessed care, they often chose traditional healers and private practitioners on account of privacy, anonymity, accessibility, and the provision of more patient-centered care. TB is highly stigmatized and has very different social repercussions for men and women. Women feared being socially ostracized and in some instances even faced the possibility of divorce, and in the case of unmarried women, experienced difficulties in finding marriage partners. In contrast, men feared more for the economic consequences of the disease (Johansson et al., 1999; Long et al., 1999). It is not surprising then that the patient–provider interaction is critical.

Long and colleagues (1999) found that in Vietnam doctor's delay (time from first contact with medical doctor to diagnosis) was significantly longer for women compared to men. Providers considered women and not factors associated with the health system or themselves to be responsible for delays in diagnosis. Women were described as "shy" and "hesitant" with "limited knowledge in health care seeking matters" and often "not following their doctor's prescription mainly because of a need to double-check these with their husband, family and neighbors." Men in comparison were described as "daring and open," "willing to follow directions and prescriptions and, being the primary breadwinners, also to have more access to money and to have a decision-making power of their own, independent of the rest of the family" (Thorson and Johansson, 2004, p. 40). An earlier study by Johansson and Winkvist (2002) reported that Vietnamese male doctors reported more difficulty in diagnosing female TB patients whilst female doctors did not report any gender-based diagnosing problems.

Depression

Gender on its own and through interaction with other structural determinants (class, ethnicity, educational levels, etc.) has also been acknowledged as an important risk factor for depression and other mental health disorders (WHO, 2001). A consistent finding in psychiatric epidemiology is that depression is almost twice as prevalent in women compared to men (WHO, 2001; Patel et al., 2004). Treatment seeking and patient care also show gender-based differences. Women seek out and receive care more often at the primary care level while men predominate in inpatient care (Bertakis et al., 2000; Astbury, 2002).

Female patients are twice as likely to be diagnosed as depressed compared to their male counterparts (Callahan et al., 1997). Higher diagnosis among women can in part be explained by the finding that with increasing number of health care visits, diagnosis of depression also increases (Cleary et al., 1990; Bertakis et al., 2001). Since men are generally less likely to seek care at the primary level, this might be an indicator of underdiagnosis of male depression. There is increasing evidence suggesting that poorer treatment seeking and underutilization of health services (particularly primary and preventive) among men might be explained by reasons linked to the stereotypes of the male identity of being "strong," "independent," and "self-reliant." Unfortunately, these values and norms embodied in such gender stereotypes can lead to comparatively poorer treatment and health outcomes for men.

While the preceding examples illustrate the impact of gender alone for care received, it is important to recognize how economic class, caste, and other social hierarchies crosscut gender. That is, while gender biases are likely to affect all women, the impact can in some instances be more harmful for women lower in the economic class and caste hierarchy. A qualitative assessment of implications of cost recovery for family planning services in Bangladesh found that poor, uneducated women perceived receiving poor quality and discriminatory care because of their social position: "We [poor people] have to buy medicine but they [rich people] get two saline instead of one. If a rich women comes they will take plenty of time to examine her, but I will not get any special favors" (Schuler et al., 2002, p. 275). Poor women felt that not only did they receive poor quality care, but that also that wealthier patients received preferential treatment. The experience of these women in the health care system arguably mirrors the values and norms of the society at large.

Differential Patterns of Care by Male and Female Health Workers

A recent meta-analytic review of 29 publications investigating the effects of physician gender in medical communication in the US found notable differences (Roter et al., 2002). Although the review found no gender differences in the biomedical information provided during the consultation, female physicians did engage in significantly more active partnership behaviors, positive talk, psychosocial counseling, psychosocial question asking, and emotionally focused talk, and spent on average two minutes (10%) longer with clients compared to male physicians. In this area of patient–provider interactions, there are two important gaps. Firstly, there is a dearth of similar studies from middle- and low-income settings investigating gender-based differential patterns of care by providers. Secondly, the authors were unable to locate studies that have directly addressed the issue of how power is altered and shaped by the gender dynamics between the patient and provider. For instance, are patients more passive in their interaction with male providers compared to female providers? Also, how does the interaction of gender with class and ethnicity of the provider influence the interaction? Alternatively, are there instances where it is more important for patients to consult with providers of their own race and ethnicity and gender is of secondary importance?

The significance of provider gender has in all probability received more attention in the areas of obstetric-gynecology than elsewhere. Here again, much of this data emerges from developed countries. Studies carried out in the US have found that only a minority of women felt strongly about their provider's gender and provider choice was more a function of the provider's attributes, including experience, communication style, and technical expertise (Howell et al., 2002; Plunkett et al., 2002; Zuckerman et al., 2002).

However, in highly patriarchal societies, the importance of gender concordance between provider and patient is important because of socio-cultural and/or religious norms and practices, which not only demarcate gender roles but also restrict social and physical contact between men and women (Holroyd et al., 2004; Rizk et al., 2005). A qualitative study carried out in Cuba, Thailand, Saudi Arabia, and Argentina examined the experiences of women seeking antenatal care and found that female doctors were more highly preferred by Saudi and Thai women (Nigenda et al., 2003). Interestingly, although Cuban women indicated being equally comfortable with male and female doctors, they were warned against male doctors: "the general practitioner (a woman) told me that in my visit to the specialist (a man) I have to take with me a piece of cloth to cover my body, otherwise the doctor (. . .) will not take his eyes away from you" (Nigenda et al., 2003, p. 17).

Globally, lower level frontline positions (e.g., nurses) are staffed by predominantly women and more senior positions (e.g., doctors) of influence and power are filled mainly by men (WHO, 2006). Hartigan (2001, p. 10) argues that this suggests that "The gendered division of labor within the health system reflects the gender division of labor within society." Poor salaries and unsatisfactory working conditions (weak and/or absent support and supervision structures), particularly for frontline providers, often leaves them feeling isolated, disempowered, and unappreciated, and has been documented in numerous studies.

In societies marked by deep gender inequities, these women experience discrimination within the workplace and the society at large. A qualitative study of the experience of female community-level workers in Pakistan reported hierarchical management and abuse of power, disrespect from male colleagues and sexual harassment, lack of sensitivity to women's gender-based cultural, hostile community, and family attitudes, all of which suggests that health care institutions not only reflect but can maintain harmful and discriminatory societal norms and values (Mumtaz et al., 2003). The frustrations and discrimination that female workers experienced influenced their interaction with patients:

> When I leave home to come to the Basic Health Unit I need to travel by local transport, and there are men who offer a lift or pass comments. I feel so bad and insulted that when I reach the Basic Health Unit I misbehave with my patients (LHV, age 24, 12 years education). (Mumtaz et al., 2003, p. 264)

There is a considerable body of literature that will not be dealt with in this chapter that deals with the abuse of health care workers, particularly female nurses by senior medical staff, and the general sexual harassment of junior staff. It is not unlikely that health care workers who are themselves harassed and do not feel safe and are not helped and supported are likely to pass on their frustrations. Research also found that health care workers often have problems of abuse in their own lives independent of their position as nurses.

Abuse of Patients

The abuse of patients by health care providers is a critical issue that is receiving increasing attention and deserves special mention. An underlying implicit assumption in many of the previous sections is that health care providers intend to provide good quality care to patients but a range of factors including gender stereotyping interfere with the quality of these interactions between providers and patients. In such a relationship all patients, but especially women, and women who are socioeconomically disadvantaged in other ways, be it poverty, race, class, or age, are particularly vulnerable to abuse.

Sexual Abuse of Patients

One of the most severe forms of abuse of the health care provider–patient relationship is that of sexual abuse. Exactly what constitutes sexual abuse in the provider–patient relationship is contested. Most medical professional boards define sexual abuse of patients as any sexual intercourse or other forms of sexual relations, touching of a sexual nature, or behavior or remarks of a sexual nature with a patient, regardless of whether or not the patient gave consent for the relationships, arguing that any relationship is "almost always harmful" (Fahy and Fisher, 1992; Health Professions Regulatory Advisory Council, 2000). There is some debate, particularly in terms of the severity of sanctions, about whether the fact that the relationship is broadly consensual makes a difference, with some medical professional groups arguing that forced sexual violation deserves the strongest sanction and others arguing for a policy of zero-tolerance for any sexual relationship between health care providers and patients (Thomasson, 1999).

Because of the prohibited nature of the sexual abuse there is little evidence beyond the anecdotal from most of the world on the exact extent to which sexual abuse of patients by providers is a problem.

Anonymous postal surveys carried out among doctors in developed countries with a range of different practitioners consistently find around 3% to 4% of practitioners admitting to having had sexual contact with patients (Wilbers et al., 1992; Lamont and Woodward, 1994). Studies on doctors' attitudes towards sexual contact between doctors and patients also consistently find that female doctors support stronger sanctions against sexual transgression and sexual violation than the male doctors and state that female doctors are more likely to be prepared to report colleagues and act as whistle-blowers (Wilbers et al., 1992; Lamont and Woodward, 1994).

Physical and Verbal Abuse of Patients

As discussed in the earlier sections on maternal health, there is also literature on physical abuse of patients in health care settings (d'Oliveira et al., 2002). In terms of physical abuse of women there is a large literature on the physical abuse of women in labor by health care workers—themselves mainly women—which has been documented around the world (Jewkes et al., 1998; UN Millennium Project, 2005). It is a sad indictment of maternal health services around the world that so much abuse is documented and appears to go unpunished. It also must go against the campaign to get more women to deliver at facilities when it is widely acknowledged that physical and verbal abuse is common in maternity services.

As discussed earlier in this chapter there is evidence from a range of countries that there is verbal abuse of patients, particularly when patients are accessing or trying to access reproductive health services—whether it is treatment for sexually transmitted infections, abortion, family planning services, or during deliveries. A study carried out in midwife-led units in South Africa found that as well as structural explanations for poor quality of care, health care workers also were in judgment of women who they felt should not be having children, for example, they are too young, unmarried, already have many children, too old, not married, etc. (Jewkes et al., 1998). Race and class differentials between health care midwives and patients was also an important explanatory factor for verbal abuse (Jewkes et al., 1998).

Work in South Africa exploring how sexual assault survivors were treated found that health care workers were often extremely judgmental and rude, and that patients rated the sympathy of health care workers alongside competence as one of the factors that mattered most to them (Christofides et al., 2006). Verbal abuse of women seems often to be linked to factors associated with health care workers presuming that women have transgressed certain gender norms. However, the same research that documents such abuse often suggests that it is health care workers own experience of abuse, either outside the health facility or by managers and other staff at the facility, that is often an explanation, with health care workers taking their frustrations out on their patients (Kim and Motsei, 2002; Christofides et al., 2005).

Economic Abuse and Over-medicalization of Patients

Many women are unable to access services, or elements of services, because of demands for under-the-counter payments for services and medications that are officially provided free of charge, as well as referrals to health care workers private practices. This is often particularly the case in non-functional health systems where basic needs of health care workers are not met (Parkhurst et al., 2005). Although the literature often does not deal with gender specifically, there is widespread anecdotal and descriptive data that suggest that because of women's access to funds and women's poverty, demanding payment can force women to rely further on men and sometimes force families into debt, and in other places make services just inaccessible to women, contributing to maternal deaths (George et al., 2005).

Related to the economic abuse of patients is over-medicalization of certain aspects of women's health. The literature suggests that over-medicalization of women's health, particularly aspects of women's reproductive health, has its roots in a range of different causes. Firstly as a result of profit motives and poor regulation of health care workers where over-medicalization is related to financial incentives for health care workers (d'Oliveira et al., 2002; Parkhurst and Rahman, 2007). Secondly as a reflection of the power dynamics between patients and providers, especially in terms of childbirth where there are studies documenting health care workers inducing labor or performing C-sections so that their social and work schedules are not interfered with (d'Oliveira et al., 2002). Thirdly due to "gender-based serotypes abut women's nature and women's bodies" (Munch, 2004). Although at times this stereotyping leads to women's illness being misdiagnosed as purely psychosomatic, these stereotypes have also resulted in the over-medicalization of natural events in women's lives, such as childbirth and menopause, partly as a result of the classification of these processes as 'diseases' (Rothman, 1982). A combination of these factors has commonly led to problems of women being submitted to "excessive or inappropriate medical treatments during childbirth" as well as over-medicalization with no real medical evidence guiding the intervention of women with infertility problems and around menopause (d'Oliveira et al., 2002).

Abuse of Health Care Providers by Patients

There is also increasing literature that documents the abuse of health care workers by patients. For example, a study of health care workers in the UK found that 12% of health care workers had experienced physical violence from patients or their relatives in 2006, with 26% reporting bullying, harassment, or abuse from patients or patients' relatives (Healthcare Commission, 2006). Nurses working in rural South Africa noted security and fear of attacks from patients as a key factor in shaping their decisions about where to work and not wanting to stay in some rural areas (Penn-Kekana et al., 2004). There is very little work that documents whether there is a gender dimension to this violence and abuse, or that documents the levels of violence and abuse in the developing world.

Impact of Gender on the Provider-Patient Relationship

There is a vast, although at times disappointing in terms of its analysis and explanatory value, literature that touches on some aspects of the way that gender impacts on the provider–patient interface. What we hope to do in this section is describe some of this literature. Due to the nature of what is being described—i.e., complex changing social phenomenon—the type of evidence that we present in this section of the chapter is mainly descriptive. Where possible we have tried to identify common themes across regions or religious groups, we have also in this section, due to the need to be selective in the information that we present, focused on certain aspects of health care, such as maternal health and treatment for sexually transmitted infections.

Besides considering how complying to gender norms impact on provider–patient relationships, it is equally important to reflect how transgressing gender norms (especially those gender norms held by health care workers) can lead to a real breakdown in provider practice. This appears to be particularly the case in reproductive health services and in the cases of women seeking help after gender-based violence (d'Oliveira et al., 2002; Kim and Motsei, 2002; Christofides et al., 2005; Chikanda, 2005; Baines, 2006). In this section we have drawn particularly from research reports and other grey material.

How Gender Influences The Patient Side Of The Interaction

There is evidence from a number of studies and evaluations that patients may avoid seeking care or care at specific facilities because of the gender of the health care workers. They may not think it acceptable, or their families might not feel it acceptable, to see a health care worker of another sex. Patients may avoid health care workers also because of the fear that health care workers will be judgmental of the medical condition for which they are seeking help (abortion, contraception, treatment for STI's, infertility, AIDS), feeling that they have transgressed some societal norms to have developed this medical condition or need this medical assistance.

Gender dynamics can also fundamentally affect the way that patient communicates with the health care workers. To avoid sanction, or because of beliefs about what it is appropriate to discuss, patients may not discuss certain symptoms that are essential for the health care worker to make a correct diagnosis. This might be about a STI or about something such as pain where studies have found that there are gendered cultural norms about the acceptability of complaining about pain. Some of these problems may be exacerbated by being treated by a health care worker of a different sex, but still exist if talking to a health care worker of the same sex.

The gender of the health care worker, and the quality of the interaction with the health care worker, will also affect patients' abilities to understand, believe, or trust what the provider says and to follow through with the treatment that the provider prescribes. This belief that the patient cannot ask questions is mediated by a range of social factors including gender. Also issues about levels of literacy and language proficiency among women who tend to be less well educated.

INTERVENTIONS FOR REDUCING GENDER BIASES AND DISCRIMINATION IN THE PATIENT–PROVIDER INTERACTION

This section takes as its starting point the six areas for intervention outlined by the Women and Gender Equity Knowledge Network (WHO CSDH). These include: (a) addressing key gender inequities that impinge on the health system from outside; (b) tackling values, norms, practices, and behavior within households and communities; (c) addressing gender-specific exposures to health risks; (d) addressing gender-specific vulnerabilities in disease and disability; (e) redressing the inequitable social and economic consequences of ill-health; and (f) engendering health systems and health research. This underscores the importance of recognizing that redressing gender biases and discrimination calls for action on multiple levels to address the complexities of the patient–provider interaction. In the following sections we will consider strategies in the following areas: (a) health systems legislation and policy, (b) integrating gender into health programs and institutions, and (c) integrating gender into health care worker training.

Health Systems Legislation and Policy

Cottingham and Myntti (2002) distinguish between legislations that have a *direct* (i.e., operate within the health care system) and those that have an *indirect* (i.e., operate outside the health care system) impact on women's health and access to quality health care. Indirect legislation and policies are those (a) that affirm and safeguard women's rights (e.g., equal rights) and guarantee their full participation in public, cultural, political, and socioeconomic life, and (b) that empower women and their ability to access health care (e.g., education of girls) (Sen and Batliwala, 2000; UN Millennium Project, 2005). Although such legislation and policy changes do not impact directly on the provider–patient interaction, they can potentially empower women to be more assertive in their interactions with providers.

Examples of more direct policies are laws pertaining to the rights of patients, decriminalization of abortion, earmarking of funds for youth-friendly health services, etc. In the next section we will consider firstly policies on the rights of the patient that have attempted to improve the patient–provider interaction and that impact gender indirectly, and secondly those policies that have more explicitly incorporated gender equity, often within a broader context of population and development policies.

The Paradigm Shift from Provider-Centered to Patient-Centered Care

At a global level, the International Declaration on the Rights of the Patient (World Medical Association, 1981) was a watershed in shifting the spotlight onto the patient–provider relationship. The Declaration not only identified a set of patient rights incorporating consent and correlative duties and responsibilities on health professionals, but also signaled an important shift away from a paternalistic model of care to one based on patient autonomy, cognizant of the balance of power between providers and patients. A Cochrane review found that training in patient-centeredness for health care providers may improve communication with patients, enable clarification of patients' concerns in consultations, and improve satisfaction with care (Lewin et al., 2005).

In late 1980s and early 1990s, international population and family planning organizations, and specifically the work of Judith Bruce and Anrudh Jaine from the Population Council, drew attention to the provider–patient interaction as an important element of quality of care within the family planning program delivery context (Bruce and Jain, 1991). In 1992, IPPF put forward a Charter on Rights of the Client that considered quality of care from the client's perspective and provided education about rights to information, access to services, choice, safety, privacy and confidentiality, dignity, comfort, and continuity of services (Huezo and Briggs, 1992). In 1994, the ICPD not only heralded a major paradigm shift in the population field towards a rights-based and social justice approach but also stressed the importance of implementation of reproductive health programs from a gender perspective. For family planning, this called for shifts towards voluntary, client-centered services (for both men and women), away from government or provider-driven targets, within a broad context of sexual and reproductive health services (Sai, 1997). The increasing use of the term 'client-centered' as opposed to 'patient-centered' care has gained currency since the former reflects an emphasis on empowerment, patient autonomy, voice, self-determination, and participation in decision-making. In this chapter, we use the terms interchangeably.

Since the seminal work of Bruce and Jain, the client-centered approach has taken root and evolved in content and focus. More recently, Murphy and Steele (2000) emphasized the importance of both *process* and *content* in the interaction. *Content* refers to the exchange of accurate information and process that create an atmosphere of trust and allow sharing between the provider and client. The "S.I.G.N.A.L. Project" in Germany is an important example of a patient-centered intervention to end violence against women (Hellbernd et al., 2005). It was initiated in 1999 and includes asking patients about abuse, assessing danger, informing and referring victims to counseling programs and women's shelters, and documenting injuries and health problems for use in legal proceedings. Nurses and physicians working in emergency departments have undergone training based on these principles.

This approach has been widely adopted by leading international family planning and reproductive organizations. These interventions go further in incorporating gender through the inclusion of men in family planning and reproductive health care, couple counseling, and providing services specifically for men (Ringheim, 2002; Kim et al., 2003a; RamaRao and Mir, 2004).

Such policies and actions that seek to empower and strengthen the political agency and autonomy of women can be limited in their reach if they are not supported by appropriate programmatic changes on the ground.

Integrating Gender into Programs and Institutions

Health literacy

A situation analysis of family planning and reproductive health services in more than 20 countries indicated that the information exchange between providers and clients is often poor or inadequate, thus compromising the ability of the patient to make an informed decision (Miller et al., 1997). An outcome of this has been an increasing emphasis on patient education and health literacy, with the latter being defined as the ability to obtain, process, and understand basic information and services needed to make appropriate decisions regarding health (Selden et al., 2000; Greenberg, 2001).

The "Smart Patient" coaching intervention in Indonesia is an example of a health literacy initiative that aimed to improve client participation through health literacy in family planning consultations. Kim and colleagues (2003b, p. 20) argue that an important outcome of this intervention was that for clients "it legitimized their right to speak." However, this was not necessarily equal for all patients: the better educated and higher-income clients gained more. Moreover, it was found that clients engaged more actively with providers from the lower socioeconomic groups, suggesting that client participation increases with a narrowing down of the social distance. This further indicates that the effectiveness of patient education is constrained by underlying structural determinants of poverty, class, and gender. In such contexts, the use of nonwritten and low literacy materials and inclusion of family members, close friends, etc., as surrogate readers are important for empowering patients. Kim and colleagues (2003b) of the Smart Patient Project also supported the idea that patient education and health literacy can be more effectively enhanced through oral communication methods and low literacy materials.

Recognizing that access to education and more specifically literacy is in many parts of the world gendered, health literacy that emphasizes reading, writing, speaking, and listening can entrench gender biases in health care and patient–provider interaction. Therefore, complementary policies that improve access to education and improved literacy especially for girls are critical (Nutbeam and Kickbusch, 2000).

Women- and Men-Centered Services

Judgmental attitudes of providers, lack of privacy and confidentiality, and in some instances denial of care, particularly in the context of sexual and reproductive health services, has been described earlier as an important barrier to access especially for unmarried women, men, and adolescents. This has contributed to the introduction of more gender- and adolescent-friendly services that can take a range of forms: youth-only and men-only clinics, women-only services within existing services, outreach and community-based services, and different hours of services within existing services.

Initiatives towards 'women-centered services' has taken a variety of forms. One example is the provision of door-to-door services for women whose mobility and hence access to services is constrained. The Lady Health Workers initiative in Pakistan is a response to meeting this need and has been effective in increasing the uptake of services, and has improved the adoption of contraceptives and improved community health (Douthwaite and Ward, 2005). The *Kumar Warmi* (Aymara for 'healthy woman') project in Bolivia illustrates how women-centered services through educational processes, shared decision-making, linking with women's groups, and drawing on nonhierarchical and nondidactic educational and communication strategies can help women overcome negative perceptions of the doctor–client relationship (Paulson et al., 1996).

Another instance is the integration of health services, which can take the form of multipurpose clinics, multipurpose staff, adding new services that serve a more diverse client population (e.g., expanding family planning services to include men and adolescents), and adding new reproductive health services (e.g., HIV/AIDS) to existing reproductive health services (e.g., MCH) (de Pinho et al., 2005). Integration has been motivated by a patient perspective in terms of time convenience (one-stop-shop), which can potentially enable access to reproductive services and simultaneously access to, for instance, child care services in the same facility. Secondly, integrating STI prevention with reproductive health services instead of separate STI services can also help to ensure privacy and reduce stigma. Although some studies have shown an improvement in the patient–provider relationship (Potter et al., 1987), others have either not examined the question of interpersonal interactions and client satisfaction (WHO, 1999), or have found little evidence of such an impact (Dehne et al., 2000).

Generally, men are poorer users of the health care system than women. Amongst the various barriers to male involvement are poor recognition and sometimes denial of ill-health, poor access (e.g., clinic hours), absence of a male provider, and provider bias against male patients (AVSC International, 1997; Hancock, 2004; Smith et al., 2006). It is increasingly recognized that the skills of health providers are often inadequate for dealing with men. Male stereotypes perpetuated by providers can create an obstacle to men's involvement (Shepard, 2004). As illustrated with studies from Brazil (Manhoso and Hoga, 2005) and South Asia (Piet-Pelon et al., 1999), providers can often fail to provide male patients with accurate information.

The ICPD's Programme of Action called for efforts and organizations to "encourage and enable men to take responsibility for their sexual and reproductive behavior" and an increasing number of organizations have increased male participation (often referring to counseling, either alone or with their female partner), particularly in reproductive health. The unequal power balance between men and women together with the recognition of men's authority within the family has propelled forward male involvement programs (Ringheim, 2002). The area of family planning has had a number of initiatives involving men, primarily so they will support partners' use of contraceptives, through improved communication; others offer reproductive health services specifically for men and, more recently, programs that attempt to reduce if not eliminate violence against women through encouraging men to examine detrimental social norms. The ReproSalud Project in Peru, which trained health workers to sensitize men on gender-based violence, is an example of such an initiative. This project had a significant impact on sensitizing men to the influence of power on the relationship between men and women and an appraisal of the project documented dramatic decreases in alcohol consumption, domestic violence, and forced sex in the project areas. A project staff member reported "The husbands who have been trained understand better. Before, they brutally forced sex. They hit, especially when they were drunk. Now, no more" (Rogow, 2000, p. 20).

Male-friendly services are promoted through separate waiting areas, male service providers, separate examination rooms, and male-only clinics. Profamilia's *Clinica Para El Hombre* in Colombia represents one of the

most successful attempts to increase men's access to comprehensive reproductive health services through the introduction of men-only clinics (AVSC
International, 1997). Quality of care and gender-sensitive patient–provider
interactions are central to the delivery of services. Staff are trained on personal and cultural beliefs about masculinity, and are encouraged to reflect
on their personal attitudes regarding gender and how gender impacts on
their interactions with patients.

Integrating Gender into Health Worker Training

Gender sensitization training

The neglect of the perspectives of providers and the complex range of factors that influence their performance and quality of care are increasingly
recognized as crucial elements in the gap between health policy and implementation. Here, we are concerned with the potential of gender sensitization strategies—which encourage providers to examine how gender norms
affect their patients' health and health-seeking behavior, how gender stereotypes impact on their interaction with patients, and how gender impacts
on their own lives within their work and home environment—for improving the patient–provider interaction.

Conventional training on interpersonal communication (IPC) and also
within the quality of care framework has often neglected the influence of
gender and other social structural determinants on the patient–provider
interaction. Health Workers for Change (HWFC) is a departure from conventional models in that it uses a participatory research-learning approach
for bringing about improvements in quality of care with emphasis on the
need for gender sensitivity in health services (Fonn and Xaba, 2001).

It is also important to understand the impact of gender, socioeconomic
status, and other structural determinants experienced by providers on their
interactions with patients. An intervention for investigating the potential role
of health workers in addressing domestic violence in South Africa started off
by seeking to understand how health workers' own experiences of gender-
based violence impacted on them professionally and personally (Kim and
Motsei, 2002). The evaluation of the intervention found that all the health
workers "reported that they had found it to be a valuable educational experience and for many, it had marked a turning point in their personal and
professional lives. All of the participants reported that they would wish to see
such training formally and more widely incorporated into the South African
nursing curriculum" (Kim and Motsei, 2002, p. 1249).

Revisiting the Medical Curriculum

A cross-sectional survey of physicians (71% male) practicing in Bal-
ochistan, Pakistan, was carried out, which assessed their knowledge,

attitude, and practices with respect to specific sexual health problems (Afsar et al., 2006). It was found that 32% reported that they were not comfortable talking personally, 44% were uncomfortable talking about frequency of sexual intercourse, and 63% found it uncomfortable to talk about partners' sexual history. Fifty-five (55%) percent of the respondents were also of the opinion that the present medical curriculum was insufficient to prepare doctors to deal with sexual health problems, particularly those in female patients. This study is an illustration of the implications of a male-centric biomedical framework that underpins the training of medical doctors across the world.

Historically, medicine and medical education has considered the male anatomy as the norm and women were and continue to be underrepresented in illustrations of nonreproductive anatomy (Giacomini et al., 1986; Lawrence and Bendixen, 1992). This has led to the neglect of the importance of gender, psychosocial, and environmental factors in explaining differences in men and women and has arguably contributed to gender-based inequities in medical treatment (kidney disease, depression, tuberculosis, etc.) (Gisbers van Wijk et al., 1996; Vlassoff and Moreno, 2002). This has ignored the reality that men and women understand, experience, and respond differently to diseases and treatment regimes.

Over the past decade, there have been efforts to integrate gender into the medical curriculum in training institutions in a range of developed and developing countries, including the Netherlands (Verdonk et al., 2005), Sweden (Hamberg, 2003), Australia (Monash University, 2007), the US (Nicolette and Jacobs, 2000), and India (Jesani and Madhiwalla, 2002).

The Gender Mainstreaming in Medical Education (GME) project, which was initiated in India in 2002, is an example from a low- to middle-income country of an important initiative that focuses not only on medical schools but also takes a broader view of gender mainstreaming through collaboration with health professionals and NGOs (Jesani and Madhiwalla, 2002; Ramanathan and Khambete, 2007).

CONCLUSION

There is clear evidence across many countries, across many medical conditions, and in terms of diagnosis, treatment as well as patient adherence and patient satisfaction, that gender has a profound impact on provider–patient interactions. The impact of gender stereotypes and biases within the provider–patient interaction has been shown to be harmful for women as well as men. With men gender norms often make it difficult for them to utilize health care, or express feelings of vulnerability (Bertakis et al., 2001; Thorson and Johansson, 2004). Much of the gender bias and discrimination that dominate the experiences of the interpersonal interactions between providers and clients can be traced to underlying structural causes (socioeconomic, political, cultural), which act out through the more intermediary factors (e.g., health system biases, exposure, vulnerability, and acknowledgment of health needs) and need to be tackled at a wider societal level.

However, while acknowledging the need to empower women and girls at the societal level, we also believe that health systems are "core social institutions" (Freedman, 2005). How people are treated in these core institutions forms an important part of the experience of what it means to be socially marginalized and disempowered. Provider attitudes and practices that discriminate on the basis of gender, class, ethnicity, and caste thereby deepen inequity. This is illustrated by the examples described in this chapter of poor and young women's experience of verbal and sometimes physical abuse in childbirth; or young women's experience of verbal abuse and scolding when they try and access contraceptive services; or poor black women in the United States being made to feel like welfare cheats and therefore constantly changing providers.

Because health facilities are core social institutions we would also argue that there is a responsibility to try and challenge gender norms that are harmful to the health of women, and in some cases men. Although often unspoken in much of the literature, there exists a tension between trying to provide 'culturally accessible' health services that recognize the gender norms that exist in the society and make it possible for women who are constrained by these norms to seek health care, and to try and challenge these gender norms. This tension is best illustrated by the work of Mumtaz and colleagues (2003) in Pakistan. The Pakistan government in recognition of women's constraints in accessing services trained a cadre of women community health care workers who were meant to meet the needs of women. The problem was that these women themselves were subjected to the very same constraints as the women they were appointed to serve. We would argue that instead of trying to merely reflect the gender norms that exist in society, there is need for the health system to start to challenge them.

Gender sensitization that challenges workers' gender stereotypes needs to happen alongside redressing gender biases that they themselves face in the work environment and the health care system. It would be futile if providers are expected to reorient their practices but at the same time continue to face gender-based biases and discrimination from their colleagues and the communities in which they work (Onyango-Ouma et al., 2001). By valuing, caring, and respecting them, they are more likely to provide client-centered and better quality of care services.

Being made aware of these biases, and how these biases result in colleagues giving different treatment to different patients for no clinical reason, may start to make health workers more reflective about their practice. Work such as that done in the HWFC program shows the powerful impact of interventions that simultaneously explore patient and provider issues (Fonn and Xaba, 2001). Health workers also need to be made aware of the gender dynamics that exist, which impact on how and when men and women seek care, and how they talk about their symptoms in interactions with health care workers. Using the example from Vietnam discussed earlier, health care workers should be aware of the constraints that women face in terms of seeking care, aware of how organization of the health care will impact on women, and aware of the social stigma that is attached to the illness for women, and this will enable them to provide better care (Thorson and Johansson, 2004). Health workers also need to be educated on issues around sexual abuse of patients, as well as the rights of patients.

As well as working with health care workers, there have also been a number of interventions that show that empowering patients also can have a significant impact on the nature of the patient–provider interaction. A systematic review of the evidence on effectiveness of empowerment to improve health by Wallerstein (2006, p. 4) found that "women's empowering interventions, integrated with the economic, educational, and political sectors, should have the greatest impact on women's quality of life, autonomy and authority and on policy changes, and on improved child and family health." The study also found that patients' empowerment strategies had led to improved health outcomes and quality of life, particularly among the chronically ill. There are a number of interventions that have attempted to do this. The limited results show that it is obviously not a simple task, but has to be a worthwhile one. When reviewing all the interventions that have tried to empower women as 'clients' it was clear that they were often one-off, small-scale interventions that were not sufficiently funded, supported, or evaluated. That may be the explanation for their limited success.

There is an increasing movement internationally that has looked at empowering patients through a range of methods, including patients' rights charters and health literacy programs, that intend to raise awareness and empower patient in their interactions with providers. We would argue that gender, and the different needs and challenges faced by women and men in such programs, need to be researched and documented in more detail.

In the quality of care literature and in the attempts to improve the quality of care in facilities across the globe the use of clinical audits and other measures of quality of care are increasingly being used. These processes rarely take account of gender. When gender audits are done, these are often one-off events and gender needs to be fundamentally integrated into these processes.

In conclusion, in this chapter we have illustrated that sexual and reproductive health services are particularly impacted by gender bias and discrimination. Gender norms around sex and reproduction are particularly strong, and there is also evidence that being seen to transgress gender norms in terms of sex and reproduction bring on particularly strong sanction from health care workers. We would therefore suggest that health workers working in these services are those that particularly need training and ongoing support on issues around gender. These are also services where there seems to be evidence that separate clinics and other services for men and women may be appropriate. In maternal health services more work needs to be done to involve men in services. The special needs of those seeking sexual and reproductive health services and the challenges of providing the services in a supportive, accessible, and nonjudgmental way that does not compromise the patient–provider relationship need to be taken into consideration when considering integrating these services into mainstream services.

REFERENCES

Afsar, H.A., S. Sohani, M. Younus, and S. Mohamad. 2006. Integration of sexual and reproductive health in the medical curriculum in Pakistan. *J Coll Physicians Surg Pak* 16 (1): 27–30.

Astbury, Jill. 2002. Mental health. In *Engendering International Health—The Challenge of Equity*, edited by G. Sen, A. George, and P. Östlin. Cambridge: MIT Press: 143–166.

AVSC International. 1997. *Profamilia's Clinics for Men: A Case Study*. New York: AVSC.

Baines, D. 2006. Staying with people who slap us around: Gender, juggling responsibilities and violence in paid (and unpaid) care work. *Gender, Work and Organization* 13 (2): 129–151.

Begum, V., P. de Colombani, S. Das Gupta, A.H. Salim, H. Hussain, M. Pietroni, S. Rahman, D. Pahan, and M. W. Borgdorff. 2001. Tuberculosis and patient gender in Bangladesh: Sex differences in diagnosis and treatment outcome. *International Journal of Tuberculosis and Lung Disease* 5 (7): 604–610.

Bertakis, K.D., R. Azari, L.J. Helms, E.J. Callahan, and J.A. Robbins. 2000. Gender differences in the utilization of health care services. *Journal of Family Practice* 49 (2): 147–152.

Bertakis, K.D., L.J. Helms, E.J. Callahan, R. Azari, P. Leigh, and J.A. Robbins. 2001. Patient gender differences in the diagnosis of depression in primary care. *Journal of Women's Health and Gender-Based Medicine* 10 (7): 689–698.

Blaauw, D., M. Ambegaokar, L. Penn-Kekana, C. Hongoro, and B. McPake. 2006. Neither robots nor angels: The 'dynamic responses' of health care workers and the unintended effects. *HSD Working Paper HSD/WP/09/06*. London: Health System Development Programme.

Bruce, J., and A. Jain. 1991. Improving the quality of care through operations research. *Prog Clin Biol Res* 371: 259–282.

Callahan, E.J, K.D. Bertakis, R. Azari, L.J. Helms, and J.A. Robbins. 1997. Depression in primary care: Patient factors that influence recognition. *Fam Med* 29 (3): 172–176.

Chikanda, A. 2005. Nurse migration from Zimbabwe: Analysis of recent trends and impacts. *Nurse Inq* 12 (3): 162–174.

Christofides, N.J., R.K. Jewkes, N. Webster, L. Penn-Kekana, N. Abrahams, and L.J. Martin. 2005. "Other patients are really in need of medical attention"— The quality of health services for rape survivors in South Africa. *Bulletin of the World Health Organization* 83 (7): 481–560.

Christofides, N.J., D. Muirhead, R.K. Jewkes, L. Penn-Kekana, and D.N. Conco. 2006. Women's experiences of and preferences for services after rape in South Africa: Interview study. *BMJ* 332: 209–213.

Cleary, P.D., B.J. Burns, and G.R. Nycz. 1990. The identification of psychiatry illness by primary care physicians: The effect of patient gender. *J Gen Intern Med* 5: 355–560.

Cottingham, J., and C. Myntti. 2002. Reproductive health: Conceptual mapping and evidence. In *Engendering International Health: The Challenge of Equity*, edited by G. Sen, A. George, and P. Östlin. Cambridge: MIT Press: 83–109.

d'Oliveira, A.F.P.L., S.G. Diniz, and L.B. Schraiber. 2002. Violence against women in health-care institutions: An emerging problem. *The Lancet* 359 (9318): 1681–1685.

de Pinho, H., R. Murthy, J. Moorman, and S. Weller. 2005. Integration of health services. In *The Right Reforms? Health Sector Reforms and Sexual and Reproductive Health*, edited by T.K.S. Ravindran and H. de Pinho. Johannesburg: Women's Health Project School of Public Health, University of the Witwatersrand: 215–263.

Dehne, K.L., R. Snow, and K.R. O'Reilly. 2000. Integration of prevention and care of sexually transmitted infections with family planning services: What is the evidence for public health benefits? *Bull World Health Organ* 78 (5): 628–639.

Dolin, P. 1998. Tuberculosis epidemiology from a gender perspective. In *Gender and Tuberculosis*, edited by V.K. Diwan, A. Thorson, and A. Winkvist. Göteborg: Nordic School of Public Health: 29–40.

Douthwaite, M., and P. Ward. 2005. Increasing contraceptive use in rural Pakistan: An evaluation of the Lady Health Worker Programme. *Health Policy and Planning* 20 (2): 117–123.

Fahy, T., and N. Fisher. 1992. Sexual contact between doctors and patients. *BMJ* 304 (6841): 1519–1520.

Fonn, S., and M. Xaba. 2001. Health Workers for Change: Developing the initiative. *Health Policy and Planning* 16: 13–18.

Freedman, L.P. 2005. Achieving the MDGs: Health systems as core social institutions. *Development* 48 (1): 19–24.

George, A., A. Iyer, and G. Sen. 2005. Gendered health systems biased against maternal survival: Preliminary findings from Koppal, Karnataka and India. *IDS Working Paper No 253*. Brighton: University of Sussex, Institute of Development Studies.

Giacomini, M., P. Rozee-Koker, and F. Pepitone-Arreola-Rockwell. 1986. Gender bias in human anatomy textbook illustrations. *Psychology of Women Quarterly* 10: 41–420.

Gisbers van Wijk, C.M.T., K.P. van Vliet, and A.M. Kolk. 1996. Gender perspectives and quality of care: Towards appropriate and adequate health care for women. *Social Science and Medicine* 43: 707–720.

Greenberg, D. 2001. A critical look at health literacy. *Adult Basic Education* 11: 67–79.

Gregory, R. 1999. Social capital theory and administrative reform: Maintaining ethical probity in public service. *Public Administration Review* 59: 63–75.

Hamberg, K. 2003. Few and sporadic gender elements in the medical curriculum at Umea. Physicians play a key role when implementing suggestions for improvement. *Lakartidningen* 100 (49): 4084–4085.

Hancock, J. 2004. Can mainstream services learn from male only sexual health pilot projects? *Sex Transm Infect* 80 (6): 484–487.

Hartigan, P. 2001. The importance of gender in defining and improving quality of care: Some conceptual issues. *Health Policy And Planning* 16 (1): 7–12.

Hausmann-Muela, S., J.M. Ribera, and I. Nyamongo. 2003. Health-seeking behaviour and the health system response. *DCPP Working Paper No. 14*. London: London School of Hygiene and Tropical Medicine.

Health Professions Regulatory Advisory Council. 2000. *Final Report to the Minister of Health and Long-Term Care: Effectiveness of Colleges' Complaints and Discipline Procedures for Professional Misconduct of a Sexual Nature.* Toronto: Health Professions Regulatory Advisory Council.

Healthcare Commission. 2006. *National Survey of NHS Staff 2006.* United Kingdom: Healthcare Commission.

Hellbernd, H., P. Brzank, A. May, and U. Maschewsky-Schneider. 2005. The S.I.G.N.A.L.-Intervention Project to combat violence against women. *Bundesgesundheitsblatt Gesundheitsforschung Gesundheitsschutz* 48 (3): 329–336.

Holroyd, E., S. Twinn, and P. Adab. 2004. Socio-cultural influences on Chinese women's attendance for cervical screening. *Journal of Advanced Nursing* 46 (1): 42–52.

Howell, E.A., B. Gardiner, and J. Concato. 2002. Do women prefer female obstetricians? *Obstet Gynecol* 99: 1031–1035.

Huezo, C.M., and C. Briggs. 1992. *Medical and Service Guidelines for Family Planning.* London: International Planned Parenthood Federation.

Jesani, A., and N. Madhiwalla. 2002. *Gender and Medical Education: Report of a National Consultation and Background Material.* Mumbai: Cehat for AMCHSS.

Jewkes, R., N. Abrahams, and Z. Mvo. 1998. Why do nurses abuse patients? Reflections from South African obstetric services. *Social Science and Medicine* 47 (11): 1781–1795.

Johansson, E., N.H. Long, V.K. Diwan, and A. Winkvist. 1999. Attitudes to compliance with tuberculosis treatment among women and men in Vietnam. *International Journal of Tuberculosis and Lung Disease* 3 (10): 862–868.

———. 2000. Gender and tuberculosis control: Perspectives on health seeking behaviour among men and women in Vietnam. *Health Policy* 52 (1): 33–51.

Johansson, E., and A. Winkvist. 2002. Trust and transparency in human encounters in tuberculosis control: Lessons learned from Vietnam. *Qualitative Health Research* 12 (4): 473–491.

Kim, J., and M. Motsei. 2002. "Women enjoy punishment": Attitudes and experiences of gender-based violence among PHC nurses in rural South Africa. *Social Science and Medicine* 54 (8): 1243–1254.

Kim, Y.M., A. Kols, F. Putjuk, M. Heerey, and W. Rinehart. 2003a. Participation by clients and nurse midwives in family planning decision making in Indonesia. *Patient Education and Counseling* 50 (3): 295–302.

Kim, Y.M., F. Putjuk, E. Basuki, and A. Kols. 2003b. *Increasing Client Participation in Family Planning Consultations: "Smart Patient" Coaching in Indonesia.* Baltimore: Johns Hopkins University Center for Communication Programs.

Lamont, J.A., and C. Woodward. 1994. Patient-physician sexual involvement: A Canadian survey of obstetrician-gynecologists. *CMAJ* 150: 1433–1439.

Lawrence, S.C., and K. Bendixen. 1992. His and hers: Male and female anatomy in anatomy texts for US medical students 1890–1989. *Social Science and Medicine* 35 (7): 925–934.

Lewin, S.A., J. Dick, P. Pond, M. Zwarenstein, G. Aja, B. van Wyk, X. Bosch-Capblanch, and M. Patrick. 2005. *Lay Health Workers in Primary and Community Health Care.* Cochrane Database Of Systematic Reviews. Cape Town: Health System Research Unit, Medical Research, Council of South Africa.

Long, N.H., E. Johansson, K. Lonnroth, B. Eriksson, A. Winkvist, and V.K. Diwan. 1999. Longer delays in tuberculosis diagnosis among women in Vietnam. *International Journal of Tuberculosis and Lung Disease* 3 (5): 388–393.

Manhoso, F.R., and L.A.K. Hoga. 2005. Men's experiences of vasectomy in the Brazilian Public Health Service. *International Nursing Review* 52: 101–108.

Miller, R., A. Fisher, K. Miller, L. Ndhlovu, M.B. Ndugga, I. Askew, D. Sanogo, and P. Tapsoba. 1997. *The Situation Analysis Approach to Assessing Family Planning And Reproductive Health Services: A Handbook.* New York: Population Council.

Monash University. 2007. Gender and medicine. Clayton: Gender and Medicine Research Unit, Monash Institute of Health Services Research, Monash Medical Centre. www.med.monash.edu.au/gendermed/gendermed.html.

Mumtaz, Z., S. Salway, M. Waseem, and N. Umer. 2003. Gender-based barriers to primary health care provision in Pakistan: The experience of female providers. *Health Policy and Planning* 18 (3): 261–269.

Munch, S. 2004. Gender-biased diagnosing of women's medical complaints: Contributions of feminist thought, 1970–1995. *Women and Health* 40 (1): 101–121.

Murphy, E., and C. Steele. 2000. *Client–Provider Interactions in Family Planning Services: Guidance from Research and Program Experience*. Washington, DC: United States Agency for International Development [USAID], Office of Population, Research Division, Maximizing Access and Quality Initiative [MAQ]: 11.

Nicolette, J.D., and M.D. Jacobs. 2000. Integration of women's health into an internal medicine core curriculum for medical students. *Academic Medicine* 75 (11): 1061–1065.

Nigenda, G., A. Langer, C. Kuchaisit, M. Romero, G. Rojas, M. Al-Osimy, J. Villar, J. Garcia, J. Al-Mazrou, H. Ba'aqee, G. Carroli, U. Farnot, P. Lumbiganon, J. Belizán, P. Bergsjo, L. Bakketeig, and G. Lindmark. 2003. Women's opinions on antenatal care in developing countries: Results of a study in Cuba, Thailand, Saudi Arabia and Argentina. *BMC Public Health* 3: 17.

Nutbeam, D., and I. Kickbusch. 2000. Advancing health literacy: A global challenge for the 21st century. *Health Promotion International* 15 (3): 183–184.

Onyango-Ouma, W., R. Laisser, M. Mbilima, M. Araoye, P. Pittman, I. Agyepong, M. Zakari, S. Fonn, M. Tanner, and C. Vlassoff. 2001. An evaluation of Health Workers for Change in seven settings: A useful management and health system development tool. *Health Policy and Planning* 16: 24–32.

Osika, I., B. Evengard, L. Waernulf, and F. Nyberg. 2005. The laundry-basket project—gender differences to the very skin. Different treatment of some common diseases in men and women. *Lakartidningen* 102 (40): 2846–2848.

Parkhurst, J.O., L. Penn-Kekana, D. Blaauw, D. Balabanova, K. Danishevski, S.A. Rahman, V. Onama, and F. Ssengooba. 2005. Health systems factors influencing maternal health services: A four-country comparison. *Health Policy* 73 (2): 127–138.

Parkhurst, J.O., and S.A. Rahman. 2007. Life saving or money wasting? Perceptions of caesarean sections among users of services in rural Bangladesh. *Health Policy* 80 (3): 392–401.

Patel, V., R. Araya, and P. Bolton. 2004. Treating depression in developing countries. *Trop Med Int Health* 9 (5): 539–541.

Paulson, S., M.E. Gisbert, and M. Quiton. 1996. *Case Studies of Two Women's Health Projects in Bolivia*. North Carolina, USA: Family Health International, Research Triangle Park.

Penn-Kekana, L., D. Blaauw, and H. Schneider. 2004. 'It makes me want to run away to Saudi Arabia': Management and implementation challenges for public financing reforms from a maternity ward perspective. *Health Policy and Planning* 19 (1): i71–i77.

Piet-Pelon, N.J., U. Rob, and M.E. Khan. 1999. *Men in India, Bangladesh and Pakistan: Reproductive Health Issues*. Dhaka: Kashraf Publishers.

Plunkett, B.A., P. Kohli, and M.P. Milad. 2002. The importance of physician gender in the selection of an obstetrician or a gynecologist. *American Journal of Obstetrics and Gynecology* 186 (5): 926–928.

Potter, J.E., O. Mojarro, and L. Nunez. 1987. The influence of health care on contraceptive acceptance in rural Mexico. *Studies in Family Planning* 18 (3): 144–156.

Raikes, A. 1992. Gender, PHC and the production of health-care services—issues For women's roles in health development for the next decade. *Ids Bulletin-Institute Of Development Studies* 23 (1): 19–28.

Rajeswari, R., V. Chandrasekaran, M. Suhadev, S. Sivasubramaniam, G. Sudha, and G. Renu. 2002. Factors associated with patient and health system delays in the diagnosis of tuberculosis in South India. *International Journal of Tuberculosis and Lung Disease* 6 (9): 789–795.

Ramanathan, M., and A.K. Khambete. 2007. *Case Study: The Gender Mainstreaming in Medical Education—The Indian Initiative.* Trivandrum, India: Achutha Menon Centre for Health Science Studies, Sree Chitra Tirunal Institute for Medical Sciences and Technology.

RamaRao, S., and A.M. Mir. 2004. *Transforming Relationships in Pakistani Villages.* New York: Quality/Calidad/Qualité Population Council.

Ringheim, K. 2002. When the client is male: Client–provider interaction from a gender perspective. *International Family Planning Perspectives* 28 (3): 170–175.

Rizk, D.E.E., M.A. El-Zubeir, A.M. Al-Dhaheri, F.R. Al-Mansouri, and H.S. Al-Jenaibi. 2005. Determinants of women's choice of their obstetrician and gynecologist provider in the UAE. *Acta Obstetricia et Gynecologica Scandinavica* 84 (1): 48–53.

Roter, D.L., J.A. Hall, and Y. Aoki. 2002. Physician gender effects in medical communication: A meta-analytic review. *Journal of the American Medical Association* 288 (6): 756–764.

Rogow, D. 2000. Alone you are nobody, together we float: the Manuela Ramos movement. Quality/Calidad/Qualité. New York: Population Council.

Rothman, B.K. 1982. *In Labor: Women and Power in the Birthplace.* New York: W.W. Norton and Company.

Sai, F.T. 1997. The ICPD program of action: Pious hope or a workable guide? *Health Transition Review* 7 (4): 1–55.

Schuler, S.R., L.M. Bates, and K. Islam. 2002. Paying for reproductive health services in Bangladesh: Intersections between costs, quality and culture. *Health Policy and Planning* 17 (3): 273–280.

Selden, C.R., M. Zorn, S.C. Ratzan, and R.M. Parker. 2000. *National Library of Medicine Current Bibliographies in Medicine: Health Literacy.* Bethesda, MD: National Institutes of Health, US Department of Health and Human Services.

Sen, G., and S. Batliwala. 2000. Empowering women for reproductive rights. In *Women's Empowerment and Demographic Processes: Moving Beyond Cairo*, edited by H.B. Presser and G. Sen. Oxford: Oxford University Press: 440.

Shepard, B.L. 2004. Addressing gender issues with men and couples: Involving men in sexual and reproductive health services in APROFE, Ecuador. *International Journal of Men's Health* 3 (3): 155–172.

Simmons, R., and C. Elias. 1994. The study of client–provider interactions—a review of methodological issues. *Studies in Family Planning* 25 (1): 1–17.

Smith, J.A., A. Braunack-Mayer, and G. Wittert. 2006. What do we know about men's help-seeking and health service use? *Medical journal of Australia* 184 (2): 81–83.

Sudha, G., C. Nirupa, M. Rajasakthivel, S. Sivasusbramanian, V. Sundaram, S. Bhatt, K. Subramaniam, E. Thiruvalluvan, R. Mathew, G. Renu, and T. Santha. 2003. Factors influencing the care-seeking behaviour of chest symptomatics: A community-based study involving rural and urban population in Tamil Nadu, South India. *Tropical Medicine and International Health* 8 (4): 336–341.

Thomasson, G.O. 1999. Educating physicians to prevent sex-related contact with patients. *JAMA* 281 (5): 419–420.

Thorson, A., N.P. Hoa, N.H. Long, P. Allebeck, and V.K. Diwan. 2004. Do women with tuberculosis have a lower likelihood of getting diagnosed? Prevalence and case detection of sputum smear positive pulmonary TB, a population-based study from Vietnam. *J Clin Epidemiol* 57 (4): 398–402.

Thorson, A., and E. Johansson. 2004. Equality or equity in health care access: A qualitative study of doctors' explanations to a longer doctors' delay among female TB patients in Vietnam. *Health Policy* 68 (1): 37–46.

UN Millennium Project. 2005. *Who's Got the Power? Transforming Health Systems for Women and Children. Summary Version of the Report of the Task Force on Child Health and Maternal Health.* New York: United Nations Development Programme.

Verdonk, P., L.J.L. Mans, and A.L.M. Lagro-Janssen. 2005. Integrating gender into a basic medical curriculum. *Medical Education* 39 (11): 1118–1125.

Vlassoff, C., and C. Garcia Moreno. 2002. Placing gender at the centre of health programming: Challenges and limitations. *Soc Sci Med* 54 (11): 1713–1723.

Wallerstein, N. 2006. What is the evidence on effectiveness of empowerment to improve health? *Health Evidence Network Report.* Copenhagen: WHO Regional Office for Europe.

WHO. 1999. *Integrating STI Management into Family Planning Services: What Are the Benefits?* Geneva: WHO.

———. 2000. *Global Tuberculosis Control: WHO Report 2000.* Geneva: WHO.

———. 2001. *The World Health Report 2001. Mental Health: New Understanding. New Hope.* Geneva: WHO.

———. 2006. *The World Health Report 2006. Working Together for Health.* Geneva: WHO.

Wilbers, D., G. Veenstra, H.B. van de Wiel, and W.C. Weijmar Schultz. 1992. Sexual contact in the doctor–patient relationship in the Netherlands. *BMJ* 304 (6841): 1531–1534.

World Medical Association. 1981. Declaration of Lisbon: The rights of a patient. http://www.wma.net. Cern, France.

Zuckerman, M., N. Navizedeh, J. Feldman, S. McCalla, and H. Minkoff. 2002. Determinants of women's choice of obstetrician/gynecologist. *J Womens Health Gend Based Med* 11: 175–180.

8 Exploring the Gendered Dimensions of Human Resources for Health

Asha George

INTRODUCTION

The World Health Report (WHR) 2006 puts forward an inclusive definition of health workers:

> "Health workers are all people primarily engaged in actions with the primary intent of enhancing health." This is consistent with the WHO definition of health systems as comprising all activities with the primary goal of improving health—inclusive of family caregivers, patient–provider partners, part-time workers (especially women), health volunteers and community workers. (WHO, 2006, p. xvi)

The plurality of health workers mentioned reflects the broad and diverse nature of health care tasks that exist, integrated by the division of medical labor specific to each country's health system. The hierarchies that mark and coordinate such a diverse health workforce are determined by technical needs, but also reflect power relations that structure health systems.

Gender,[1] as one among other power relations, plays a critical role in influencing the structural location of women and men in the health labor force and their subjective experience of that location. It affects how work is recognized, valued, and supported with differential consequences at the professional level (career trajectories, pay, training and other technical resources, professional networks) and at the personal level (personal safety, stress, health, autonomy, self-esteem, family, and other social relationships).

Nonetheless the gendered nature of human resources for health has not figured largely in health research or policy, despite current attention to the crisis in human resources for health.[2] This lack of attention is significant considering the dominant role that women play in health service delivery (Wirth, 2008). In 10 OECD countries and the Russian Federation between 1993 and 1997, women made up between 62–85% of the health labor force (Gupta et al., 2003, p. 7). In the USA, frontline[3] health workers are 79% female and were the fastest growing segment of all health care occupations and of all occupations in the economy in 2003 (Schindel et al., 2006, pp. 11, 13). Yet despite women's numerical presence in the health labor force, sex as a variable is often not reported in health labor-force surveys or in human resources studies, making a gender analysis impossible.

In addition to undertaking sex-disaggregated analysis to count women's presence in the health labor force, a gender analysis also examines how the health work is conceptualized. Health labor-force statistics rarely incorporate part-time work, paid work that is informally arranged, or unpaid work; spheres of work where women are overrepresented. In undercounting women's health work these gender biases in description fundamentally conceal how health systems function on the basis of female labor.

In addition to hiding women's contribution to health work, gender bias also stratifies their location across and within health occupations. Health occupations that require fewer years of education, earn lower earnings, and face more insecurities during health sector reform processes, also have higher proportions of women working in them (Standing, 1997) (Table 8.1 and 8.2). Within the same occupation, gender bias results in women earning less than men. Although the WHR 2006 suggests that there are few differences in male and female pay in the health sector (WHO, 2006), other research differs from this assessment (Robinson, 2001, cited by Di Martino, 2003; Adams, 2005; Yutzie et al., 2005; Halford and Savage, 1997; Reichenbach, 2007; Kanchanachitra et al., 2007).

Gender as a power relation, apart from determining the structural location of women and men in the health labor force, also defines the subjective evaluation and experience of that location. Women are more likely to be stereotyped as caring health personnel than men. This not only excludes,

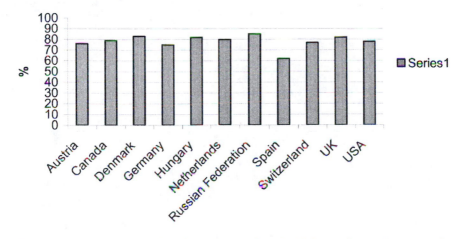

Figure 8.1   Percentage of female health workers in 11 Luxembourg income study countries, 1993–1997, adapted from Gupta et al. (2003).

Table 8.1   Health Professions in British Columbia, Canada

Category	Female	Post-Secondary Education in Years	Approximate Average Annual Earnings 1986	Total Number 1989–1990
Certified dental assistants	99.8%	0.85	CAN 21,000	3,606
Registered nurses	97.6%	2–4	CAN 25,000	30,140
Dental hygienists	97.3%	2	CAN 21,000	880
Occupational therapists	96.7%	4	CAN 23,000	448
Licensed practical nurses	93.8%	0.85	CAN 20,000	6,387
Physiotherapists	86.9%	4	CAN 28,000	1,575
Registered psychiatric nurses	73.7%	2		2,087
Pharmacists	44.9%	5	CAN 34,000	2,379
Psychologists	43.1%	7–9		788
Physicians	19.0%	8+	CAN 90,000	6,421
Optometrists	17.6%	5–6		227
Dentists	10.9%	7–8	CAN 73,000	2,002
Podiatrists	3.7%	6+		54

Source: Kazanjian (1993), citing data from Job Futures British Columbia, Employment and Immigration Canada, and the Cooperative Database, Health Human Resources Unit, University of British Columbia.

Table 8.2   Health Professions in Nicaragua

	Female	Unemployed	Earning less than 300 USD	Rely on single employment	In public sector
Nurses	95%	6%	52%	95%	95%
Pharmacists	79%	2%	14%	70%	24%
Technicians	73%	8%	29%	82%	90%
Dentists	65%	4%	16%	71%	56%
Doctors	41%	1%	19%	60%	81%

Source: Adapted from Nigenda and Machado (2000), citing data from Labour Market of Health Workforce in Nicaragua 1996. Ministry of Health/World Bank/Funsalud.

or even worse excuses, men, but also presents a homogenized, static understanding of women's capacities. At the same time, the specific needs of women health workers are often not addressed, whether it is child care or protection from violence. These problems are seen as caused by women, rather than by how health services are organized.

Many gender distortions in the organization of health systems, whether in terms of child care, sexual harassment, home care, or unintentional skill mixing, are absorbed by women through individual adjustments at times to the detriment of their work and for some even to their own health and livelihoods. While the availability of female health professionals is an important demand from female patients, a gendered division of labor that primarily places women in restricted, low-valued, and insecure work situations, makes it less likely for them to exert the autonomy required to improve service delivery and champion patient's interests.

Throughout this review chapter I further detail the gender analysis presented in this introduction through an examination of gender dynamics in medicine, nursing, community health workers, and home carers. I also examine from a gender perspective current issues concerning delegation, migration, and violence, which cut across these categories of health workers. I conclude with brief policy recommendations for each section.

EVIDENCE BASE FOR THIS REVIEW

As this chapter represents a summarized subsection of a larger review on gender and human resources in health (George, 2007a), interested readers are encouraged to refer to that commissioned paper. The terms of reference for this chapter were to review both formal and informal aspects of human resources for health to highlight themes, concerns, and key policy recommendations based on the existing literature. During the final quarter of 2006, 534 journal articles, book chapters, and Internet reports were compiled into an EndNote database. Web sites and search engines were used, bibliographies of articles checked, and correspondence with other experts undertaken. Although most of the literature reviewed was in English, some of it was also in Spanish and Portuguese. Despite the large amount of literature compiled, the information generated is skewed. Most research on gender aspects of human resources for health is descriptive with very little evaluation of interventions, programs, or policies. OECD countries generate most of the available research on gender and human resources for health, with the US being the most prolific. In contrast for many non-OECD countries, information on gender issues in human resources for health is derived from a single article. Most publications focus on the dominant profession—medicine—with less research and documentation of other kinds of health workers. Many research articles did not provide sex-disaggregated data and instead presented data by health worker category. In addition, health workers are not classified uniformly across the world. This complexity complicates efforts to systematically compile information about human resources for health internationally, let alone undertake a gender analysis of human resources for health.

GENDERED EXPERIENCES IN HUMAN RESOURCES FOR HEALTH

This section applies a gender analysis to a few occupational groups like medicine, nursing, health workers at the community level, and home carers. As health systems vary dramatically across nations, the occupational meaning of a doctor or a nurse cannot be assumed to be universally valid. While this review cannot detail the contextual details of every national health system mentioned, it does mention the national contexts from which examples are drawn.

As not all health professions are covered, this review will not provide a comprehensive gender analysis of the diverse forms of work that the health labor force undertakes. While the literature on gender dimensions of certain health occupations, like dentistry, pharmacists, and other technicians, is not available at a global level, the literature on midwifery is already well represented in international health debates and too heterogeneous to summarize within the space constraints of this review.

Medicine

Medicine is the premier health occupation that rules the division of labor within health care. In this section, I briefly review how medicine is feminizing before discussing various kinds of occupational biases that work against women in medicine, with reference largely to doctors but not exclusively so. As discussed in the introduction, more details are provided with respect to how the position of women in medicine is structurally disadvantaged, as well as subjectively biased through stereotypical assumptions.

Although overall female representation in medicine is only just beginning to reach 50%[4] in some countries, some projections for the future are optimistic given that female medical students currently equal or surpass male medical students. The increasing female representation among doctors has sparked debate about the consequences of medicine feminizing. Reactions range from concerns about a decline in the medical profession, as well as hopes that women will promote a more humane workplace and improved quality of care. The concerns expressed are likely to be overreactions and the hopes premature (Riska, 2001), with the attention paid reflecting anxiety about women beginning to approach parity in medicine, the most elite health profession dominating the clinical hierarchy of health systems.

Although the numbers of women entering medicine is reaching parity, the empirical reality indicates that women are far from taking over the reigns of power within medicine as a profession. Female doctors are less likely to specialize and more likely to be under- and unemployed in comparison to their male colleagues (Frenk et al., 1999; Nigenda and Machado, 2000; Kassak et al., 2006; Kanchanachitra et al., 2007). Although women are increasingly entering medicine, they do so on terms that are not equal with their male colleagues. While this is also due to the contradictory forces of specialization and cost-rationalization that are internally dividing health professions (Friedson, 1986; Annandale et al., 2004; Adams, 2005), the gender biases faced by women entering medicine remain substantial. Consequently, women are in extremely few positions of leadership in medicine in the US (Tesch et al., 1995; Magrane et al., 2005; Jagsi et al., 2006). The contrast between women forming the base of the health sector but not being represented in policy or other leadership positions is also found in low-income countries (UNIDO, 1989, cited by Standing, 2000; Dwisetyani Utomo et al., 2006).

Occupational Gender Biases

One form of gender bias is expressed through the differences in working hours between female and male doctors (Knaul et al., 2000; Kassak et al., 2006), although these differences are neither static (Dedobbeleer et al., 1995) nor universal (Gupta et al., 2003). From a gender lens, the small difference in working hours between women and men that seems to favor women might in fact disfavor women once domestic responsibilities are considered (De Koninck et al., 1993; Grandis et al., 2004). Indeed some of the gender differences in working hours are more apparent between single and married medical professionals, with the brunt being borne by married females (Carr et al., 1998; Adams, 2005).

In the absence of adequate support, women make informed decisions that may constrain their professional capacity in order to balance their professional and personal lives (Elston, 1993). Some female doctors consequently select specializations that enable them to have a family life, rather than specializations in 'urgentology.' These efforts remain invisible to management, contributing to biased statements from male colleagues like "You women do not plan your career adequately" (De Koninck et al., 1997, p. 1829).

In balancing these double work burdens, offering part-time working hours may not necessarily resolve gender inequities. Several studies found that while women in medicine chose part-time work or consider leaving full-time work due to family responsibilities, men do so due to private practice or higher salaries elsewhere (Levinson et al., 1993; Foster et al., 2000; Mayorova et al., 2005; Fox et al., 2006). Some of these dynamics may be changing across generations (Warde et al., 1996).

In Switzerland, although part-time specialist training was more readily taken up by women (33%) than men (6%), 10 years after the recommendation to initiate part-time training had been passed for all specialties these part-time training opportunities were more likely to be found in female-dominated specialties than in male dominated specialties (Heuss and Hanggeli, 2003). This suggests that it is not enough to ensure that part-time or family leave is more available within medical practice, but that it must also be done in ways that doesn't retrench gender stereotypes in medicine. In Sweden, although parents can decide who takes the majority of parental leave, in light of research that showed that women mostly did this, a certain proportion of it is now reserved exclusively for fathers (Bergman and Hobson, 2002).

As important as gender equitable family leave policies are, sex differences still remain even when controlling for the time constraints of balancing family responsibilities and professional lives (Tesch et al., 1995; Halford and Savage, 1997; Schroen et al., 2004). This implies significant gender discrimination, which medical school faculty members in the US report that they were poorly prepared to handle (Foster et al., 2000; Carr et al., 2000, 2003). One successful effort that helped to counteract such bias in the US, leading to an increase in 4 to 20 female associate professors in three years, involved updating female faculty members about promotion criteria annually and providing a yearly assessment about each faculty member's appropriateness for promotion (Fried et al., 1996).

Although these focused interventions are important in boosting women's advancement in medicine, in order to succeed on a longer-term basis, efforts must also address gender biases that permeate the everyday working cultures of medical practice (Reichenbach and Brown, 2004). Hamel and colleagues (2006) note that a culture of working 60 to 70 hours per week, meetings held outside of traditional working hours, and tenure clocks disfavor faculty members in medicine who have family responsibilities. For this reason, Standing and Baume (2001) argue that although focused affirmative action measures might achieve targets, this by itself is not enough. Moreover, a focus on targets alone might lead to backlash, as it focuses on the individual that is promoted rather than changing the organization or on the management's responsibility for integrating diversity (McCourt, 2000, cited by Standing and Baume, 2001).

Female faculty in the US identified strategic measures that are required to improve female representation in academic medicine (McGuire et al., 2004). More action-oriented research needs to be carried out with health professionals to identify the strategic measures required to promote gender equality in their own work environments. Bickel (2000) concludes that the reasons for women not advancing in medicine are multiple, leading to cumulative disadvantages. They include women's strategic choices, sexism, cultural stereotypes, constraints in combining family responsibilities with professional opportunities, and lack of effective mentoring. Multiple interventions are required to address these various forms of gender bias, which include but also go beyond improved family leave policies.

Stereotyped Gender Assumptions

Although many studies in the US also conclude by recommending mentoring for women, mentoring alone cannot address all the forms of gender discrimination at play, nor does it address the pervasiveness of male norms and male working models. Women physicians in Quebec, Canada, reflected, "You have to act like they do. They can have a sex, but not us." Another female physician in the same study said, "I felt as if I were asexual because being a woman made no difference, as long as I did not get pregnant" (De Koninck et al., 1997, p. 1828). Equality becomes understood as conforming to male norms.

Does the increase of women in general practice challenge gender stereotypes in medicine? A UK study found that many women entered general practice expecting to be generalists, but find themselves facing expectations to focus on women's health (reproductive health, pediatrics, and psychosocial work) (Brooks, 1998). Some female doctors took on a more 'caring' approach to their work. Nonetheless, despite being doctors, because of their more 'caring' work, they also felt more threatened by nurse practitioners. In contrast, women physicians who wanted to stay as generalists sought to work in practices with other nurses or nurse practitioners in order to retain their doctor role. They were hostile to female patients who did not respect their professional boundaries, which they interpreted as a lack of respect for their professional achievement. Furthermore, they were unhappier if working part-time or with other men, as then they could not avoid the gendering of their work.

Brooks (1998) concludes that both strategies followed by women general practitioners in the UK are problematic, as they both reinforce conservative gender stereotypes. They also do not contest a gendered form of accountability (West, 1993), where women are expected to have both technical and emotional skills (help manage the practice and office personnel, as well as their patients), while men are only expected to be technical. Due to these gendered expectations of women being more emotionally sensitive to patients and to office personnel, female doctors are more likely to disappoint their colleagues and patients, even if they are behaving the same as their male colleagues (Brooks, 1998).

A gender analysis reveals that interpretations of women's roles as either being inherently problematic or essentially caring serve to deflect attention from "the social processes that naturalise and depoliticise the different positions of women and men in the organisation of health care" (Wegar, 1993, p. 173). These social processes also reflect power relations enacted through professional socialization, organization, and practice. A study in the US found that while female nurses viewed their gender as an important link to female residents, female residents placed more primacy on their occupational status than their gender in relating to female nurses (Wear and Keck-McNulty, 2004).

Nursing

In contrast to medicine, nursing has always been female dominated. The following section reviews the historical evolution of nursing. This serves as a useful background for contemporary discussions about delegation, as it places in context the professional struggles that shape the division of labor in health care.

Divided Histories of Nursing

Despite being a female-dominated profession, from its origins gender bias constrained the location of nursing within the division of labor in health care in the UK. Nurses were stereotyped as innately qualified to undertake the caring, nurturing, and menial tasks required to complement male doctor's curative roles (Maggs, 1983; Carpenter, 1993). It is in this context that nursing emerged as an occupation secondary to and supportive of medicine. Over time as medicine continued to specialize, the changing division of labor in health care meant that certain groups of nurses began to acquire elements of medical knowledge, although nursing was largely still rooted in hygiene and housekeeping. By the 1960s in the UK the resulting differences were firmly established between untrained nursing auxiliaries and assistants, enrolled nurses with a two-year practically based training, and registered nurses with three years of more academically focused training. These social divisions continue today, as clinical nursing in particular seeks to professionalize in ways that exclude its lower ranks (Carpenter, 1993).

Considering these divisions, the managerial reforms, and the cost-rationalization pressures on the NHS, Carpenter is cautious about assumptions that female nurses are natural allies to or advocates for patients. Instead he suggests that the more divisions occur that mimic curative hierarchies in medicine, the more likely it is for lower-level ranks of nursing to fall behind and be less sympathetic to patients (1993, p. 112). Hagbaghery and colleagues (2004) similarly argue that in Iran today, nurses avoid independent caring roles even though they may have the knowledge and skills to attend to patients, as their authority and self-confidence is undermined by the physician-centered and routine-oriented hospital culture they are located in.

Manley (1995) similarly reflects on the social divisions that mark nursing in the US historically and currently. In addition, Manley (1995) notes how similar tactics deployed by occupational groups led to different outcomes due to their social position, rather than by what their occupations contributed to society. While the 1910 Flexner report reformed medicine in the US by eliminating the three-year medical degree, raising medical school standards, and restricting entry into medicine, the 1923 Goldmark report failed to do the same for nursing. Doctors, as a socially more powerful group, framed nursing as instrumental in nature and thus influenced the compromises made in the Goldmark report. As a result, nursing emerged as a stratified profession divided between highly educated registered professional nurses and vocationally trained practical nurses. These divisions have continued as government funding enabled minority women to train for lower levels of nursing, but not for baccalaureate training, which determines teaching and leadership positions (Table 8.3).

As seen in the UK and US, embedded within the histories of nursing are the markers of social divisions that continue today. In South Africa, nursing not only evolved as a profession along Apartheid segregationist lines, but also along class lines (Rispel and Schneider, 1990). Currently, enrolled nurses feel alienated as they are lost in routine activities, misused, materialized, and domesticated in contrast to registered nurses (van der Merwe, 1999). At the same time race, class, and gender dynamics also disenfranchised native medical aides trained in battlefields and in the mines of South Africa. They failed to get recognition as nurses and were relegated into preventive work for sexually transmitted and tropical diseases, plague, and rodent control (Burns, 1998).

In Thailand, nursing is similarly characterized by various social groups that serve different roles (Muecke and Srisuphan, 1989). An elite professional cadre exists with little in common with provincial nurses or auxiliaries trained for basic patient care. Male nurses differentiate themselves from female nurses by self-selecting into areas that confirm ideals of masculinity, for instance, orthopedic nursing (large motor skills), in anesthesia, operating rooms, emergency units, and intensive care units (high-technology and high-risk mortality), for Buddhist monks (taboo for women), or in community nursing (great independence).

Other countries reflect similar findings. In Ghana, Malawi, Zambia, and Kenya professional nurses succeeded in banning the training of less-qualified enrolled nurses (Dovlo, 2004). In Nicaragua, 50% of nurses are called professionals, although the majority have no university degree (Nigenda and Machado, 2000). In India, private sector nurses who are informally

Table 8.3 Occupational Position of African Americans within Nursing from 1970s to 1990s

Nursing Categories	*African-American Nurses*		
	1970	*1980*	*1990*
Registered Nurses	6.2%	6.9%	7.4%
Licensed Practical Nurses	21.6%	17.3%	17.6%
Nursing Aides	21.0%	23.3%	30.7%

Source: Manley (1995, p. 307) and unpublished data from Patrica Roos, US Bureau of Labour Statistics (1991).

trained are the worst off, as they earn the lowest wages and have few labor rights (Iyer and Jesani, 1995; Baru, 2005). These axes of differentiation in terms of education, roles, and career paths make it hard for nurses to galvanize collective professional power.

Although medicine is also increasingly stratified, its professional power hinges on its ability to retain discretion and judgment. The essence of medicine is treasured as an indeterminate art of healing that cannot be standardized or generalized (Jamous and Peloille, 1970). Although women's history as healers of the sick and reducers of risk during delivery exists, it is largely obscured. DeVries notes that women are stereotypically seen to "care for the sick. But the care they give is palliative care. They are a presence during uncertain episodes of sickness, but they do not alter its course or reduce its impact through intervention" (1993, p. 144). Gender bias therefore plays a critical role in stereotyping medicine as curative from nursing, which is perceived to be caring in ways that are instrumental and routinized. Nonetheless, as discussed in the next section, current pressures affecting health systems has led to increasing differentiation within medicine and nursing, at times blurring and at other times reinforcing the historical struggles between them.

Delegation

The histories and policy pressures that foreground the blurring of professional boundaries through substitution and delegation are specific to the health sectors they belong to. They encompass war and conflict situations, cost containment pressures, and efforts to expand health service delivery. The gender dynamics of delegation also need to be considered on a contextual basis. For example, in Malawi as nurses with internationally recognized degrees depart for better financed health systems, reforms in 2001 created parallel cadres with opportunities for men, rather than women, that ensured retention by withdrawing international recognition (Palmer, 2006).

In other contexts, efforts to delegate tasks to female-dominated professions have met with resistance from male-dominated professions. In Bangladesh, in efforts to scale up emergency obstetric training, nurses face resistance whether in normal deliveries or in more skilled activities due to biased attitudes against them and competition from trainee doctors (Tajul Islam et al., 2006). In Brazil, obstetric nurses face resistance from managers and doctors who fear reputational and financial losses if they let nurses attend normal births. These current organizational tensions have revived historical differences between nurses and doctors, left professional differences about the knowledge and management of birth processes unresolved, and impeded service delivery reforms in Brazil (Corrêa and Piola, 2003).

These professional tensions are not insurmountable. In Mozambique, initial hostility to delegation efforts changed to collaboration and mutual recognition as professional boundaries changed (Bergstrom, 1998, cited by Dovlo, 2004). In Ghana, leadership from influential obstetric-gynecologists supported the enhanced role of midwives in postabortion care (Karolinska Institute, 2001, cited by Dovlo, 2004). Reduced workloads and increased time for higher professional skills are key incentives for professionals to aide delegation efforts (Dovlo, 2004). However, transitions need political skills to manage, even when benefits to higher-level professionals and to health service delivery more broadly are objectively detailed. In Brazil, nurses were enlisted as supervisors to community health agents, helping to neutralize their resistance to this new cadre (Tendler and Freedheim, 1994).

A key gender concern is that the professional reordering of health occupations restructures health systems to do more in different ways, rather than to stretch further on a cheaper basis, resorting to underpaid and unsupported female labor. In the absence of intentional delegation, unintentional skill mixing is the informal norm (Gerein et al., 2006). In the UK, nurses were equivocal about undertaking doctor's tasks by unofficially prescribing, diagnosing, taking blood, and putting in cannulas, as it drew them away from their traditional roles as nurses and overburdened them with the low status, menial aspects of medical work. Yet the tacit acceptance of these blurred boundaries, "ensured that patients got symptomatic relief, tests were carried out on time, treatment continued without interruptions" (Allen, 2004, p. 256). By unofficially taking on greater responsibilities and risks, nurses protected patients from the turbulent processes of coordinating care in large hospitals and smoothed organizational tensions (Allen, 2004). Paid home care workers in the US (Stacey, 2006) and auxiliary staff in India (Iyer and Jesani, 1995) similarly take on greater responsibilities and risks than their formal designations, with tacit understanding from management and policy makers that without doing so patient care would suffer and health services would stall. In order to succeed substitution, delegation efforts need to assess how gender hierarchies among the health occupations are formally and informally sustained and subverted, in order to alleviate rather than exacerbate current gender inequalities.

Community Health Workers

Community health workers are not a uniform category. They include volunteers, auxiliaries, and even nurses depending on the health systems they belong to. This section discusses the gender biases these rural health workers face at multiple levels that undermine the appropriateness and effectiveness of their behavior both at a personal and professional level.

For many female health workers questions about the legitimacy of their work start at home, though this is open to change even in conservative rural contexts like in Pakistan (Mumtaz et al., 2003). In India, similar experiences were reported by female auxiliary health staff; however, gender still colored how support was viewed and valued (George, 2007b). Several female staff reported that the main reason for not going for training, a requisite for promotion, was the lack of household support. Male colleagues also based their household status on their earning power, but they saw household support as an entitlement rather than as something conditional.

At the community level, female auxiliary health staff are often deployed to deliver services that are closely intertwined with the gendered beliefs and practices that form an intimate part of community identities. In South Asia, their work draws them into contentious discussions about family size, raising the age of marriage, where and how birth should take place (Blum et al., 2006; George, 2007b). Being female alone does not mean that these gender norms are contested. In Brazil, Portella and Gouveia (1997) argue that by relying on only female staff the female health agent program reinforced the assumption that only women can provide maternal health advice. It failed to contest conservative gender relations that excused men from taking responsibility for child care, failed to sanction forms of male sexuality that increased STI risk among their wives, and failed to question norms around domestic violence that inhibited women from talking to male health workers in their homes.

In Indonesia, community-based female volunteers were women who were village elite role models. As such their social status helped to further the success of the family planning program; however, it also reinforced stereotypical roles of female domesticity, voluntarism, and caregiving in reproductive roles (Dwisetyani Utomo et al., 2006). Reflecting on a South African lay health worker program that relied on volunteer female labor, Daniels and colleagues (2005) conclude that although it opened up spaces and aspirations for women, more effort was required to avoid the partial retrenching of gender stereotypes.

Gender bias that idealizes women's volunteer labor and devalues their skilled professional needs can combine with service delivery biases. In India, as auxiliary health staff working at the community level, female health workers are responsible for health education and promotive and preventive health care tasks. Yet in increasingly commercialized health systems, communities want curative commodities like tablets and injections, rather than health education that encourages self-reliance measures. As one respondent in Thailand noted, with respect to village volunteers, "They know nothing, they're not necessary because the village is so close to town. When people are ill, they go to the private hospital outside of town for good service and technology" (Kauffman and Myers, 1997, p. 253).

Without curative symbols to aid them or functioning referral systems to back them, female auxiliary staff in India are sometimes referred to by communities as a *dai* (traditional birth attendant). In contrast, male auxiliary health staff are referred to as 'malaria doctors' because they deploy health care commodities in the form of blood smear slides and malaria tablets. Preexisting social hierarchies are reinforced, as male village elites or male peddlers can take on the role of village doctors, but lower caste, female birth attendants or volunteers do not dare to entertain such aspirations, despite at times having training and linkages with government or NGO programs (Pinto, 2004).

As one respondent from Pakistan noted, "Compared to men, women must work harder to be accepted as serious and responsible workers. They first have to overcome the image of being *seedi-saadi* (simple-minded) housewives and then prove themselves as professionals" (Mumtaz et al., 2003, p. 265). This also explains why nurses in Zimbabwe persisted in the use of weighing scales in antenatal care checkups, although guidelines reduced the number of visits and eliminated the weighing scale. The clinical symbolism of the weighing scale and multiple visits served a more powerful purpose in the patient–provider interaction than what was rationalized by the clinical evidence base behind the policy change (Mathole et al., 2005). Female staff whose professionalism and social status is questioned due to gender biases may rely on such clinical symbols more than male counterparts.

While these family, community, and health system pressures undermine the credibility of female health staff, they face discrimination from management hierarchies within government administration. In India, male auxiliary health staff can unofficially assume senior supervisory positions at the PHC level, but such informal promotion is not allowed for female auxiliary health staff. Instead they are more likely to be scapegoated for problems in service delivery than their male peers (George, 2007b). In India, with limited educational backgrounds and with teaching as the only other rural salaried occupation open to women, female auxiliary health workers are not in a position to bargain for better working conditions (Iyer and Jesani, 1995).

The gendered challenges to female health staff working at the community level are not insurmountable. In Matlab, Bangladesh, the personal prestige of female health staff was delicately negotiated in ways that redefined the meaning of *purdah* (seclusion) for female staff and the communities they worked in. The success of the program relied not only on its accommodative approach to redefining gender norms to affirm the personal prestige of female staff, but also due to its twinning of personal prestige with professional prestige (Simmons et al., 1992).

After gaining the initial approval of village elites, female auxiliary health staff also gained respect because they gave out medicines and injections and came to be seen as the 'little doctor' linked to 'big doctor' through referral systems that were adequately resourced. When senior staff visited them in the field they symbolically showed signs of respect to their more junior, female colleagues rather than reprimanding them in public. By combining perseverance with these multiple supports, female health workers over time assumed increasingly influential and respected roles in the villages they worked in (Simmons et al., 1992). Community-based female lay health workers in South Africa and Brazil were similarly supported through multiple relationships that ensured their continued performance and motivation (Daniels et al., 2005; Tendler and Freedheim, 1994). Although these system-wide improvements will benefit all health workers at the community level, it is notable how these systemic improvements are often undertaken in a gender-blind manner, if at all. Too often community-based health workers are expected to improve health outcomes, despite the lack of functioning health systems, reflecting false expectations that are themselves gendered.

Home Carers

Self-care and home care form the base of health care systems with women primarily carrying out home care, whether paid or unpaid, formally regulated or informally arranged. This section reviews literature that documents the extent of home care; its gender dimensions and its consequences for women themselves and for health systems more broadly.

It is estimated that 90% of illness care is provided within the home (WHO, 2000; Uys, 2003, cited by Ogden et al., 2006). Not only are women numerically more involved in care work within families and homes (Taylor et al., 1996, cited by Ogden et al., 2006; Sugiura et al., 2004; Lopez-Ortega et al., 2007), but significant gender differences exist between male and female carers in terms of their social background, kind of patients looked after, and support received in undertaking their care work. In the US, informal female caregivers are more likely than informal male caregivers to be age 65 or older, African-American, married, unemployed, and primary caregivers, and yet provide more intensive and complex care (Navaie-Waliser et al., 2002). Furthermore, female caregivers face more difficulties with care provision and struggle more in balancing caregiving with other family and employment responsibilities than male caregivers (Navaie-Waliser et al., 2002; Tiegs et al., 2006). In Japan, recipients of female caregivers tended to be older and have more cognitive disorders than the recipients of male caregivers. While female caregivers spent more time providing care and undertook more care activities, male caregivers were more likely to use the home helper service provided by the insurance scheme (Sugiura et al., 2004).

Caregiving at home goes beyond assisting with curative or palliative health care to include basic services of a broad variety. A study in Chile found that only 40 minutes out of 9 hours of daily care was spent on administering medicines, physiotherapy exercises, giving injections, dressing wounds, and inserting catheters. A third of the time was spent on domestic labor. Most importantly, half of the time was spent keeping the sick person company, maintaining their comfort, and observing their possible needs. Most informal family carers slept in the same room or very near the ill person (Reca et al., 2002). In this sense, the great majority of home care requires constant attendance, since it cannot be regularly scheduled. It also entails substantial emotional involvement (Bunting, 2001).

While the time spent on such disparate activities and the emotional work involved may not be valued by formal health systems, both are seen as critical nurturing activities by caregivers themselves. Although formal caregivers were paid poorly and looked down upon by others due to menial aspects of their work, they themselves drew a strong sense of pride from their work. They felt that they directly contributed to their patient's comfort and dignity and knew more about the patient than other more skilled health workers who depended on them. Many of them had also turned to home care as a more humane and autonomous alternative to providing care in formal care institutions, where they felt that working conditions and quality of care were unsupportable (Stacey, 2006).

Care work, while critical to societies and valued by recipients and caregivers alike, continues to be marginalized by legal and labor systems. While the Fair Labor Standards Act in the US was amended in 1974 to include domestic workers, so they can claim the right to a minimum wage and to overtime pay, paid domestic caregivers were exempted because they are largely seen as 'companions' to the elderly and disabled, rather than as 'workers' (Biklen, 2003, cited by Stacey, 2006). In the US, long-term care providers, of which home care aides are a subset, are among the lowest wage earners in the health system, with the smallest wage gain in the past four years and the highest percentage of minority workers (almost 50%; Schindel et al., 2006, p. 70). Moreover, 40% to 45% of home care aides in the US lack health insurance (Lipson and Carol, 2004). High levels of turnover are reported in this sector, although little research has been undertaken to document it (Schindel et al., 2006).

Studies across the world noted that most female carers cope by internalizing stereotypical female roles defined by self-sacrifice, silent suffering, altruism, piety, holding up against the odds, keeping harmony rather than asking for help, and turning to religion. The consequences for women are not benign. Female carers in Japan had higher scores for work burden and depression than their male counterparts (Sugiura et al., 2004) and in the US they suffered from poorer emotional health than male carers (Navaie-Waliser et al., 2002). In Chile, carers reported insomnia, stress, stomach ailments, oversensitivity, anxiety, sadness, depression, loneliness, anguish, and worry. Yet few consulted doctors about their needs and even fewer undertook treatment or therapy (Reca et al., 2002).

In Canada, a study on women in nursing, medicine, physiotherapy, and social work who also care for elderly relatives at home, found that the boundaries between their professional and personal lives were frequently blurred and eroded beyond their coping strategies, resulting in feelings of isolation, tension, and extreme physical and mental exhaustion (Ward-Griffin et al., 2005). In Thailand, women providing care for HIV positive patients felt split as they could not always provide care, but felt obligated to do so (Songwathana, 2001). In Botswana, among family caregivers, older women felt overwhelmed with the magnitude and multiplicity of the tasks to be done, felt exhausted, malnourished, depressed, and neglected their own health. Younger girls missed school and were more at risk of sexual and physical abuse and depression (Lindsey et al., 2003). The lack of support and skills in caregiving left families in Botswana, South Africa, and India in social isolation, stigmatized, pauperized, and in psychological distress (Lindsey et al., 2003; Orner, 2007). In Spain, unpaid care work for young, elderly, and disabled family members was mainly done by less educated and poorer women who, due to their care work, were less able to undertake paid work, maintain social relations with friends and other family members, and bore increased mental and physical health risks (Garcia-Calvente et al., 1999). In Mexico, not only was care work for the elderly gendered with a disproportionate burden on women, it was poor and less educated women specifically (Lopez-Ortega et al., 2007).

Ogden and colleagues (2006) conclude that women's efforts subsidize the formal economy, sometimes at great costs to women themselves in terms of forgone paid work, schooling, and other health-producing activities. Although these costs may not be easily measured or monetized, women's unsupported care efforts cannot be seen as a cheaper option for health systems (Columbia University, 2004). In fact, one could argue that research highlighting the medical poverty trap and the pauperizing effects of paying for health care has yet to consider how much women's informal care buffers these iatrogenic health system effects.

Nonetheless, UN frameworks for community home-based care (WHO, 2002) detail the kinds of care that need to be carried out within the home, without specifying who is to provide such care, the consequences of doing so, or the support needs for doing so (Ogden et al., 2006). This is striking considering extensive feminist research that revealed households to be dynamic, heterogeneous sites of unequal power relations. Efforts to support home-based care must therefore take into consideration who in the household shoulders the burden of home care in terms of gender and age.

The challenges of doing so in poor households where access to basic needs is compromised can be substantial. In order to care for one HIV positive person, up to 24 buckets of water are required per day to wash the sick person, to clean soiled sheets, to wash dishes, and to prepare food (Columbia University, 2004, cited by Ogden et al., 2006, p. 336). Support needs to integrate various kinds of social services beyond the formal health care sector to encompass social protection, employment, water, sanitation, agriculture, nutrition, and housing, keeping in mind the perspectives of women as primary home carers (Ogden et al., 2006).

GENDERED ISSUES IN HUMAN RESOURCES FOR HEALTH

Three crosscutting themes emerged from this desk review. While issues with respect to delegation have been discussed within the section on nursing due to its links to issues around professional boundaries, issues related to migration and violence are discussed in the following section.

Migration

The international migration of health workers is today one of the most contentious policy issues concerning human resources in health. While the proportion of the world's population that are international migrants has only risen from 2.3% in 1965 to 2.9% in 2000, this still translates into a doubling of people living outside of their country at any one time since 1965 (United Nations Population Division, 2002, cited by Stilwell et al., 2004, p. 595). Within these global flows, women are playing an increasing role. In 2000, UK work permit data indicated that female occupations were the fastest growing segments of migrant employment (Piper, 2005, p. 7).

In the health sector, more nurses and health professionals other than doctors are currently leading migration flows, in contrast to 30 years ago when the first studies of global migration of the health labor force were undertaken (Bach, 2004). In addition, the scale of migration has magnified. Between 1998 and 2002 the percentage of nursing applicants from abroad in the UK increased from 25% to 50% (Buchan and Sochalski, 2004). Between 1996 and 2001, the number of nurses leaving the Philippines increased from 4,500 nurses to over 12,000. In South Africa, from 1995 to 2000, requests for verification of nursing qualifications (an indicator of intent to move) increased fivefold from 511 to over 2,500 (Vujicic et al., 2004, p. 2).

The drivers of health worker migration are varied. At a broad level, the resort to migrant labor reflects global processes of economic restructuring (Van Eyck, 2004, p. 4). Ageing populations, rising incomes, underfunded health systems, and the feminization of the workforce are put forward as reasons fuelling the demand for female health workers from low-income countries. Nonetheless, research also indicates that the surge in demand is directly related to specific policy changes in OECD countries that facilitate the migration of health personnel (Pond and McPake, 2006). Although some of these migration flows reflect established cultures of medical out-migration (Hagopian et al., 2005), its current force also draws from a latent pool of discontented, underemployed, or unemployed health workers in both source and recipient countries. In response, to improve the retention of nurses in Botswana, reforms have introduced overtime allowance, part-time employment, flextime, and housing. In Zambia, financial support from donors has enabled the doubling of nurse salaries in 2001 (SEW, 2002, cited by Gerein and Green, 2006). However, more must be done in high-income countries to address the high levels of burnout and turnover among local nursing staff, rather than resort to cheaper migrant nursing labor.

The migration of health workers further stratifies health labor markets in both source and recipient countries. As skilled labor is drawn to more formal, better financed, and functioning health systems, lower level health workers, who are more likely to be women, whether paid or not, are expected to shoulder the burden of sustaining local health systems that are already ailing. In the UK, 60% of immigrant nurses came from sub-Saharan Africa, a region that can ill afford the absence of such skilled personnel (Buchan et al., 2006).

Those most qualified and experienced are those most able to migrate, yet they often immigrate into jobs below their formal qualifications (Hagopian et al., 2005; Packer et al., 2006). Hence the global migration of health personnel is not just a 'brain drain' and a perverse subsidy (Packer et al., 2006) from health systems that are severely underresourced, but also a 'brain waste,' as health personnel are not efficiently incorporated into recipient health systems (Gerein and Green, 2006). Efforts to counteract such deprofessionalization include, for example, those by the Filipino Nurses Support Group, which organized review classes for nurses to pass licensing exams and lobbied to ensure that Filipino nurses would not be penalized for breaking their live-in caregiver agreements if they found nursing positions instead (Van Eyck, 2004).

The personal consequences for women involved in global migration are mixed. Research studies on migrant nurses document ambivalent experiences (Winkelmann-Gleed and Seeley, 2005) reflecting both distress and accomplishment (Yi and Jezewski, 2000). Migrants face a contradictory class positioning through the "simultaneous experience of upward and downward mobility in migration, which is not necessarily the same for men and women. Discrimination, loss of status, and erosion of skills in destination areas may be combined with upward mobility at home, as remittances are invested in small businesses, housing and children's education" (Piper, 2005, p. 2).

Migration has the potential to reconfigure gender relations, although little research exists on the gender implications of remittances[5] and the role of female migrants in diasporas (Piper, 2005). Nurses report struggling with social isolation, abusive practices by recruiting agencies, and the strain from working several low-paying jobs to break even, with 30% incurring higher debts than previously expected (Van Eyck, 2004, p. 6). Although negative effects are reported on families and communities, as skilled migrant women leave behind their children in source countries to be looked after by extended families, more research is required to move the evidence base beyond anecdotal accounts. More research is also required to examine the gender effects of migration for health professionals as they encounter immigration point and licensing systems, are denied labor rights when they migrate as secondary dependents, struggle to assimilate into health careers as well as integrate families into new contexts, and maintain extended family links abroad (Shuval, 2000; Iredale, 2005; Purkayastha, 2005).

Some source countries have set up government departments to address the migration problems faced by nurses (Packer et al., 2006). For example, the Filipino government set up the Philippine Overseas Employment Administration, an agency that markets Filipino workers, negotiates agreements, regulates private recruiting agencies, inspects contracts prior to departure, maximizes remittances, and helps to safeguard worker's rights. Research that evaluates the functioning and effectiveness of these government efforts to manage migration is required, especially since they encourage nurse migration in countries that also face domestic nurse shortages.

Violence

Violence in the health sector is significant, but still not adequately recognized. In advanced economies, like Sweden, it may constitute almost a quarter of all violence at work (Nordin, 1995, cited by Di Martino, 2002). Results from a broad study of violence in the health sector across several countries revealed that both physical and psychological forms of violence are more prevalent than previously understood, with the latter being more frequently reported (Table 8.4). Women, and younger women in particular, are at greater risk as they are more likely to be victims of violence and to suffer longer health and psychosocial consequences than men from the violence (Di Martino, 2002, 2003). When one considers the informal sector, which is overrepresented by less-qualified, female health workers often working in illegal conditions, the rates of violence could be higher.

Little research exists on gender-based forms of violence targeted at health personnel, including that related to sexual harassment. Except for the research studies in the US, most of the evidence on sexual harassment against health personnel is anecdotal. In the US, research findings indicate that sexual harassment in medical schools is widespread, with significant effects on student's specialty choices and residency rankings (Carr et al., 2000; Stratton et al., 2005). This suggests that despite the increasing female presence among medical students and in medicine in general, harassment is still a very common experience in the US.

Despite the prevalence of gender discrimination and sexual harassment, research seems to indicate that women currently just cope with such inequities (Carr et al., 2000). Hinze (2004) examined the everyday lives and coping strategies of women in medical schools with regard to sexual harassment in the US. Incidents were reframed as one of women's sensitivity or relegated as inconsequential. Hinze (2004) concludes that both tactics of resistance fail because they individualize the problem of sexual harassment. In doing so, they deflect attention from systemic gender inequalities that permit the continuation of such forms of behavior.

A striking finding from South Africa was that nurses were at greater risk of abuse due to their professional status (Kim and Motsei, 2002). Many

Table 8.4 Incidence of Violence in Health Sectors

In the previous year	Portugal Health Centre	Portugal Hospital	Bulgaria	Lebanon	S. Africa Public	S. Africa Private	Thailand	Australia	Brazil
N	221	277	508	1016		1018	1090	400	1569
N % Women	77	79.9	80.3	69.8		78	72.7	68.5	70.46
Any violence	60	37	75.8		71.1	51.6	54	67.2	46.7
Physically attacked	3	3	7.5	5.8	17	9	10.5		6.4
Verbally abused	51	27.4	32.2	40.9	60.1		47.7	67	39.5
Being bullied/ mobbed	23	16.5	30.9	22.1	20.6		10.7	10.5	15.2

Source: Di Martino (2002).

of them relied on their husbands in order to attend nursing school. As a result, they felt obliged to hand over their salaries to their spouses at the end of the month, leaving them with little control over their own finances. Tension and violence in the house was reported due to their spouses feeling threatened by their professional, income-earning status and because of their interactions with male colleagues.

Just as in South Africa, the transgression of gender norms also lies at the heart of threats to personal security made against female health workers in South Asia. In Bangladesh, "women who break gender norms are ridiculed not so much because they harm themselves, but because the loss of their prestige undermines the very foundations of society" (Simmons et al., 1992, p. 100). Female health workers can be seen as immoral due to their involvement in delicate subjects like family planning, their interactions with male colleagues and their unchaperoned travel across villages. The backlash against them can target their sexuality. As one villager commented, "They call themselves doctors; they are not doctors but prostitutes" (Simmons et al., 1992, p. 101). In extreme cases, this can justify violence against community-based female staff.

With respect to personal security, female auxiliary health staff in India reported being afraid to walk on their own in between villages, coping with remotely located housing with inadequate lighting, facing harassment from villagers, and not trusting villagers when called out to help at odd hours. In contrast only one male auxiliary health worker answered the question about personal security. His response was, "Personally, there is no problem, because I have all-round support. There is no problem" (George, 2007b, p. 138).

These responses show that the lack of infrastructural support, in terms of transport, housing, and lighting, has gendered consequences for female health workers, most intimately embodied in their personal security. Although supervisors informally acknowledge these problems, they do not see them as part of their official managerial remit (Mohan et al., 2003). In the absence of managerial support to counter these security problems, female health staff in India rely on spouses or cultivate support among local people to accompany them to households for night deliveries. These efforts reflect informal adjustments and individual private coping strategies to problems of gender bias that require collective, public acknowledgment and resolution.

Although responses to personal security and sexual harassment require better reporting, investigating, and security personnel in the short term, longer-term prevention measures require broader strategies that address gender norms, interpersonal relations among staff, and working environments. For example, Brazilian health workers identified prevention strategies that linked the incidence of violence in the health workplace to social problems of inequality in society, their lack of working conditions, which have a direct effect on quality of care for patients, and their lack of worker's rights in the health sector (Di Martino, 2002).

CONCLUSIONS

As discussed in this chapter, gender, as a social construct enforced by power relations, affects how health work is conceptualized, valued, and supported with differential impacts on the professional and personal lives of health workers, the services they deliver, and the health systems they belong to. It consequently determines the structural location of women and men across and within health occupations, as well as the subjective experiences of these locations. Although gender biases have distortionary effects on both women and men that are contextually dependent, in general, women tend to be disproportionately disadvantaged while men tend to be disproportionately privileged.

These gender biases are inequitable, as they are in and of themselves unfair. But their power resonates through various other distortions. They can be invisible due to description biases that affect how we view and understand the nature of health work and health systems. They can be ingrained as they affirm forms of privilege that resist change and marginalize those that seek change, with gender tensions often being resolved through private, individual adjustments rather than through public, collective transformations. They are also inefficient or unproductive as they restrain the true capacity of individuals working in health systems. Finally, they are iatrogenic, as those least supported, trained, and rewarded absorb the contradictions of gender-biased and resource-constrained health systems at great cost to their own health and livelihoods.

In conclusion, a gender analysis of human resources in health reveals that although health systems are themselves meant to provide a source of healing and a social safety net for society, it can replicate and exacerbate many of the social inequalities it is meant to address and itself be immune from. Health systems rely on a foundation of health workers who are often informal, poorly paid or not paid at all, poorly supported, and disproportionately female. Even among formally recognized sections of the health labor force, significant forms of gender bias exist across and within health occupations. Despite the prevalence of such structural and subjective biases, they are neither static nor universal, but actively contested, negotiated, and adjusted to at the individual level. These individual efforts by women and men must be constructively and collectively amplified through policy and program efforts at higher and broader levels in health systems. Such policy and program efforts would result not only in more gender equality in the health labor force, but also in improved health system functioning more broadly.

Important policy and program measures include:

1. Sex-disaggregated data and analysis along with more accurate measurement of the diverse range of health care tasks that make up health work must be supported so that women's contributions to health work can more accurately be represented and recognized.

2. Delegation must be seen as part of long-term planning and investment efforts that skillfully restructure health systems to do more in different ways, rather than as a means to stretch further on a cheaper basis, often falling back on unsupported female labor. The gender effects of delegation must be analyzed on a contextual basis so as to avoid exacerbating gender inequalities.

3. Individual strategies to address gender inequalities based on affirmative action and training must couple with broader measures that address how health work is organized. This means:

- improving access to family leave or child care provisions in a gender equitable manner
- resolving gender differences in access to strategic resources like mentoring and supervision, administrative and infrastructural support, secure funding sources and employment contracts, formal and informal networking
- reviewing gender biases in measuring, rewarding, and supporting work
- addressing gendered vulnerabilities to sexual harassment and other forms of violence experienced by health workers
- neutralizing gender stereotypes that assume that women are more nurturing or sexually provocative and thus serve to distract attention from important organizational biases

4. Addressing the gender biases that question the legitimacy of female community health workers requires attention to personal and professional prestige by:

- supporting the questioning and reinterpretation of gender norms in a constructive manner
- allowing them to assume broader roles than the original simple health care tasks they are charged with
- guiding them with continuous training and supervision
- linking them with functioning referral systems
- acknowledging them through positive relationships with peer groups, community members, other health professionals, and managers

5. Home-based care efforts must recognize who in the household shoulders the burden of home care in terms of gender and age. Support needs to integrate various kinds of social services beyond the formal health care sector to encompass social protection, employment, water, sanitation, agriculture, nutrition, and housing, keeping in mind the perspectives of women as primary home carers, without stereotyping women as the only ones who can undertake care work.

6. As skilled labor is drawn to more formal, better financed, and functioning health systems, lower-level health workers, who are more

likely to be women, whether paid or not, cannot be expected to shoulder the burden of sustaining crumbling health systems in source countries. More must be done in both source and recipient countries to retain local nursing staff, who in the absence of support either quit or migrate to better work environments. More research is also required to understand the specific opportunities and vulnerabilities faced by migrating health workers from a gender perspective.

7. Violence in the health workplace must be recognized as an important priority. Interventions must address both the normative values that naturalize and sanction such violence, as well as the organizational biases that place female health workers at greater risk through poor working conditions and gender-blind management practices.

ACKNOWLEDGMENTS

I thank Gita Sen for encouraging me to do this review. This chapter is a summarized version of a larger paper written with the aid of a grant from the World Health Organization and the International Development Research Centre, Ottawa, Canada, and undertaken as work for the Women and Gender Equity and Health Systems Knowledge Networks established as part of the WHO Commission on the Social Determinants of Health. The views presented in this chapter are those of the author and do not necessarily represent the decisions, policy, or views of IRDC, WHO, or Commissioners.

NOTES

1. Gender is understood here as the learned social characteristics that distinguish males and females in society. By reflecting normative power relations it can sustain social inequalities between women and men. Other normative power relations that create social inequalities include those relating to social class, race, age, sexual orientation, etc.
2. With the exception of Standing (2000) and Reichenbach (2007).
3. A frontline worker was defined by the authors as doing work that entails a high level of direct patient care or care delivery support services, median annual wages of approximately US$40,000 or less, and work that required educational training of a bachelor's degree or below (Schindel et al., 2006, p. 3).
4. The exceptions are Mongolia, Russia, the former Soviet republics, and Sudan (WHO, 2006).
5. Remittances for most of the 1990s exceeded official development aid for source health worker countries (Stillwell et al., 2004).

REFERENCES

Adams, T.L. 2005. Feminization of professions: The case of women in dentistry. *Canadian Journal of Sociology—Cahiers Canadiens De Sociologie* 30 (1): 71–94.

Allen, D. 2004. The nursing-medical boundary: A negotiated order? In *Medical Work, Medical Knowledge and Health Care*, edited by E. Annandale, M.A. Elston, and L. Prior. Oxford: Blackwell: 243–264.

Annandale, E., M.A. Elston, and L. Prior. 2004. *Medical Work, Medical Knowledge and Health Care*. Oxford: Blackwell.

Bach, S. 2004. Migration patterns of physicians and nurses: Still the same story? *Bulletin of the World Health Organisation* 82 (8): 624–625.

Baru, R. 2005. Gender and social characteristics of the labour force in health services. In *Exploring Gender Equations: Colonial and Post Colonial India*, edited by S. Kak and B. Pati. New Delhi: Nehru Memorial Museum and Library: 281–299.

Bergman, H., and B. Hobson. 2002. *Compulsory Fatherhood: The Coding of Fatherhood in the Swedish Welfare State*. Cambridge: Cambridge University Press.

Bergstrom, S. 1998. *Issue Paper on Maternal Health Care*. Stockholm: SIDA.

Bickel, J. 2000. Women in academic medicine. *Journal of American Women's Medical Association* 55 (1): 10–13.

Biklen, M. 2003. Health care in the home: Re-examining the companionship services exemption to the Fair Labor Standards Act 35. *Columbia Human Rights Law Review* 113.

Blum, L.S., T. Sharmin, C. Ronsmans. 2006. Attending home vs. clinic-based deliveries: perspectives of skilled birth attendants in Matlab, Bangladesh. *Reprod Health Matters* 14 (27): 51–60.

Brooks, F. 1998. Women in general practice: Responding to the sexual division of labour? *Social Science and Medicine* 47 (2): 181–193.

Buchan, J., R. Jobanputra, P. Gough, and R. Hutt. 2006. Internationally recruited nurses in London: A survey of career paths and plans. *Human Resources for Health* 4 (1): 14.

Buchan, J., and J. Sochalski. 2004. The migration of nurses: Trends and policies. *Bulletin of the World Health Organisation* 82 (8): 587–594.

Bunting, S. 2001. Sustaining the relationship: Women's caregiving in the context of HIV disease. *Health Care Women International* 22 (1–2): 131–148.

Burns, C. 1998. 'A man is a clumsy thing who does not know how to handle a sick person': Aspects of the history of masculinity and race in the shaping of male nursing in South Africa, 1900–1950. *Journal of Southern African Studies* 24 (4): 695–717.

Carpenter, M. 1993. The subordination of nurses in health care: Towards a social divisions approach. In *Gender, Work and Medicine: Women and the Medical Division of Labour*, edited by E. Riska and K. Wegar. London: Sage: 95–130.

Carr, P.L., A.S. Ash, R.H. Friedman, A. Scaramucci, R.C. Barnett, L. Szalacha, A. Palepu, and M.A. Moskowitz. 1998. Relation of family responsibilities and gender to the productivity and career satisfaction of medical faculty. *Annals of Internal Medicine* 129 (7): 532–538.

Carr, P.L., A.S. Ash, R. Friedman, L. Szalacha, R.C. Barnett, A. Palepu, and M.A. Moskowitz. 2000. Faculty perceptions of gender discrimination and sexual harassment in academic medicine. *Annals of Internal Medicine* 132 (11): 889–896.

Carr, P.L., L. Szalacha, R. Barnett, C. Caswelland, and T. Inui. 2003. A "ton of feathers": Gender discrimination in academic medical careers and how to manage it. *Journal of Women's Health* 12 (10): 1009–1018.

Columbia University. 2004. Costing the care economy. *A Report Commissioned by the United Nations Development Programme, Prepared by the Columbia University School of International and Public Affairs*. New York: Columbia University.

Corrêa, S., and S. Piola. 2003. *Area Tecnica de Suade da Mulher -Balanco 1998–2002: Aspectos Estrategicos*. Programaticos e Financieros Brasilia: Ministerio de Saude.

Daniels, K., H.H. Van Zyl, M. Clarke, J. Dick, and E. Johansson. 2005. Ear to the ground: Listening to farm dwellers talk about the experience of becoming lay health workers. *Health Policy and Planning* 73: 92–103.

De Koninck, M., P. Bergeron, and R. Bourbonnais. 1997. Women physicians in Quebec. *Social Science and Medicine* 44 (12): 1825–1832.

De Koninck, M., H. Guay, R. Bourbonnais, P. Bergeron, and M.-A. Tremblay. 1993. *Femmes et medicine: Enquete aupres des medicins du Quebec sur leur formation, leur pratique et leur sante*. Quebec: Corporation Professionelle des Medecins.

Dedobbeleer, N., A. Contandriopoulos, and S. Desjardins. 1995. Convergence or divergence of male and female physicians' hours of work and income. *Medical Care* 33 (8): 796–805.

DeVries, R.G. 1993. A cross-national view of the status of midwives. In *Gender, Work and Medicine: Women and the Medical Division of Labour*, edited by E. Riska and K. Wegar. London: Sage: 131–146.

Di Martino, V. 2002. *Workplace Violence in the Health Sector: Country Case Studies: Brazil, Bulgaria, Lebanon, Portugal, South Africa, Thailand, and an Additional Australian Study (p. 42): ILO / ICN / WHO / PSI Joint Programme on Workplace Violence in the Health Sector*. Geneva: ILO, ICN, WHO, and PSI.

———. 2003. *Workplace Violence in the Health Sector: Relationship between Work Stress and Workplace Violence in the Health Sector*. Geneva: ILO, ICN, WHO, and PSI.

Dovlo, D. 2004. Using mid-level cadres as substitutes for internationally mobile health professionals in Africa: A desk review. *Human Resources for Health* 2 (1): 7.

Dwisetyani Utomo, I., S.S. Arsyad, and E. Nurul Hasmi. 2006. Village family planning volunteers in Indonesia: Their role in the family planning programme. *Reproductive Health Matters* 14 (27): 83–90.

Elston, M.A. 1993. Women doctors in a changing profession: The case of Britain. In *Gender, Work and Medicine: Women and the Medical Division of Labour*, edited by E. Riska and K. Wegar. London: Sage: 27–61.

Foster, S., J. McMurray, M. Linzer, J. Leavitt, M. Rosenberg, and M. Carnes. 2000. Results of a gender-climate and work-environment survey at a midwestern academic health center. *Academic Medicine* 75 (6): 653–660.

Fox, G., A. Schwartz, and K.M. Hart. 2006. Work–family balance and academic advancement in medical schools. *Academic Psychiatry* 30 (3): 227–234.

Frenk, J., F. Knaul, L. Vazquez-Segovia, and G. Nigenda. 1999. Trends in medical employment: Persistent imbalances in urban Mexico. *American Journal of Public Health* 89 (7): 1054–1058.

Fried, L., C. Francomano, and S. MacDonald. 1996. Career development of women in academic medicine: Multiple interventions in a department of medicine. *Jama-Journal of the American Medical Association* 276: 898–905.

Friedson, E. 1986. *Professional Powers*. Chicago: University of Chicago Press.

Garcia-Calvente, M., I. Mateo, and P. Gutierrez. 1999. *Cuidados y cuidadores en el sistema informal de salud Grenada*. Grenada: Escuela Analuza de Salud Publica e Instituto Andaluz de la Mujer.

George, A. 2007a. Human resources for health: A gender analysis. *Background Paper Prepared for the Women and Gender Equity Knowledge Network and the Health Systems Knowledge Network of the WHO Commission on Social Determinants of Health*. Geneva: WHO.

————. 2007b. *The Outrageous as Ordinary: Maternal Mortality and Primary Health Care Workers' Perspectives on Accountability in Koppal District, Karnataka State, India. Institute of Development Studies (p. 283)*. Brighton: Sussex University.

Gerein, N., and A. Green. 2006. Midwifery and nursing migration: Implications of trade liberalisation for maternal health in low income countries. In *Trading Women's Health and Rights: Trade Liberalisation and Reproductive Health in Developing Economies*, edited by C. Grown, E. Braunstein, and A. Malhotra. London: Zed: 235–254.

Gerein, N., A. Green, and S. Pearson. 2006. The implications of shortages of health professionals for maternal health in sub-Saharan Africa. *Reproductive Health Matters* 14 (27): 40–50.

Grandis, J.R., W.E. Gooding, B.A. Zamboni, M.M. Wagener, S.D. Drenning, L. Miller, K. Doyle, S.E. Mackinnon, and R.L. Wagner. 2004. The gender gap in a surgical subspecialty—Analysis of career and lifestyle factors. *Archives of Otolaryngology-Head and Neck Surgery* 130 (6): 695–702.

Gupta, N., K. Diallo, P. Zurn, and M. Dal Poz. 2003. Assessing human resources for health: What can be learned from labour force surveys? *Human Resources for Health* 1 (5).

Hagbaghery, M.A., M. Salsali, and F. Ahmadi. 2004. A qualitative study of Iranian nurses' understanding and experiences of professional power. *Human Resources for Health* 2 (9).

Hagopian, A., A. Ofosu, A. Fatusi, R. Biritwum, A. Essel, L. Gary Hart, and C. Watts. 2005. The flight of physicians from West Africa: Views of African physicians and implications for policy. *Social Science and Medicine* 61 (8): 1750–1760.

Halford, S., and M. Savage. 1997. *Gender, Careers and Organisations. Current Developments in Banking, Nursing and Local Government*. Basingstoke: Macmillan Press.

Hamel, M.B., J.R. Ingelfinger, E. Phimister, and C.G. Solomon. 2006. Women in academic medicine—Progress and challenges. *New England Journal of Medicine* 355 (3): 310–312.

Heuss, L.T., and C. Hanggeli. 2003. Open access to part-time specialist training the Swiss experience. *Swiss Medical Weekly* 133 (17–18): 263–266.

Hinze, S.W. 2004. 'Am I being oversensitive?' Women's experience of sexual harassment during medical training. *Health* 8 (1): 101–127.

Iredale, R. 2005. Gender immigration policies and accreditation: valuing the skills of professional women migrants. *Geoforum* 36 (2): 155–166.

Iyer, A., A. Jesani, with A. Fernandes, S. Hirani, and S. Khanvilkar. 1995. *Women in Health Care*. Mumbai: Foundation for Research in Community Health.

Jagsi, R., E.A. Guancial, C.C. Worobey, L.E. Henault, Y.C. Chang, R. Starr, N.J. Tarbelland, and E.M. Hylek. 2006. The "gender gap" in authorship of Academic Medical Literature—A 35-year perspective. *New England Journal of Medicine* 355 (3): 281–287.

Jamous, H.P., and B. Peloille. 1970. Changes in the French university-hospital system. In *Professions and Professionalisation*, edited by J. Jackson. Cambridge: Cambridge University Press: 111–152.

Kanchanachitra, C., S. Wibulpolprasert, and T. Thammarangsi. 2007. Gender and physician mobility in Thailand. In *Exploring the Gender Dimensions of the Global Health Workforce*, edited by L. Reichenbach. Boston: Global Equity Initiative, Harvard University: 153–184.

Karolinska Institute. 2001. *Issues in Abortion Care, Deciding Women's Lives Are Worth Saving: Expanding the Role of Midlevel Providers in Safe Abortion Care*. Stockholm: IPAS IHCAR.

Kassak, K.M., H.M. Ghomrawi, A.M.A. Osseiran, and H. Kobeissi. 2006. The providers of health services in Lebanon: A survey of physicians. *Human Resources for Health* 4 (4).

Kauffman, K., and D. Myers. 1997. The changing role of village health volunteers in northeast Thailand: An ethnographic field study. *International Journal of Nursing Studies* 34 (4): 249–255.

Kazanjian, A. 1993. Health-manpower planning or gender relations? The obvious and the oblique. In *Gender, Work and Medicine: Women and the Medical Division of Labour,* edited by E. Riska and K. Wegar. London: Sage: 147–171.

Kim, J., and M. Motsei. 2002. "Women enjoy punishment": Attitudes and experiences of gender-based violence among PHC nurses in rural South Africa. *Social Science and Medicine* 54 (8): 1243–1254.

Knaul, F., J. Frenk, and A. Aguilar. 2000. The gender composition of the medical profession in Mexico: Implications for employment patterns and physician labour supply. *J Am Med Women's Assoc* 55 (1): 32–35.

Levinson, W., K. Kaufman, and J. Bickel. 1993. Part-time faculty in academic medicine: Present status and future challenges. *Ann Intern Med* 119 (3): 220–225.

Lindsey, E., M. Hirschfeld, and S. Tlou. 2003. Home-based care in Botswana: Experiences of older women and young girls. *Health Care Women International* 24 (6): 486–501.

Lipson, D., and R. Carol. 2004. *Health Insurance Coverage for Direct-Care Workers: Riding Out the Storm, 1 (3).* Washington, DC: Institute for the Future of Aging Services.

Lopez-Ortega, M., C. Matarazzo, and G. Nigenda. 2007. Household care for the elderly and the ill in Mexico: An analysis from a gender perspective. In *Exploring the Gender Dimensions of the Global Health Workforce,* edited by L. Reichenbach. Boston: Global Equity Initiative, Harvard University: 59–90.

Maggs, C.H. 1983. *The Origins of General Nursing.* London: Croon Helm.

Magrane, D., J. Lang, and H. Alexander. 2005. *Women in US Academic Medicine: Statistics and Medical School Benchmarks.* Washington, D.C.: Association of American Medical Colleges.

Manley, J.E. 1995. Sex-segregated work in the system of professions—the development and stratification of nursing. *Sociological Quarterly* 36 (2): 297–314.

Mathole, T., G. Lindmark, and B. Ahlberg. 2005. Dilemmas and paradoxes in providing and changing antenatal care: A study of nurses and midwives in rural Zimbabwe. *Health Policy and Planning* 20 (6): 385–393.

Mayorova, T., F. Stevens, A. Scherpbier, L. van der Velden, and J. van der Zee. 2005. Gender-related differences in general practice preferences: Longitudinal evidence from the Netherlands 1982–2001. *Health Policy* 72 (1): 73–80.

McCourt, W. 2000. Human resource management in the UK public service: Its practice and its relevance to public reformers in South Africa. *Human Resources in Development Working Paper Series 8.* Manchester: Institute for Development Policy and Management.

McGuire, L.K. M.R. Bergen, and M.L. Polan. 2004. Career advancement for women faculty in a US school of medicine: Perceived needs. *Academic Medicine* 79 (4): 319–325.

Mohan, P., S.D. Iyengar, S.B. Mohan, and K. Sen. 2003. Auxiliary nurse midwife: What determines her place of residence? *Journal of Health and Population in Developing Countries.* http://www.jhpdc.unc/edu.

Muecke, M.A., and W. Srisuphan. 1989. Born female: The development of nursing in Thailand. *Social Science and Medicine* 29 (5): 643–652.

Mumtaz, Z., S. Salway, M. Waseem, and N. Umer. 2003. Gender-based barriers to primary health care provision in Pakistan: the experience of female providers. *Health Policy and Planning* 18 (3): 261–269.

Navaie-Waliser, M., A. Spriggs, and P. Feldman. 2002. Informal caregiving: Differential experiences by gender. *Medical Care* 40 (12): 1249–1259.

Nigenda, G., and M.H. Machado. 2000. From state to market: The Nicaraguan labour market for health personnel. *Health Policy and Planning* 15 (3): 312–318.

Nordin, H. 1995. *Fakta om vaold och hot i arbetet Solna.* Solna: Occupational Injury Information System, Swedish Board of Occupational Safety and Health.

Ogden, J., S. Esim, and C. Grown. 2006. Expanding the care continuum for HIV/AIDS: Bringing carers into focus. *Health Policy and Planning* 21 (5): 333–342.

Orner, P. 2007. The psychosocial impacts on primary household-based caregivers of people with AIDS: Gender implications for policy and programs. In *Exploring the Gender Dimensions of the Global Health Workforce*, edited by L. Reichenbach. Boston: Global Equity Initiative, Harvard University: 91–128.

Packer, C., R. Labonte, and D. Spitzer. 2006. Globalisation and the health worker migration crisis. *Draft Paper for the WHO Commission for Social Determinants of Health.* Geneva: WHO.

Palmer, D. 2006. Tackling Malawi's human resource crisis. *Reproductive Health Matters* 14 (27): 27–39.

Pinto, S. 2004. Development without institutions: Ersatz medicine and the politics of everyday life in rural north India. *Cultural Anthropology* 19 (3): 337–364.

Piper, N. 2005. *Gender and Migration.* Geneva: Global Commission on International Migration.

Pond, B., and B. McPake. 2006. The health migration crisis: The role of four Organisation for Economic Cooperation and Development countries. *The Lancet* 367 (9520): 1448–1455.

Portella, A.P., and T. Gouveia. 1997. *Social Health Policies: A Question of Gender? The Case of Community Health Agents from Camaragibe Municipality.* Pernambuco State Recife: SOS CORPO.

Purkayastha, B. 2005. Skilled migration and cumulative disadvantage: The case of highly qualified Asian Indian Immigrant women in the US. *Geoforum* 36 (2): 181–196.

Reca, I.C., M. Alvarez, and M.E. Tijoux. 2002. *The Hidden Costs of Home Care: A Research Methodology for Case Studies.* Chile: PAHO.

Reichenbach, L. 2007. The overlooked dimension: Gender and the global health workforce. In *Exploring the Gender Dimensions of the Global Health Workforce*, edited by L. Reichenbach. Boston: Global Equity Initiative, Harvard University: 1–14.

Reichenbach, L., and H. Brown. 2004. Gender and academic medicine: Impacts on the health workforce. *British Medical Journal* 329 (7469): 792–795.

Riska, E. 2001. *Medical Careers and Feminist Agendas: American, Scandinavian and Russian Women Physicians.* New York: Aldine de Gruyter.

Rispel, L., and H. Schneider. 1990. Professionalisation of South African nursing: Who benefits? In *Nursing at the Crossroads: Organisation, Professionalisation and Politicisation. Symposium Proceedings*, edited by L. Rispel. Johannesburg: The Centre for Health Policy, University of Witwatersrand.

Robinson, D. 2001. Differences in occupational earnings by sex. In *Women, Gender and Work*, edited by M. Loutfi. Geneva: International Labour Office.

Schindel, J., D. Cherner, E. O'Neil, K. Solomon, B. Iammartino, and J. Santimauro. 2006. *Workers Who Care: A Graphical Profile of the Frontline Health and Health Care Workforce.* San Francisco: Robert Wood Johnson Foundation and Health Workforce Solutions.

Schroen, A.T., M.R. Brownstein, and G.F. Sheldon. 2004. Women in academic general surgery. *Academic Medicine* 79 (4): 310–318.

SEW. 2002. *Newsletter of the International Council of Nurses, January–March.*

Shuval, J. 2000. The reconstruction of professional identity among immigrant physicians in three societies. *Journal of Immigration and Health* 2(4): 191–202.

Simmons, R., R. Mita, and M. Koenig. 1992. Employment in family planning and women's status in Bangladesh. *Family Planning* 23 (2): 97–108.

Songwathana, P. 2001. Women and AIDS caregiving: Women's work? *Health Care Women International* 22 (3): 263–279.

Stacey, C.L. 2006. Finding dignity in dirty work: The constraints and rewards of low-wage home care labour. *Sociology of Health and Illness* 27 (6): 831–854.

Standing, H. 1997. Gender and equity in health sector reform programmes: A review. *Health Policy and Planning* 12 (1): 1–18.

———. 2000. Gender—A missing dimension in human resource policy and planning for health reforms. *Human Resources for Health Development Journal* 4 (1): 27–42.

Standing, H., and E. Baume. 2001. Equity, equal opportunities, gender and organisation performance. *Presented at the Workshop on Global Health Workforce Strategy.* Annecy, France: World Health Organization.

Stilwell, B., K. Diallo, and P. Zurn. 2004. Migration of health-care workers from developing countries: Strategic approaches to its management. *Bulletin of the World Health Organisation* 82 (8): 595–600.

Stratton, T., M. McLaughlin, F. Witte, S. Fosson, and L. Nora. 2005. Does students' exposure to gender discrimination and sexual harassment in medical school affect specialty choice and residency program selection? *Academic Medicine* 80 (4): 400–408.

Sugiura, K., M. Ito, and H. Mikami. 2004. Evaluation of gender differences of family caregivers with reference to the mode of caregiving at home and caregiver distress in Japan. *Nippon Koshu Eisei Zasshi* 51 (4): 240–251.

Tajul Islam, M., Y. Ali Haque, R. Waxman, and A. Bayes Bhuiyan. 2006. Implementation of emergency obstetric care training in Bangladesh: Lessons learned. *Reproductive Health Matters* 14 (27): 61–72.

Taylor, L., J. Seeley, and E. Kajura. 1996. Informal care for illness in rural southwest Uganda: The central role that women play. *Health Transition Review* 6: 49–56.

Tendler, J., and S. Freedheim. 1994. Trust in a rent-seeking world: Health and government transformed in Northeast Brazil. *World Development* 22: 1771–1791.

Tesch, B., H. Wood, A. Helwig, and A.B. Nattinger. 1995. Promotion of women physicians in academic medicine: Glass ceiling or sticky floor? *Journal of the American Medical Association* 273: 1022–1025.

Tiegs, T., M. Heesacker, T. Ketterson, D. Pekich, M. Rittman, J. Rosenbek, B. Stidham, and L. Gonzalez-Rothi. 2006. Coping by stroke caregivers: Sex similarities and differences. *Top Stroke Rehabilitation* 13 (1): 52–62.

UNIDO. 1989. *Human Resources in Zimbabwe's Industrial Development: The Current and Prospective Contribution of Women.* Regional and Country Studies Branch Industrial Policy and Perspectives Division. Geneva: UNIDO.

United Nations Population Division. 2002. *Population Database 2002.* New York: United Nations Population Division.

Uys, L. 2003. Guest editorial: Longer-term aid to combat AIDS. *Journal of Advanced Nursing* 44: 1–2.

van der Merwe, A.S. 1999. The power of women as nurses in South Africa. *Journal of Advanced Nursing* 30 (6): 1272–1279.

Van Eyck, K. 2004. *Women and International Migration in the Health Sector.* Ferney-Voltaire, France: Public Services International.

Vujicic, M., P. Zurn, K. Diallo, O. Adams, and M. Dal Poz. 2004. The role of wages in migration of health care professionals from developing countries. *Human Resources for Health* 2 (3).

Warde, C., W. Allen, and L. Gelberg. 1996. Physician role conflict and resulting career changes. Gender and generational differences. *J Gen Intern Med* 11 (12): 729–735.

Ward-Griffin, C., J.B. Brown, A. Vandervoort, S. McNair, and I. Dashnay. 2005. Double-duty caregiving: Women in the health professions. *Canadian Journal on Aging—Revue Canadienne Du Vieillissement* 24 (4): 379–394.

Wear, D., and C. Keck-McNulty. 2004. Attitudes of female nurses and female residents toward each other: A qualitative study in one US teaching hospital. *Academic Medicine* 79 (4): 291–301.

Wegar, K. 1993. Conclusions. In *Gender, Work and Medicine: Women and the Medical Division of Labour*, edited by E. Riska and K. Wegar. London: Sage: 173–188.

West, C. 1993. Reconceptualising gender in physician patient relationships. *Social Science and Medicine* 36 (1): 57–66.

Winkelmann-Gleed, A.M., and J. Seeley. 2005. Strangers in a British world? Integration of international nurses. *British Journal of Nursing* 14 (18): 954–961.

Wirth, M. 2008. Professionals with delivery skills: Backbone of the health system and key to reaching the maternal health millennium development goal. *Croatian Medical Journal* 49: 318–333.

WHO. 2000. *Fact Sheets on HIV/AIDS for Nurses and Midwives*. Geneva: WHO.

———. 2002. *Community Home-Based Care in Resource-Limited Settings: A Framework for Action*. Geneva: WHO.

———. 2006. *The World Health Report 2006: Working Together for Health*. Geneva: WHO.

Yi, M., and M. Jezewski. 2000. Korean nurses' adjustment to hospitals in the United States of America. *Journal of Advanced Nursing* 32 (3): 721–729.

Yutzie, J.D., J.L. Shellito, S.D. Helmer, and F.C. Chang. 2005. Gender differences in general surgical careers: Results of a post-residency survey. American Journal Of Surgery 190 (6): 955–959.

9 Accountability to Citizens on Gender and Health

Ranjani K. Murthy

INTRODUCTION

It is nearly three decades since the adoption of the 1979 United Nations Convention on the Elimination of All Forms of Discrimination against Women (CEDAW), and nearly a decade since General Comments to the International Covenant on Economic and Social and Cultural Rights on the right to the highest standard on health (irrespective of sex/gender and other identities) was passed (United Nations, 2000).

Gender inequalities in health access and outcomes, however, continue throughout the developing world (Sen et al., 2007; Goetz, 2008). Gender inequalities in health mainly discriminate against women, girls, and transgender people, but at times they disadvantage men and boys (Macklin, 2006). Persistence of gender biases within the health sector as well as within communities and households is one of the important reasons for the persistence of gender inequalities in health.

In this context, it is essential to strengthen accountability of power holders in the health sector to reduce gender inequalities in health access and outcomes and to address gender-specific health needs and rights of women, men, and transgender people (in short, accountability on gender and health). Such accountability processes should ideally involve citizens, including women, marginalized men, and transgender people.

The main aims of this chapter are to review the concept of accountability to citizens on gender and health, review the practice of accountability to/with citizens on gender and health, learn lessons, assess gaps in practice, and suggest strategies for strengthening accountability processes. The following sections of this chapter address each of these aims.

At the outset it must be stressed that literature on citizens' pressing for accountability on gender and health is scarce. There is more literature on citizens' pressing for health accountability in general (see case studies in Potts, 2008; United Nations, 2005, 2006, 2007, and 2008), than on citizens pressing for accountability on gender and health. Further, much of the available literature on accountability on gender and health pertains to government's internal mechanisms, and not citizens' initiatives (see Murthy et al., 2005; Root et al., 2008). Nevertheless, it is hoped that the review attempted in this chapter will offer some insights on accountability to/with citizens on gender and health.

CONCEPTS OF ACCOUNTABILITY

This section discusses concepts of accountability to citizens, health accountability, and accountability to citizens on gender and health.

Accountability to Citizens

Two definitions of accountability shape the concept of accountability adopted by this chapter. Goetz (2008) sees accountability processes as consisting of two elements: *answerability* and *enforcement*. *Answerability* refers to how power holders give an account of what they do/did with public trust and national revenue, and *enforcement* refers to corrective action taken (on power holders) in instances of performance failure (Goetz, 2008).

Caseley (2003) sees *engagement* and *responsiveness* as two key elements of accountability. *Engagement* refers to a reciprocal relationship between two actors whereby demands are articulated by one actor in a transparent manner to the other. *Responsiveness* refers to the extent to which the party on which demands are placed acts on the demands. Responsiveness, in turn, is seen by Caseley as comprising of one or more of the following three elements: answerability, enforcement, and organization change (Caseley, 2003).

This chapter combines elements of both definitions, and sees accountability to citizens as including elements of engagement of citizens with power holders, answerability of power holders to citizens, and enforcement of action by power holders.

Accountability to Citizens on Health

Health accountability experiences can be explored from the different angles listed here:

- Who is accountable?
- To whom?
- With regard to what?
- When?
- How is accountability operationalized?
  (George, 2003; Murthy et al., 2005)

Power holders in the health sector could range from health policy makers, health donors, health managers, health providers, to health workers.

They could be from the public or private health sector or a combination of both (e.g., Global Fund for Fighting AIDS, Tuberculosis and Malaria). This chapter will examine who within the health sector is held accountable and who is not.

Health accountability can be 'internal' in the sense to colleagues, to higher-ups within the health sector, or to health professional bodies, or 'external' in the sense to citizens' groups, judiciary, quasi-judicial organizations (e.g., national human rights commissions), international treaty monitoring bodies, or treaty monitoring officials (e.g., Special Rapporteur on the right of everyone to the enjoyment of the highest standards of physical and mental health[1]). This chapter is concerned with external accountability and in particular with accountability to citizens that involve the participation of citizens.

Health accountability can be with regard to legislation, policies, budgets, expenditure, service provision, or human rights violations by power holders in the health sector. One of the concerns of this chapter would be to examine to what aspect health accountability to citizens is promoted.

Health accountability can be prospective or retrospective (Potts, 2008). Prospective accountability implies accountability before taking or implementing decisions. The purpose is to prevent errors or respond to health needs and interests. Retrospective accountability refers to accountability after decisions are taken or implemented. The purpose of retrospective accountability is to detect and correct errors. One of the concerns of this chapter is to examine when health accountability is promoted.

In short, this chapter is concerned with accountability of all power holders in the health sector to citizens, with regard to aspects ranging from health legislation and policy formulation to service delivery, prospectively and retrospectively, and through any means that involve citizens' participation.

Accountability to Citizens on Gender and Health

Accountability to citizens on gender and health refers to accountability processes (to citizens) that involve citizens and reduce gender inequalities in health and address gender-specific health concerns and rights of women and men (See Box 9.1).

As observed by Sen and colleagues (2007), gender differences lead to different exposure of men and women to health risks (together with sexual differences), different vulnerability of men and women to diseases and disability (together with sexual differences), different access of men and women to health services, different abilities of men and women to adhere to advised treatment, and different consequences to men and women of ill-health. Women in developing countries are more disadvantaged than men with regard to the last three, while men and women face different kinds of exposure and vulnerabilities, leading at times to different sex/gender-specific health needs. For example, incidence of mental depression and breast

Accountability to citizens on gender and health refers to processes by which power holders in the health sectors engage with and answer to women, men and transgender people who make demands on it, and enforce actions in such a manner to reduce gender inequalities in health and address gender-specific health concerns and rights of women, men and transgender people.

Box 9.1   Defining accountability to citizens on gender and health.

cancer is higher amongst women than men, while incidence of substance use disorder and injuries due to traffic accidents is higher amongst men than women (WHO, 2004). The gender-specific health needs of transgender people may include issues like access to sex-change operation and hormone therapy. Thus an important concern of the chapter is to examine whether accountability practices (to/with citizens) reviewed in this chapter have reduced unequal health access, adherence to treatment, and consequences to women, and addressed sex/gender-specific health concerns of women, men, and transgender people.

Some of the gender-specific health needs of women, men and transgender people are controversial and/or low priority, while others are noncontroversial and/or high priority. What is controversial and low priority varies from context to context. Provision of safe abortion services for women where they are illegal (e.g., Philippines) may be controversial, while they may not be controversial in contexts where they are legal (e.g., South Africa). There may be nothing controversial about treatment for reproductive cancer or alcohol use disorder amongst men, but they may be of low priority given national goals and resources available (Murthy et al., 2005). An important focus of this chapter is to examine whether accountability practices (to citizens) have strengthened addressing controversial and low-priority gender-specific health needs of women, men, and transgender people, in addition to the noncontroversial and high-priority ones.

ACCOUNTABILITY IN PRACTICE TO CITIZENS ON GENDER AND HEALTH

The available literature points to five broad *strategies* that have been used by citizens for demanding accountability to gender and health:

1. using international human rights instruments, agreements, and human rights monitoring positions

2. using spaces for citizens' participation in new aid infrastructure (e.g., Poverty Reduction Strategy Papers) from within, as well as critiquing outcomes of new aid architecture from outside
3. using progressive national legislation on rights of citizens to accountability
4. using, protecting, and demanding gender-sensitive health legislation, policies, programs, and structures
5. using community-level health structures, funds, and health audit tools

This section outlines 15 experiences of citizens using these five broad strategies from Asia, Africa, and Latin America to press for accountability on gender and health (including social determinants). When case studies fall into more than one of the five strategies, they have been allocated to one according to the main emphasis. Successful/partially successful (12) and unsuccessful experiences (three[2]) on promoting accountability to/with citizens on gender and health have been included with the objective of drawing out lessons.

Human Rights Instruments, International Agreements, and Accountability to Gender and Health

The CEDAW, the International Covenant on Economic, Social and Cultural Rights (ICESCR), the International Covenant on Civil and Political Rights (ICCPR), and the official position of the Special Rapporteur on the right to health have been used by citizens in the demanding of accountability of power holders in the health sector on gender and health. Citizens have also used the 1994 Program of Action, drawn at the end of the International Conference on Population and Development (ICPD) Cairo towards similar ends. Three case studies, listed here, illustrating such use are examined in this chapter:

A. Peru: the first case study describes how women's organizations and the Ombudsmen Centre in Peru successfully held a doctor who carried out a fatal sterilization operation on a woman to account using the CEDAW, the ICESCR, and the ICCPR, and advocated the removal of the policy of forced sterilization.
B. Egypt: the second case study documents how civil society actors used the 1994 ICPD commitments to ensure that the progressive legislation against female genital mutilation is not repealed.
C. Global Fund in Myanmar: the third case study outlines how the Special Rapporteur on the right to health attempted, unsuccessfully, to hold the Global Fund to Fight Aids, Tuberculosis and Malaria (Global Fund in short) to account for suddenly withdrawing support to Myanmar in 2005 based on complaints received.

(A) Peru: Using human rights instruments for demanding answerability on the policy of forced sterilization and death of a woman in hospital

Between 1996 and 2000, several Peruvian women underwent forced sterilization as part of the public health policy on population control during the period of the ex-President Alberto Fujimori (Macklin, 2006; Boyd, 2001). Women were being misled, bribed, or physically coerced into having sterilizations. One woman died on the operation table when she was undergoing sterilization. The Peruvian Ombudsman Centre, with the help of human rights and women's rights organizations, documented the case and submitted it to the Inter-American Human Rights Commission, stating that forced sterilization and her death was a violation of her human rights and a case of gender discrimination under the ICESCR and the CEDAW. The Commission held the government responsible for her death, and asked the government to compensate her (Macklin, 2006).

What occurred in response, however, was restriction of contraceptive and abortion services by the government. Between 2000 and 2004 contraceptive prevalence rate for modern methods declined from 50% to 40%, and rates of illegal abortion increased from 350,000 to 410,000 (United Nations Population Fund, 2005). In September, 2002, the Ombudsman Centre filed another case with the Inter-American Human Rights Commission stating that the new policy, like the earlier one, also discriminated against women (Macklin, 2006). Due to pressure from civil society groups and other quarters, the government now promotes emergency contraception as well as a wider range of contraceptive methods, but without adopting coercive means (United Nations Population Fund, 2005). However, problems have emerged from other quarters. The USAID has now requested government and NGOs and their partners in Peru to not promote emergency contraception through their activities (Chavez and Coe, 2007).

(B) Egypt: Using Cairo, ICPD Follow-Up Structures, and Processes as a Tool for Protecting Pro-Women's Health Legislation

As early as 1959, the Ministry of Health, Egypt, had passed a decree prohibiting health professionals and public hospitals from performing the procedure of female genital mutilation (FGM) in Egypt. A national law made it a crime to permanently mutilate anyone (Nelson, 2006). During the 1994 ICPD conference in Cairo, the Population and Family Welfare Minister vowed that Egypt was going to work towards the elimination of FGM at the community level. But some members of Egypt's religious community saw this proclamation as a form of Western imperialism and challenged the then-secular government. In response, the minister issued a decree permitting medical doctors to do the procedure of FGM in public health institutions for a fee (Nelson, 2006).

The Egyptian Task force against FGM, constituted in late 1994 under the auspices of the Egyptian National NGO Commission on Population and Development (organized to follow up ICPD implementation), was successfully able to advocate for the reversal of the new decree, and reaffirm the earlier decree banning the practice of FGM. They backed their advocacy by citing data on the deaths of several young women who underwent FGM in hospitals and the fact that the government had endorsed the Program of Action drafted at the end of the 1994 ICPD. The declaration of a progressive religious leader who stated that the practice had no sanction in Islam, and the appointment of a new sympathetic Minister of Health also helped in this reversal.

In spite of the legislation banning the practice, FGM continued in 1995. Young women saw the practice as a passport for social acceptance, while their mothers saw it as necessary to gain marriage alliances for their daughters. Concerted community-level campaigns and empowerment programs through its Task Force member organizations followed. According to a study in the late 1990s, the practice has declined amongst girls in the 10 to 14 age-group in the post-ICPD period (Petchesky, 2005).

(C) Pressure through Special Rapporteur on the Global Fund not to withdraw from Myanmar

The Global Fund suddenly withdrew from Myanmar on November 15, 2005 (United Nations, 2006). This severely hampered people's access to services related to the three communicable diseases, and in particular access of poor women to health care services. Women were particularly vulnerable to HIV/AIDS, as the incidence of rape by armed forces, forced marriages, and sexual exploitation was high (United Nations, 2006). Upon receiving and validating citizens' complaints and other reports about the withdrawal of Global Fund from Myanmar, the Special Rapporteur sent a communication to the Global Fund on November 15, 2005, expressing that this withdrawal would violate rights of vulnerable groups to the highest standards of health (United Nations, 2006). The Global Fund replied on February 2, 2006, stating that the provision of three grants to the United Nations Development Program in Myanmar (its recipient in the country) was based on "access to project sites" and the government had tightened access of all donor agencies. It hence withdrew from the country (United Nations, 2007). The Rapporteur responded on April 20, 2006, that restriction of access to project sites was only temporary, and asked whether it had communicated to the government about its plan to withdraw and received any response. He also asked the Global Fund whether the 60 days notice as per the agreement was issued to UNDP about its withdrawal. The Rapporteur did not receive a reply until December 2007 (United Nations, 2007, 2008). In a separate communication to the Myanmar government, the Rapporteur raised the issue of violations of health and sexual rights of women and girls by armed forces to which, again, it has not received any reply (United Nations, 2006).

New Aid Architecture, Country-Level Programming, and Accountability to Gender and Health

Citizens groups have used new aid architecture like Poverty Reduction Strategy Papers (PRSPs) and sector-wide approaches (SWAPs) to health, which emerged in the 1990s and early 2000s, to press for accountability on gender and health. When the new aid architecture has not reflected a rights-based perspective, they have critiqued it from outside. Three case studies, listed in the following, illustrating these strategies are described in greater detail.

A. Rwanda: the first case study is of how women's rights groups' participation in the first PRSP process led to engendering of the first PRSP, including the health component.
B. Bangladesh: the second case study describes how women's health rights groups in Bangladesh engaged with the design of the SWAPs to health, and the mixed impact of the same.
C. India: the third case study is on the Independent People's Tribunal of the World Bank in India, which included a critique of World Bank's state-specific health systems development projects. However, a year after the Tribunal, changes in World Bank's health policies are not visible.

(A) Rwanda: Using PRSPs to Promote Accountability to Citizens on Gender and Health

The Interim Rwanda PRSP, 2000, led by the Ministry of Finance and Planning, was not considered particularly gender sensitive or an example of civil society participation (Zucherman, 2001). The Ministry of Gender and Women and Development (MIGEPROFE) hence decided to take the lead in mainstreaming gender into the final PRSP and hold consultations with women's NGOs.

The Ministry, with the support of Department for International Development (DFID), invited an external gender consultant to facilitate the process. With the help of the consultant, the MIGEPROFE and Ministry of Finance and Planning held a PRSP engendering workshop, at the end of which a PRSP engendering committee was formed. Leaders of women's NGOs were represented in the workshop and in the engendering committee. As some of the senior staffs of the MIGEPROFE were honorary heads of NGOs, NGO inputs were taken seriously (Zucherman, 2001). Sectoral-specific gender teams were constituted, including one on gender and health. The PRSP Engendering Committee reviewed existing sex-disaggregated government data and carried out new surveys to fill data gaps (Zucherman, 2001).

The Rwanda PRSP document that evolved through this process included a gender analysis of household poverty and the gender-specific reasons women slip into poverty. The PRSP recommended that budget be allocated to address women's gender-specific needs, like women's rights to land, improved access to fuel and fodder, and female literacy. Legal strategies for ending post-genocide problems like polygamy, nonlegal marriages, and prostitution were outlined. In addition, the PRSP report outlined strategies to address sex/gender-specific health needs of women and men. These included improving maternal health care (including for delivery), improving contraceptive choice and services for women, improving access of women to health care, and strengthening prevention of HIV/AIDS (Zucherman and Garett, 2003). However, conspicuous by its absence was male responsibility with regard to contraception.

An evaluation of the implementation of Rwanda PRSP (Phase I) notes that while access of the poor to health services has improved, maternal and child mortality continue to be high. Further, improvement in education indicators has been faster than health, because a three times greater budget was allocated to education in 2005 (International Monetary Fund and International Development Association, 2006).

(B) Bangladesh: Engendering Sector-Wide Approaches in Health

The Bangladesh case study illustrates the potential and limitations of citizen's engagement with SWAPS in health to engender them. In Bangladesh, as part of formulating the Health and Population Sector Strategy (HPSS) 1996, and Health and Population Sector Programme: 1998–2003 (HPSP), a 40-member task force was constituted that included women and men from communities, health providers, health policy makers, important donors, health NGOs, media, political parties, and religious leaders (World Bank, 2001).

The stakeholders prioritized reproductive and child health (family planning, basic emergency obstetric care, and prevention and control of STIs/RTIs and infertility), communicable disease control, and limited curative care as part of the Essential Service Package (ESP). These services were to be implemented through one-stop clinics at the village level, and more comprehensive health services at the *Upazilla* (subdistrict) level. The government also adopted a Patient Charter of Rights, which was to be enforced during implementation of the HPSS/HPSP. To institutionalize stakeholder participation in implementation, the MOHFW established a National Steering Committee. At the clinic level, community groups were to be established to oversee construction, maintenance, and functioning, comprising of local elected representatives, local health providers, and influential leaders. At the Upazilla level, Community Health Watch Groups were to be set up consisting of citizens, NGOs, providers, elected representatives, and health administrators. These health watch groups were to monitor the quality of service and client-needs satisfaction (World Bank, 2001; Mahmud, 2006).

While the World Bank sees stakeholder participation as a success story, researchers have critiqued it on several accounts. Murthy and colleagues (2005) noted that rights-based women's organizations were not initially invited for consultations and had to demand that they be invited. Treatment for health complications due to violence against women has been kept outside the ESP, though provided for in a few urban-based hospitals. Jahan (2003) points out that while the HPSS/HPSP was designed in a participatory manner, citizens were not involved in overseeing the implementation. Implementation has been better with regard to the child health component when compared to maternal health component. Mahmud (2006) observes that the clinic community groups did not perform any oversight functions and became defunct. The health watch groups performed oversight roles only when supported by rights-based organizations (Mahmud, 2006). To strengthen accountability with regard to implementation of HPSS, civil society actors have recently formed 'Health Watch,' Bangladesh.[3]

(C) Using the Independent People's Tribunal of the World Bank in India to Press for Accountability to Gender and Health

In contrast to Bangladesh, most of the nine health systems development projects (HSDPs) of the World Bank in India have been formulated without a broad-based consultative process. Between September 21 and September 24, 2007, several human/women's rights organizations and activists together convened an Independent People's Tribunal of the World Bank in India. The 13 member jury (including four women) comprising of renowned human rights activists, sensitive retired members of judiciary and government, and academicians heard 150 testimonies (50% from women) from across the country and the opinions of experts on the impact of World Bank groups' interventions in India in different sectors, including the health sector (World Bank Tribunal Secretariat, 2008).

Assessing the impact of the nine state-level HSDPs operational/completed[4] in India as of 2007, health activists and economists who took part in the Tribunal observed that these projects had led to a shift from universal public health services to targeted health services with user fees being levied at secondary and tertiary hospitals. Poor women's access to health services was more price elastic than that of poor men as they were more in the informal sector. Data on four[5] of the six states where HSDPs were completed suggests that the proportion of pregnant women seeking delivery care in public facilities had fallen during the project period despite substantial investment in infrastructure improvements, while figures show an increase in numbers of users of private facilities. This was also borne out in testimonies. A majority of the budget in completed projects went towards HIV/AIDS, ignoring other health priorities (Ravindran, 2007; World Bank Tribunal Secretariat, 2008). The jury demanded that the World Bank compensate the poor whose rights had been violated, and institutionalize an independent audit of World Bank policies and activities in the country. World Bank backed out of participation in the Tribunal at the last minute, but posted a rebuttal in its Web site (World Bank Tribunal Secretariat, 2008). No changes in policies of the World Bank are yet visible.

Making Use of Accountability Legislation to Press for Accountability to Citizens on Health

Citizens' groups have used general (not specific to gender and health) accountability legislation like right to participation, right to information, and public interest litigation to demand accountability on gender and health. Three case studies, listed here, illustrating these strategies are described in greater detail.

A. South Africa: this case study illustrates how civil society organizations have used the constitutional clause on right to participation to successfully advocate for liberal abortion laws.

B. Brazil and Argentina: the second case study is on the mandatory Brazilian Policy Councils and Argentinean participatory budgeting, and how these have been used by citizens for influencing health policy (Brazil) and demanding that adequate budget be allocated for child care (Argentina).

C. Nepal: the third case study is on how groups working for the rights of lesbian, gay, bisexual, transgender, and intersexual (LGBTI) people in Nepal have used the mechanism of public interest litigation for decriminalization of homosexuality and promotion of laws to prevent discrimination against them.

(A) South Africa: Making use of the Constitution Mandate on Right to Public Involvement in Legislation and Policy Formulation for Legalizing Access to Abortion

The African National Congress, when it won the elections in 1994, invited public inputs into the new constitution through placing advertisements in diverse local language media asking for inputs. The Clause 59.1 of the constitution, which emerged through this process, requires that that the parliament facilitate public involvement in the legislation and other processes of the assembly and its committees. By the year 2002, this consultative process had become ad hoc, depending on the interests of particular politicians or bureaucrats concerned. But once laws get to the parliament, there is an established practice of public hearings at which any individual or group in civil society can ask to present their concerns (Klugman, 2002).

The Congress of South Africa Trade Unions (COSATU) established an office with the specific brief of keeping watch on parliamentary processes and ensuring that union members' voices are heard. NGOs involved in health and women's rights have used this space for advocating progressive policies, including favorable policies on abortion and violence against women (Klugman, 2002).

These NGOs allied with the Medical Research Council and presented evidence that liberalizing abortion laws could reduce costs to the government and improve the country's performance with respect to reduction of maternal mortality. Women who had borne the brunt of unsafe illegal abortion were also mobilized to speak before parliament, and the support of the mass-based organization COSATU and the African National Congress Women's League was solicited on this issue. The presence of allies within the Parliamentary Committee and the Ministry of Health significantly helped to push through the controversial policy on liberalizing the abortion law. The present law is one of the most liberal in the world: it permits abortion on request in the first trimester and allows adolescents to access abortion without requiring parental consent (Klugman, 2002).

(B) Brazil and Argentina: Policy Councils and Participatory Budgets and Issues of Accountability to Gender and Health

After 21 years of military rule, civil rule was restored in 1985 in Brazil. A new constitution that supports democratic elections and universal suffrage followed in 1988. The (new) constitutionally mandated policy councils and the practice of participatory budgeting implemented since 2002 in Brazil have been used by citizens for influencing health policies at the local level (in all municipalities) as well as allocation of health budgets (in some municipalities).

Health Councils are comprised of representatives of users, health workers, health managers, and elected members. Roughly 50% of those elected health councilors were women in 2003 (Cornwall, 2007). Deliberations in councils were nevertheless constrained by several factors. Cornwall (2006) observes that some users were previous contractors with municipal government and interested in securing personal gains, while others were genuinely interested in exercising their voice. Amongst the latter, there was substantial tension between those who believed that their role was holding the health council answerable for services and those who believed that they were there to deliberate on health policies.

Three concerns were expressed by users with regard to the functioning of health councils: politicization of councils, lack of effective independence of health councils (as health personnel are also represented), and de facto implementation role of health councils. Health workers pointed to the hierarchy between users/health workers in council and health managers. Health managers pointed out that elected members had an interest to get reelected and prioritized infrastructural interventions. They also felt that users were not competent to make technical decisions (Cornwall, 2006).

While literature on impact of citizen's participation in Brazilian health councils and participatory budgets on gender and health could not be found, a study from Argentina on participatory budgeting found that there were different committees on different social services, and they had to argue their proposal in a larger assembly where decisions (through voting) were taken on what to allocate resources for. In one municipality, a woman activist with prior experience in negotiating with such spaces, brought women supporters in large numbers to cast a vote for a child care program, so that women could earn income without worrying about their children (Rodgers, 2006). One could argue that better child care and income would improve the health of women and their access to health services.

(C) Nepal: Using Public Interest Litigation for Pressing for Decriminalizing Homosexuality

The system of a third party petitioning the Supreme Court directly when rights of another party or group are violated is referred to as public interest litigation (PIL). That is, the aggrieved party need not approach the court directly. Filing a PIL is also less cumbersome and expensive than a private litigation.

In Nepal, four LGBTI organizations, including the Blue Diamond Society, had filed a writ petition in April 2007 (05/01/2064) demanding the Supreme Court defend and protect equal rights of LGBTI people of Nepal. After three hearings in December 2007, in a landmark judgment, the Supreme Court of Nepal recognized LGBTI people as natural persons who should enjoy all the rights as other sexes/genders enshrined by the constitution of Nepal and by human rights conventions in which Nepal is a State Party. The Court issued directive orders to the government of Nepal to ensure rights to life according to their own identities, introduce laws providing equal rights to LGBTI people, and amend all laws that discriminate against LGBTI people. The court has ordered the formation of a committee comprising officials from health, law, and other ministries, police, and the National Human Rights Commission to address issues faced by sexual minorities (Sarkar, 2007; Pant, 2007). On the issue of same-sex marriage, the court has also issued a directive order to form a seven-member committee (a doctor appointed by the Health Ministry, one representative from the National Human Rights Commission, one from the law ministry, socialist appointed by the government of Nepal, representative from the Nepal police, representative from the ministry of population and environment, and one advocate from the LGBTI community) to conduct a study about other countries' policies on same-sex marriages (Pant, 2007).

Demanding and Using Progressive Gender and Health Policies, Programs, and Personnel for Pressing for Accountability

Citizens' groups have pressed for, and used, progressive gender and health national legislation, policies, and programs in their attempt to promote accountability on gender and health. Three case studies, listed here, are discussed that illustrate such strategies, one pertaining to the private health sector:

A. Ghana: the first case study is of how government, Women In Development structure, and a women's rights organization (headed by elite women) came together to successfully press the health department to strengthen breast cancer screening services for women in four government hospitals. However, priorities of poor women like cervical cancer were not addressed.

B. India: the second case study is of the strategies used by one campaign in the state of Tamil Nadu, India, to press for the strict enforcement of the Prohibition of Sex Selection Act, 1994, which, however, is accused of leading to lesser access of women to abortion for other legal reasons.

C. Bolivia: the third case study is from Bolivia, of strategies adopted by Help Age International with local organizations to strengthen access of older women to health insurance and health services.

(A) Ghana: Pressing Government to Provide Breast Cancer Screening Facilities

During the 1970s and 1980s, breast cancer in Ghana was addressed as a clinical issue by the medical community. Breast cancer accounted for 7.45% of all cancers treated at Korle Bu teaching hospital between 1972 and 1977. There were no screening-based studies on the incidence of breast cancer (Reichenbach, 2002).

During the 1990s, political attention to breast cancer as a public health issue increased, spearheaded by the National Council for Women in Development (NCWD) and the 31st December Women's Movement (31 DWM; a movement that mobilizes rural and urban women throughout the county). In 1996, the 31 DWM had a base of 1.5 million women. It was headed at that time by the then first lady of Ghana, which gave the organization a lot of clout. In March 1991, breast cancer was raised as an issue in one of the NCWD's regional meetings at Accra. A medical professor also released a book on breast cancer in Ghana, which received wide media publicity. The NCWD and the 31 DWM came together with the objective of creating awareness on breast cancer and to raise funds for the government to purchase mammography equipment. They arranged to receive copies of a video of a US television program with a popular American actress on her experience with breast cancer. This video was shown in beauty parlors and hair salons. The month of October was designated as the breast cancer awareness month every year. At the community level, regional rallies were held on breast cancer and to instruct villagers to perform self-examinations. Funds were raised from Ghanians and charity organizations abroad for mammography equipments. By 1996 four mammography units had been acquired and installed in three regions of the country. The Ministry of Health trained staff on using the equipment and paid for recurring costs (Reichenbach, 2002).

The advocacy by the NCWD and the 31 DWM led to the availability of screening facilities in four hospitals. However, as of 2002 breast cancer screening was yet to be institutionalized within the government health programs. While the National and Reproductive Health Service Policy and Standards discussed the prevention and management of breast cancer, it did not provide screening or treatment protocols. Mammography services were limited to four government hospitals. Treatment facilities were not readily available in government facilities, and are very expensive outside. Further, the incidence of cervical cancer amongst poor women is higher than breast cancer, as in most developing countries, but has not received the same priority by the 31 DWM or the NCWD (Reichenbach, 2002). The annual report of the Ghana Health Service for 2007 does not mention provision of breast or cervical cancer screening or treatment as part of the essential health package (Ghana Health Service, 2007).

(B) India: Pressing Government to Implement the Prohibition of Sex Selection Act

The government of India, pressurized by civil society organizations, passed legislation (the Prohibition of Sex Selection Act) in 1994 to combat the practice of disclosure of sex of the fetus by prenatal diagnostic centers and sex-selective abortion by couples. This act was amended in 2002 as the Pre-Conception and Pre-natal Diagnostic Techniques Act (PCPNDT Act).

The Campaign Against Sex Selection Abortion (CASSA) was launched in Tamil Nadu in 1998 by a coalition of child rights and women's rights groups with the mission of preventing the declining sex-ratio at birth and juvenile sex-ratio (0–6 years) while at the same time protecting and promoting the rights of women to abortion when it is for reasons other than sex selection. An innovative monitoring intervention of the campaign was to send pregnant women for scanning to private and public scanning centers/facilities and ask for information on the sex of the fetus. Through this process, they started detecting the scanning centers that violate the act and reported the matter to the district and state authorities. The campaign members also visited scanning centers to find out if they are registered under the PCPNDT Act, as was required under the law. The appropriate authorities have taken action against the unregistered prediagnostic clinics whose existence the campaign pointed to and those that were disclosing sex of the fetus after scanning. Doctors performing sex-selective abortion were also brought to account.

Due to pressure from the campaign, the government of Tamil Nadu constituted advisory committees in all the districts as required under the act, some of which included members of the campaign. The government has started collecting and monitoring data on sex-ratio at birth (natural sex-ratio at birth is supposed to be 952 females per 1000 males). Medical associations have committed themselves to work for effective enforcement of the act (CASSA, 2006). Data on sex-ratio at birth in the different districts of Tamil Nadu gathered from the government by the campaign reveals a steady increase in the same between 2001 and 2004 in 45% of the districts, and a slight increase at the state level (CASSA, 2006).

The campaign, however, has come under criticism recently from women's health rights groups as it organized a meeting this year wherein some speakers advocated that all abortions during the second trimester under the Medical Termination Pregnancy Act 1972 should be reviewed to scrutinize the reasons. Such a move would restrict access of pregnant women in the second trimester who are presently legally eligible for abortion (if the pregnancy poses threat to life of women, abnormality of fetus is detected, and if pregnancy is due to rape of women). Women's health rights groups also observed that providers are now afraid to provide legal abortion services as they feel that they could be wrongly booked under the PCPND7 act. Further, women's health rights groups observe that the borderline is thin between such campaigns (which use the term female feticide to imply that fetuses have life) and pro-life movements against abortion of all fetuses (see e-contribution of George A., Coalition—Maternal Neonatal Health Safe Abortion Solution Exchange, 2008).

(C) Bolivia: Addressing Gender Inequalities in Health Access Amongst Older Women

In Bolivia older women live longer than men, but have lower access to income. Seventy-three percent of women over 60 years in Bolivia are nonliterate, when compared to 28% of older men (cited in Goetz, 2008; data for which year unspecified). Since 1992, older people in Bolivia have had access to universal health insurance, and in 2006 the health insurance provision was redrafted to improve access in rural areas. However, older women, because of their lower literacy levels, income, and caretaking role, find it more difficult than older men to access such insurance (Goetz, 2008).

The new law hence includes a monitoring framework consisting of Committee de Vigilencia (vigilance committee), which includes older women and men and organizations representing them that identify barriers faced by older people to access health insurance. HelpAge International hence led an older citizens monitoring project that trained four older people's local organizations to monitor the financing and delivery of insurance and health services. The local organizations in turn trained older rural women on their entitlements under the health insurance, and on how to dialogue with health providers. It also trained older women members in the vigilance committee. Over a period of time shortfalls in access of older women to health insurance reduced and quality of health services improved (Goetz, 2008).

Community Health Structures and Accountability Tools, and Gender and Health Accountability

Governments, donors, and NGOs have attempted to promote accountability to citizens through devolution of health services, community health structures, and health accountability tools. Three examples listed in the following are illustrated in this section:

A. Philippines: the first case study from the Philippines discusses the adverse impact of devolution of health services on strengthening accountability to sex/gender-specific health services.
B. China/India: the second case study documents experiences of the Gender and Health Equity Network in creating community health structures in India and China from the outside to demand accountability to gender and health.
C. Uganda, Costa Rica, and Haiti: the third case study documents experiences in using provider report cards to strengthen accountability of providers to citizens on health, and gender and health.

(A) The Philippines: Devolution and Accountability to Gender and Health

Devolution is a popular mechanism used by donors and government to promote accountability to citizens on social services. The government of the Philippines embarked on devolution of health and social services after the passing of the Local Government Code of 1991. As part of the devolution in health services, 95% of its facilities, 60% of its personnel, and 45% of the budget was transferred to local government units (LGUs) at provincial, city, and municipality levels (Tadiar, 2000). Local health boards were set up in each LGU, comprising of the governor or mayor as its chairperson, municipal health officer as vice chairperson, the local councilor for health, a representative of the department of health, and a representative of a health NGO (Tadiar, 2000). Local government expenditures doubled between 1990 and 2002, with 66% going for health. However, the majority of the health expenditure was incurred at provincial levels and less at city, municipality, and *barangay* levels (World Bank and Asian Development Bank, 2005). Though this amount is in principle untied, a significant proportion went for salaries of health workers. The Local-Government Assistance and Monitoring Service (LGAMS) was established within the department of health to monitor LGU health programs and provide technical assistance. The LGAMS was also supposed to augment resources of

LGUs, if they agreed to implement national health programs, including the reproductive health program[6] (Tadiar, 2000).

Researchers have observed that the implementation of gender-aware health programs has suffered because of decentralization. Provision of a wide range of contraceptives by local clinics depended on attitudes of members elected to LGUs at different levels. This in turn led to high rates of unsafe abortions. While emergency obstetric care has been on the priority list of many LGUs, in practice such services have been affected because of weakening referral systems, as different levels of health care are being managed by different elected bodies (Lakshminarayanan, 2003). Access to diagnosis and management of HIV/AIDS is still limited and unequally distributed across rich and poor areas. Men's gender-specific health needs are often not prioritized by LGUs. By and large, curative care was given more priority over preventive care by several LGUs, as these are more visible and aid reelection. There has also been little effort to build capacities of local health boards and LGUs on their roles and responsibilities as elected members as well as on gender and health issues (Lakshminarayanan, 2003; Tadiar, 2000).

(B) Gender and Health Equity Network (GHEN): Mobilizing Women to Press for Accountability to Gender and Health in India and China

The GHEN is an international partnership demonstrating through applied research the case for taking gender equity issues into account in health policies and programming. While the first phase focused on reviewing literature on gender issues in technical areas of health, the second phase included an action research component. As part of the second phase, the GHEN partners are mobilizing women in project areas of India, China, and Mozambique for pressing for accountability to gender and health equity. Experiences from India and China have been documented (GHEN, 2007) and are summarized in the following.

In the Koppal district of Karnataka, India, it became clear to the GHEN team that the government-formed village health committees were dominated by men and not interested in promoting accountability on gender and health issues. The Network, through partnering with the government initiated *Mahila Samkahya Programme* (Women's Empowerment through Education Program) formed neighborhood groups for every 20 households. Each village has around 20 to 25 neighborhood groups, which have been trained by Mahila Samakhya to gather information on the number of pregnant women, their access to antenatal and postnatal checkups, high-risk pregnancies, and pregnant women who require immunization. This information is shared with government Auxiliary Nurse Midwives (ANMs) and doctors from primary health centers. As a result of this community-provider monitoring and dialogues, the schedule of ANMs has been reorganized by the Health Office to ensure better coverage of villages, regularity of visits, and better quality of maternal health services. Verbal autopsies of maternal deaths are also conducted by the government with the involvement of women. However, frequent transfer of district health officers poses a problem (GHEN, 2007).

Replication of this model in China posed difficulties. There are few independent NGOs or mechanisms for participation of rural women in government policy or service provision monitoring. Although the National Federation of Women exists, it is a top-down and party-led institution, and 42% of women do not participate in elections of its cadres. The GHEN hence formed gender and governance groups for strengthening gender equity integration in health planning, and for pressing of accountability of providers. The governance group consists of rural women elected by people, a representative of the National Federation of Women, a representative of Township Health Bureau, and the vice mayor in charge of health. The trained governance groups have been provided with an incentive fund to support delivery of services that address any gender inequality in health status and access. At present the gender and governance group is functioning as a health promotion group, and has yet to perform oversight roles (GHEN, 2007).

(C) Provider-specific Reports in Developing Countries: Uganda, Costa Rica, and Haiti

Provider report cards refer to any effort to compare providers within a specified geographical region on a routine basis, according to certain standards of quality performance. These report cards can be public (results made available to citizens) or private (results made available only to providers) and they can be voluntary or mandatory. When provider report cards are made public and mandatory and involve citizens, they tend to promote accountability to citizens on health (Mcnamara, 2006).

The Yellow Star Program in Uganda is one example from a developing country. It is sponsored by the government and donors. The program evaluates health care facilities (public and private) on a quarterly basis using 35 indicators that include standard of infrastructure, management systems, infection prevention, health education, interpersonal communication, clinical skills, and client services. Ratings of a provider are made available to the public. A facility in which all providers have received a 100% score for two quarters receives a yellow star, which is then posted prominently outside. If performance falls, it is removed. The average score of facilities assessed climbed from 47% in the first quarter to 65% in the second. Initially implemented in 12 of the 56 districts, plans are now afoot to expand to all the 56 districts of the country (Uganda, DISH, 2004, cited in Mcnamara, 2006).

While the Uganda report cards have not included sex/gender-specific indicators for monitoring, Costa Rica has included the criteria of existence of a mechanism to analyze maternal death and delivery complication rate. Haiti has included availability of family planning supplies as one of the indicators (Mcnamara, 2006). However, there are concerns that providers may be constrained by availability of resources or civil service rules from addressing shortcomings. The clout of the medical lobby may also get in the way of effective implementation (Mcnamara, 2006).

LESSONS ON ACCOUNTABILITY TO CITIZENS ON GENDER AND HEALTH

Several lessons on promoting accountability to citizens on gender and health flow from the practice of accountability documented in the previous section.

Accountability on Gender and Health cannot be Looked at in Isolation

A first lesson is that accountability to citizens on gender and health is closely linked to accountability to development, to health (including health financing), and to gender/social equity. In Rwanda, women's organizations' engagement with the planning process led to the first PRSP prioritizing women's right to land, women's access to fuel and fodder, and female literacy. If these plans are implemented, women's health and access to health care is likely to improve. In Argentina, poor women's involvement in participatory budgeting in a municipality led to greater budget being allocated for child care services, which is central to expanding poor women's income and access to health services. In Bolivia, improving access to information for older women and their participation in health vigilance committees improved their access to universal health insurance and health services. The Egyptian Task Force against FGM's pressure on policy makers to not repeal the anti-FGM legislation has a bearing on women's and girls' health.

Need to Engender Existing Health/Citizen Accountability Structures, Process, and Tools

At the same time, it is essential to engender health accountability processes, and weave health strongly into gender accountability processes. Otherwise gender inequalities in health access and outcomes, and gender-specific health needs of women and men, may not be addressed comprehensively. The GHEN experience in India and the Philippines devolution example, suggest that poor women may be largely absent in government-initiated community health structures and not be in a position to demand accountability to gender and health. Even when alternative structures with women are created, their representation alone is not enough. It is important to build their capacity for monitoring and demanding accountability on gender and health. The case study on provider report cards in Uganda in the public domain illustrates that quality assessments involving citizens need not automatically be gender sensitive. There is a need to include indicators of whether sex/gender-specific health needs have been addressed and whether gender inequalities in access have been reduced. Similarly, accountability processes to citizens on gender need to be made 'health' aware. The Rwanda case study shows that the effort to 'engender' PRSP through involving women's organizations led to prioritization of maternal health, contraceptive and HIV prevention services being included, but not issues like women's access to abortion, mental health services, reproductive cancer services, or treatment for violence against women.

Need to Press for Accountability at Multiple Levels

Another lesson is that accountability mechanisms on gender and health are required at multiple levels. International human rights instruments and agreements and positions of Special Rapporteurs related to development, health, and gender are essential for creation of spaces for citizens' groups to push for accountability of governments to gender and health. This is amply illustrated through the example of safeguarding anti-FGM legislation using ICPD process in Egypt and prohibiting forced sterilization in Peru through using international human rights treaties and agreements. In Myanmar the position of the Rapporteur on right to health was used to put pressure on the Global Fund, though the effort has yet to meet with success.

At the national level, legislation, policies, programs, and structures in keeping with the international agreements (and at times beyond) are important. A case in point is the legal prohibition of sex selection in India and FGM in Egypt. National legislation on right to participation and accountability are also important. The Nepal case points to how citizens can use accountability legislation like the public interest litigation to promote extension of constitutional rights to LGBTIs. In fact, as of yet, international human rights instruments on the rights of LGBTIs do not exist. In South Africa, the right to participation was used by women's organizations to demand women's and adolescent girls' rights to legal abortion. At the local level, progressive legislation, policies, and structures need to be followed up with structures, tools, and processes for promoting accountability. The health watch groups in Bangladesh, when supported by rights-based NGOs and community groups representing women and other marginalized groups, played an important role in monitoring the implementation of HPSP/HPSS (also see Naripokko and ARROW, 2006).

Need to press for accountability of multiple institutions

Accountability of multiple institutions, and the organizational forms they take, to gender and health is necessary. State is an obvious institution, and the accountability or lack of accountability of the public health sector has been much discussed since the 1990s. Several examples in this chapter have dealt with public health sector accountability. However, it is important to press for accountability of market organizations involved in health as well, like pharmaceutical companies, private clinics, and hospitals, as well as public–private partnerships that are emerging. The campaign against sex selection in Tamil Nadu has met with some degree of success in lowering this practice because it monitored both the private and the public scanning facilities and providers. Interstate organizations like the World Bank and regional development banks are other key players in health whose accountability needs to be ensured, as illustrated by citizens' engagement from inside in the case of Bangladesh HPSP/HPSS and Rwanda PRSP, and citizens engagement from outside in the case of the Independent People's Tribunal of the World Bank in India. New entities that fall in the realm of public–private partnerships also need to be held (though difficult to do) to account, as illustrated by the case of the communication between the Special Rapporteur on the right to health and the Global Fund. Bilateral donors are another set of group to be held to account, in particular USAID, which has reduced access to abortion services and emergency contraception, as illustrated by the Peru case study. Further, as illustrated by the Egyptian anti-FGM task force experience, it is important to bring gender-aware changes at the community and household level.

Need to Use Multiple Mechanisms to Press for Accountability to Citizens

Given the multiple levels, institutions, and facets at which accountability to gender and health needs to be promoted, no one accountability mechanism is adequate for all contexts and there is a need to use multiple mechanisms from a basket that includes:

- human rights agreements, instruments, and positions
- international, regional, and national courts of justice
- national legislation on right to participation
- public interest litigation
- right to information
- PRSPs
- SWAPs to health
- government ombudsmen centers
- participatory councils
- media advertisements calling for inputs

- participatory budgeting
- public hearings and tribunals
- community health structures
- community monitoring/vigilance committees
- provider/facility report cards

Not all methods would be appropriate in all contexts. If a country has not signed or ratified ICESCR it may be difficult to hold the government accountable to implementation of the right to health components. If the literacy levels are low in a country, placing of media advertisements in newspapers would not be appropriate to solicit public inputs into policies. If there is no legislation permitting public interest litigation, it cannot be used for demanding accountability. If electoral processes are weak, structures that involve elected representatives pressing for accountability may not work.

Need to Address Accountability in its Various Facets

Yet another lesson is the importance of addressing accountability in its three facets: engagement, answerability, and enforcement. Citizens' participation in the Rwanda PRSP, Brazil health councils, and Bangladesh HPSP are examples of accountability as engagement. The use of public interest litigation by LGBTIs groups in Nepal to put an end to criminalization of homosexuality is an example of accountability as answerability. The Peruvian women's groups' and Ombudsmen's Centre's use of the Inter-American Human Rights Commission to bring a provider who was negligent in the death of a woman who came in for a sterilization operation is an example of accountability as enforcement.

At times citizens have to go beyond these three facets of accountability and protect gains made. This was the case with the Egypt anti-FGM task force, which had to protect the move to dismantle the law prohibiting FGM. At times pressing for accountability on one gender and health issue may have an adverse impact on another. In the case of Peru, demands to take action against forced sterilization led to the government restricting availability of contraception and abortion services, and hence a second litigation to regain access to contraceptive (but not forced) and abortion services had to be filed. The campaigns against sex-selective abortion in India are alleged to have reduced women's access to legal abortion, though evidence on this is anecdotal.

Need to Address Power Relations

The review of accountability practices suggests that accountability is about challenging power relations. Health workers who took part in health councils in Brazil pointed to the hierarchies between managers and themselves, and managers and citizens, which came in the way of how far health councils were accountable to citizens. In Egypt and part of the Philippines, certain sections of religious leaders exercised power over government (national or local), which got in the way of accountability to citizens on gender and health. Gender-based power relations within the household and community were cited as a reason for the continuation of the practice of FGM in Egypt and sex-selection abortion in India in spite of legislation banning these practices. The Ghana breast cancer case study illustrates how at times power relations amongst women based on their economic background gets in the way of how far gender-specific health priorities of poor women get articulated and addressed through representation of civil society organizations.

Several of the case studies point to the need for alliance building between progressive actors within civil society as well as between them and gender- and health-sensitive bureaucrats, donors, and consultants to alter these power relations. The gains in terms of policy changes on gender and health in Bangladesh HPSP and RWANDA PRSP (and to some extent in Ghana) were possible due to such alliances. Further, gathering data and evidence is central for answerability and enforcement of power holders in the health sector on gender and health as illustrated by the South African and Peruvian case studies on access to abortion and removal of forced sterilization respectively.

Need for Vibrant Democracies, Political Will, and Resources

Lastly, promoting accountability to gender and health requires vibrant democracy, as well as earmarking of resources on the part of the international donor community and national governments. In rural China, independent women's organizations are few, and hence mobilizing women to press for equitable access to health care posed a challenge for the GHEN. The case of Nepal points to the need for an independent and activist judiciary to uphold the rights of people discriminated on the grounds of their sexual/gender identities. Resources are required to make health policy makers and providers sensitive to the importance of accountability to citizens, as well as on gender and health. Resources are also essential to build pressure groups of women, men, transgender, and intersexual people from below to make accountability mechanisms work and to address their specific health needs, reduce gender inequalities in health, and uphold their health rights.

GAPS IN ACCOUNTABILITY TO CITIZENS ON GENDER AND HEALTH

The review of evidence in this chapter points to the existence of a rich gamut of experiences in promoting accountability to citizens on gender and health. At the same time there are several gaps that relate to who is being held to account, to whom, how, and in relation to what issues. These gaps are discussed in this section.

Who are Citizens not Holding to Account on Gender and Health?

There are more examples of citizens holding governments to account on gender and health than of the private health sector in health. In the context of the receding role of the state, and expanding role of the private health sector, this gap is an area of great concern. Another concern is that there are few examples of citizens successfully holding multilateral financial institutions, the USAID, and global public–private partnerships to account on gender and health despite the fact that their role is increasing in the health sector. Only 4% of the correspondence of the Special Rapporteur (based on complaints received and visits made) on right to health with health actors between December 2003 and December 2007 on violations of right to health dealt with violations by nonstate actors (United Nations, 2005, 2006, 2007, 2008). None of the correspondence dealt with violations by global private health sector actors or the World Bank Group. At a more local level, examples of citizens holding traditional community organizations and male household heads to account on gender and health are largely absent; unless it is an act of physical or sexual violence.

Who is Being Left out in the Accountability to Citizens' Process?

Examples of direct accountability to marginalized women and men are rare, especially to LGBTI people. With few exceptions, accountability through government- or donor-initiated community-level structures has been stronger to the social and economic elites (often men), than to marginalized women, men, and adolescents. The Indian village health committees, Bangladesh clinic committees, Philippines health boards, and consultations in Ghana on breast cancer are examples. At provincial and national levels, accountability to citizens on gender and health has been equated by government and donors with accountability to civil society organizations working with marginalized groups, and rarely to marginalized groups directly. Marginalized women and men have rarely been invited to national-level consultations. While rights-based civil society organizations do represent the interests of marginalized groups, at times they are not called to policy dialogues by governments, as illustrated by the Bangladesh HPSP/HPSS case study. However, the voice of marginalized groups has been greater when rights-based groups have pressed for accountability on gender and health from the outside, like in the case of GHEN in India, Blue Diamond Society in Nepal, Independent Citizen's Tribunal on the World Bank in India, and the women's rights groups/Ombudsman Centre in Peru.

What Issues are Being Left out in Accountability Processes?

Government-initiated accountability processes on gender and health that involve citizens have mainly strengthened accountability to improve women's access to noncontroversial health services like maternal health care services (e.g., Costa Rica) and contraception (where antenatal policies are in place, like Haiti). Citizens' initiatives from the outside, on the other hand, have promoted legal changes on controversial gender and health issues like decriminalization of homosexuality (in Nepal) and withdrawal of policy on forced sterilization (in Peru). At times citizens' advocacy has led to good legislation (e.g., anti-FGM in Egypt) not being repealed due to pressure from the right wing.

However, citizens' groups—including rights-based groups—have rarely prioritized accountability to reduce gender inequalities in health access, and have tended to focus more on blatant violations of rights to survive, sexual and reproductive rights of women, and gender/sex-specific health needs of women in the area of maternal health, abortion, and contraception. Few have successfully pressed for greater accountability on providing cervical cancer services, infertility services, mental health services for women, and antiretroviral therapy for nonpregnant women. Gender inequalities in health outcomes disadvantaging men, like higher traffic accidents and higher substance use disorders amongst men, have again not been prioritized by citizens' groups. Accountability processes that address sex/gender-specific health needs of transgender and intersexual people (apart from the area of prevention of HIV) appears to be rare in developing countries. The example of Blue Diamond in Nepal is noteworthy in this regard. Further, at times there is conflict of interest between the girl child rights lobby and the women's health rights lobby, as illustrated by the case of CASSA in Tamil Nadu; with such conflicts yet to be resolved.

Which Preconditions for Accountability are met and which are not?

The preconditions for accountability to citizens (i.e., independent electoral process, independent media and judiciary, political will, and adequate resources) are not met in many developing countries. Several examples of accountability to citizens come from India, South Africa, and Brazil where democratic space is high, though declining recently. A survey by Freedom House (2006) on civil and political freedoms in 192 countries found that only 46% of the countries scored well on political rights (multiparty free elections) and civil liberties (including freedom of association and freedom of press). Resources are another constraint in low-income countries, limiting what the 'engagement' route to accountability can achieve in terms of policy change, and what the 'enforcement' route can achieve in terms of implementation. According to the Report on the Commissions on Macroeconomics and Health, 2001, providing minimal essential health services (major communicable diseases and maternal and perinatal conditions) would require public expenditure in 2007 of at least US$34 per capita in low-income countries. A vast majority of the least developed countries and other low-income countries spend much less than this amount (cited in Ravindran et al., 2005).

How is Accountability to Citizens Ensured?

The review of accountability practices also suggests that few health accountability mechanisms are gender aware or gender specific. Provider report cards, for example, often do not include indicators on gender sensitivity of health providers or whether providers ensure privacy (see review by Mcnamara, 2006). The community-based monitoring and evaluation of health services by the Uganda Debt Network, again, did not include indicators of gender sensitivity of health services and gender equality in utilization of health services (Uganda Debt Network, 2002).

Another gap is that not all accountability mechanisms are available in all countries. As of October 1, 2008, only 92 countries are parties to the optional protocol of CEDAW and as of March 5, 2008, only 111 countries are parties to the (first) optional protocol of the ICCPR, which empowers individuals and civil society organizations to appeal to treaty monitoring bodies when rights have been violated (information from www.ohcr.org, accessed October 15, 2008). Right to Health is part of ICESCR, and this Convention has one of the lowest numbers of countries who are parties to it,[7] and as of October 15, 2008, it does not have an optional protocol. At the national level, some countries like the Philippines have seen a reversal in access to modern contraception due to the influence of the Catholic Church. Few countries have passed legislation on rights of citizens to participate in public policy or right to health or right to gender equity.

PATHWAYS FOR THE FUTURE

The analysis of the practice of accountability to citizens on gender and health and the gaps and lessons therein suggest five pathways to strengthen accountability to citizens on gender and health in the future. These pathways are elaborated in the following.

Pathway 1: Strengthen Accountability of all Health Actors on Gender and Health

The accountability strategies and mechanisms that have been documented in this chapter with regard to the public sector should be extended to the private health sector and multilateral financial institutions, and all public–private partnerships in health and donors, as well as new ones appropriate to each actor, should be identified. For example, the right of citizens to participate should apply to not only formulation and monitoring of public health policies and budgets, but also to formulation and monitoring of policies of donors, public–private partnerships, and multilateral financial institutions involved in health in a country. Citizens' right to participation should also extend to their participation in regulation of the private health sector. Right to information should include the rights of citizens to information not only from the government, but also the other stakeholders in the health sector. It may be made compulsory for private hospitals and public–private partnerships to have representatives of civil society organizations on their boards, to institutionalize grievance redress mechanisms, and to make all quality assessment reports available to the public.

Citizens groups need to be made aware that the position of the Special Rapporteur on the right to health could be used to hold public–private partnerships and UN agencies to account (at least regarding answerability). It is not clear if the Special Rapporteur on the right to health can hold global private health actors (e.g., global pharmaceutical companies) or the World Bank Group to account if he/she receives a complaint that they have violated a right to health. If not, powers of the Special Rapporteur on the right to health need to be broadened in this direction.

Pathway 2: Strengthen Direct Accountability to Women, Marginalized Men, and Transgender/Intersexual People

It is crucial that all health policy, program, and budget documents be translated into local languages and made accessible to women and other marginalized groups through mass print, audio, and visual media. Mechanisms for proportionate representation of marginalized groups in government-initiated health accountability structures at local, district, and provincial levels may be promoted. At the same time, monitoring and vigilance structures independent of government may be formed of these constituencies so that they can put pressure from outside on health accountability structures (see GHEN, 2007). Capacities of women and other marginalized groups on negotiation, health, and gender issues need to be strengthened. These independent health structures should ideally be federated at district, provincial, and national levels, to input into national policies. Resources may be allocated by governments and donors for building capacities of different stakeholders to make these accountability structures work in favor of marginalized women, marginalized men, transgender, and intersexual people.

Pathway 3: Strengthen Accountability on Gender Equity in Health and on all Gender and Health Issues

It is important to bring issues of gender/sex inequalities in health access and outcomes (disadvantaging women, transgender, and intersexual people), lack of legal access to abortion and contraception in some countries, criminaliza-tion of homosexuals in many countries, poor implementation of legal access to abortion where they exist, weak policies on breast, cervical cancer, and infertility treatment, inadequate access to treatment for gender-based vio-lence, and gender-specific health needs of men, transgender, and intersexual people into public debate in the first place. Sensitization of media, religious leaders, health providers, managers, and elected government representatives on these issues is a must. Mechanisms of health priority setting at national levels that go beyond cost-effectiveness models may need to be adopted, as these principles lead to the exclusion of equity goals and gender and health needs listed earlier that do not fall under the 'public good' category. Donors may promote civil society initiatives to use CEDAW and the right to the highest standard on health (General Comment 2000 on ICESCR) to press for accountability of health actors on neglected issues discussed earlier.

Pathway 4: Strengthen Democratic Spaces, Political Will, and Resources

In countries where electoral democracies exist, democratic spaces need to be deepened through strengthening the ability of the poor women and men to contest and win elections, as well as creating legislation and structures for participation in policy formulation, budgeting, and local governance along the lines attempted in Brazil and Argentina. An independent and activist press and judiciary is crucial if citizens are to press for accountability, includ-ing accountability to gender and health. Low- and lower-middle-income countries need to increase resources for health through increased flow of funds from donors and greater allocation of government budget to health.

Pathway 5: Addressing Challenges in Using the Five Possible Accountability Strategies

International and national pressure should be put on national governments that have not signed the ICESCR, ICCPR, or CEDAW, and the optional protocols to do so without reservations. Shadow reports by health and women's rights groups monitoring progress towards Cairo, ICPD, Mil-lennium Development Goals, and the Beijing Platform for Action need to continue, along with advocacy for policy and legal changes where neces-sary (at national and provincial levels). Advocacy for national legislation on the right to health (irrespective of identities) and to gender equality is essential. It is imperative that WHO and health donors support initia-tives to engender health accountability structures and tools, and weave health issues into gender accountability structures and tools.

Traveling on the road of these pathways is crucial for strengthening account-ability to reduce gender inequalities in health, and to address gender-specific health concerns of women, men, transgender, and intersexual people.

ACKNOWLEDGMENTS

The author is grateful to Gita Sen and Piroska Östlin for suggestions on how to take the WGEKN version of the accountability paper forward for this volume. She is also grateful to the Asia Pacific Research and Resource on Women, Malaysia, and Asha George, UNICEF, New York, for accessing recent materials on the topic.

NOTES

1. Referred to, in short, in this chapter as the Special Rapporteur on the right to health.
2. The pressure by the Special Rapporteur (based on complaints received) on the right to health on the Global Fund to give an explanation on its withdrawal from Myanmar and the call of the Citizens' World Bank Tribunal in India to the World Bank to change its anti-poverty policies and institutionalize accountability process did not yield any results. The impact of devolution in the Philippines on the sexual and reproductive health of women is noted to not have been positive.
3. Correspondence of the author (November 2006) with Rounaq Jahan, Senior Research Scholar and Adjunct Professor, Southern Asia Institute, Colombia University.
4. Completed in the states of Andhra Pradesh, West Bengal, Karnataka, Punjab, Maharashtra, and Orissa, and ongoing in the states of Rajasthan, Uttar Pradesh, and Tamil Nadu.
5. The four states refer to Karnataka, West Bengal, Punjab, and Andhra Pradesh.
6. The reproductive health program in the Philippines includes services to improve contraceptive choice and access, maternal and child health and nutrition, prevention and management of abortion complications, prevention and treatment of reproductive tract infections and sexually transmitted infections, including HIV/AIDS, education and counseling on sexuality and sexual health, detection and treatment of breast and reproductive tract cancers, men's and adolescents' reproductive health, care and counseling for victims of violence against women, and prevention and treatment of infertility and sexual disorders (Tadiar, 2000).
7. As of September 26, 2008, 159 countries are parties to ICESCR, compared to 185 in the case of the CEDAW (as of February 15, 2008) and 162 in the case of ICCPR (September 26, 2008).

REFERENCES

Boyd, S. 2001. Peru sterilisation scandal 'swept under the carpet' in *Illuminating Voices*. January 1, 2001. London: Panos.

Campaign Against Sex Selective Abortion (CASSA). 2006. Notes on the mission, objective, activities and outcome of the campaign. Madurai/Chennai: CASSA Secretariat (mimeo).

Caseley, J. 2003. Blocked drains and open minds: Multiple accountability relationships and improved service delivery performance in Indian city. *Working Paper 211*. Brighton, UK: Institute of Development Studies.

Chaver, S., and A.B. Coe. 2007. Donor policies and influences. *Reproductive Health Matters* 15 (29): 139–148.

Cornwall, A. 2007. Negotiating participation in Brazilian health council. In *Spaces for Change? The Politics of Citizen Participation in New Democratic Spaces*, edited by A. Cornwall and V.S. Coelho. London and New York: Zed Books: 155–179.

———. 2007. Deliberating democracy: Scenes from a Brazilian municipal health council. *Working Paper 292*. UK: Institute of Development Studies.

Freedom House. 2006. *Freedom in the World 2006*. Columbia: Freedom House.

GHEN. 2007. *GHEN News Issue 5, January 2007*. Brighton, UK: Institute of Development Studies.

George, A. 2003. Issues in current policy, using accountability to improve reproductive health care. *Reproductive Health Matters* 11 (21): 161–170.

Ghana Health Service. 2007. *Annual Report Ghana Health Service 2007*. Accra: Ghana Health Service.

Goetz, A.M. 2008. *Progress of the World's Women: 2008/2009, Who Answers to Women? Gender and Accountability*. New York: UNIFEM.

International Monetary Fund and International Development Association 2006. *Joint staff advisory note of the poverty reduction strategy paper. Annual Progress Report*. Washington: International Monetary Fund.

Jahan, R. 2003. Restructuring health systems: Experiences of advocates for gender equity in Bangladesh. *Reproductive Health Matters* 11 (21): 183–191.

Klugman, B. 2002. Africa accountability paper. *Paper Prepared for the Initiative for Sexual and Reproductive Rights in Health Reforms*. Johannesburg: Women's Health Project, School of Public Health.

Lakshminarayanan, R. 2003. Decentralization and its implication for reproductive health: The Philippines experience. *Reproductive Health Matters* 11 (21): 96–107.

Macklin, R. 2006. Women's health: Are global inequalities greater than those for men. *Paper Presented at the 6th International Congress on Feminist Approaches to Bioethics—Gender Justice and Women's Rights in Health Care, August 4–6, 2006*. Beijing, China: Albert Einstein College of Medicine: International Network on Feminist Approaches to Bio-ethics, Coordinated from London (Ontario) and Adelaide.

Mahmud, S. 2006. Space for participation in health systems in rural Bangladesh, the experience of stakeholder community groups. In *Spaces for Change? The Politics of Citizen Participation in New Democratic Space*, edited by A. Cornwall and V.S. Coelho. London and New York: Zed Books: 55–75.

Mcnamara, P. 2006. Provider specific report cards: A tool for health sector accountability in developing countries. *Health Policy and Planning* 21 (2):101–109.

Murthy, R.K., B. Klugman, and S. Weller, with L. Aizenberg. 2005. Service accountability and community participation. In *The Right Reforms? Health Sector Reforms and Sexual and Reproductive Health*, edited by T.K.S. Ravindran and H. de Pinho. Johannesburg: The Women's Health Project, School of Public Health: 264–317.

Naripokkho, and ARROW. 2006. *Women's Health and Rights Advocacy Partnership Completion Report: 2003–2006. Internal Document*. Malaysia: Asia Pacific Research and Resource Centre on Women.

Nelson, T., n.d. Violence Against women, Washington: Worldwatch Institute. http://www.phenomenologycenter.org/course/violence.htm (last accessed 24th June, 2009).

Pant, S. 2007. Great Victory for Nepalese LGBTI! In *Take Action. Nepal: IGLHRC Congratulates Nepali LGBTI Organizations on Supreme Court Victory*.

12/21/2007. New York: International Gay and Lesbian Human Rights Commission. http://www.iglhrc.org/cgi-bin/iowa/article/takeaction/resourcecenter/322.html (Last Accessed June 23rd 2009).

Petchesky, R.P. 2005. *Global Prescriptions: Gendering Health and Human Rights.* London and New York: Zed Books.

Potts, H. 2008. Accountability and the Right to the Highest Attainable Standard of Health. Colchester: University of Essex. http://www2.essex.ac.uk/human_rights_centre/rth/project (accessed October 10, 2008).

Ravindran, T.K.S. 2007. Health sector development projects (HSDPs) of the World Bank. *Paper Presented at the Independent People's Tribunal on the World Bank in India, September 21–24.* New Delhi: Independent People's Tribunal on the World Bank.

Ravindran, T.K.S., D. Maciera, and D. Kikomba. 2005. Health financing reforms. In *The Right Reforms? Health Sector Reforms and Sexual and Reproductive Health,* edited by T.K.S. Ravindran and H. de Pinho. Johannesburg: The Women's Health Project, School of Public Health: 26–89.

Reichenbach, L.J. 2002. The politics of priority setting for reproductive health: Breast and cervical cancer in Ghana. *Reproductive Health Matters* 10 (20): 47–58.

Rodgers, D. 2006. "Subverting the spaces of invitation? Local politics and participatory budgeting in post-crisis Buenos Aires". in *Spaces for Change: The Politics of Participation in New Democratic Arenas,* edited by A. Cornwall and V.S. Coelho (eds.). London and New York: Zed.

Root, B., I. Levine, and J.J. Amon. 2008. Counting and accountability. *The Lancet* 371 (9607): 113.

Sarkar, S. 2007. Nepal's sexual minorities emerge as 2007's winters. *NERVEWS of India,* December 22, 2007. http://www.nerve.in/news (accessed October 15, 2008).

Sen, G., A. George, and P. Östlin. 2007. Unequal, unfair, ineffective and inefficient: Gender inequality in health: Why it exists and how we can change them. *Final Report of the Knowledge Network on Women and Gender Equity in Health, Commission on Social Determinants on Health.* Bangalore and Stockholm: Indian Institute of Management/ Karolinska Institute.

Solution Exchange. 2008. Solution Exchange for the Maternal and Child Health Community: E Discussion Summary. Issue Date: 5 May, 2008. Delhi: United Nations. http://www.solutionexchange-un.net.in/health/cr/cr-se-mch-07020801.pdf (Accessed June 24, 2009).

Tadiar, F.M. 2000. *Reproductive Health Programmes under Health Reform: The Philippines Case.* Malaysia: International Council on Management of Population Programmes. http://www.icomp.org.my/Country/inno7b.html (accessed June 26, 2007).

Uganda Debt Network. 2002. *The Community Based Monitoring and Evaluation system (CBMES) Pilot Test in Kamuli District, 11th to 13th April.* Kampala: Uganda Debt Network.

United Nations. 2000. The right to the highest attainable standard of health. *E/C.12/2000/4 (General Comments). Committee on the Economic and Social Cultural Rights, Twenty-Second Session, April 25–May 12.* Geneva: UN.

———. 2005. Report of the Special Rapporteur on the right of everyone to the enjoyment the highest standard of physical and mental health. *Paul Hunt, Addendum Summary of Communications Transmitted to Government and Replies Received. E/CN//4/2005/51/Add.1. February 2.* New York: Commission on Human Rights.

———. 2006. Report of the Special Rapporteur on the right of everyone to the enjoyment the highest standard of physical and mental health. *Paul Hunt,*

Addendum Summary of Communications Sent to and Replies Received from Governments and Other Actors: December 2004–December 2005. E/CN./4/2006/48/Add.1. December 22. New York: Commission on Human Rights.

———. 2007. Report of the Special Rapporteur on the right of everyone to the enjoyment the highest standard of physical and mental health. *Paul Hunt, Addendum Summary of Cases Transmitted to Government and Replies Received. A/HRC//4/28/Add.1. February 23.* New York: Office of the Human Rights Council, UN.

———. 2008. Report of the Special Rapporteur on the right of everyone to the enjoyment the highest standard of physical and mental health. *Paul Hunt, Addendum Summary of Communications Sent to and Received from Government and Other Actors. A/HRC//7/11/Add.1. March 4.* New York: Commission on Human Rights.

United Nations Population Fund. 2005. *Country Program Document for Peru.* New York: United Nations.

World Bank. 2001. *Empowering the Vulnerable Through Participation: Bangladesh Health and Population Program Project. Social Development Notes, No. 63, July.* Washington, DC: World Bank.

World Bank and Asian Development Bank. 2005. *Decentralization in the Philippines: Strengthening Local Government Financing and Resource Management in the Short Run.* Washington, DC: World Bank.

World Bank Tribunal Secretariat. 2008. *Findings of the Jury: Independent People's Tribunal on the World Bank in India.* Mumbai: World Bank Tribunal Secretariat.

WHO. 2004. *Gender in Mental Health.* Geneva: World Health Organization, Department of Gender, Women and Health.

Zucherman, E. 2001. Why engendering PRSPs reduce poverty, the case of Rwanda. *Discussion Paper, 2001/112.* Helsinki, United Nations University: World Institute for Development Economic Research.

Zucherman, E., and A. Garett. 2003. *Do poverty reduction strategy papers address gender?* A Gender Action Publication. Washington: Gender Action. http://www.genderaction.org/images/2002_PRSP&Gender.pdf (last accessed 24th June, 2009).

10 Gender Mainstreaming in Health
The Emperor's New Clothes?

T.K.S. Ravindran and A. Kelkar-Khambete

GENDER MAINSTREAMING IN HEALTH— DEFINITIONS AND CONCEPTS

Background

The concept of 'gender mainstreaming' evolved from attempts to improve women's share of the gains of development in the early 1970s. In the years following the International Conference on Population and Development (ICPD) in 1994 and the Fourth World Conference on Women in Beijing in 1995, the agenda shifted from an exclusive focus on women to 'mainstreaming,' or 'integrating' gender into the mainstream in all sectors. This was in response to the realization that the approach of the earlier decades had led to the 'ghettoization' of women's projects, and to the mere addition of a few services, without fundamental changes in the way programs are formulated and service is delivered.

This chapter is an attempt to draw on recent (since 1995) experiences in gender mainstreaming in health across regions and at various levels, in order to understand what has been achieved, what the challenges have been, and to discuss how we may move the agenda forward. The chapter is constrained by the limited availability of information. The authors were able to use only published work in English. The literature search was mainly Web-based. The search yielded less than 100 articles and publications dealing with gender mainstreaming in health. All, except a very small number (less than 10), were either how-to manuals, descriptions of projects, or reflections by implementers on barriers to gender mainstreaming. Information on the process of implementation, and evaluations of gender mainstreaming efforts, was very limited. Consequently, this chapter depends much on perspectives of implementers and on the authors' own experiences to formulate tentative hypotheses on the reasons for the apparently limited progress of gender mainstreaming efforts in health.

The chapter is structured as follows. This first section introduces concepts related to gender mainstreaming in health. The second section presents an overview of examples of 'operational' gender mainstreaming—mainstreaming gender in health policies, programs, and projects, in health research and training of health providers. Experiences with 'institutional' mainstreaming, both within the national health sector and within international organizations, are presented in section three. Section four presents the summary and raises some questions on how we may move the agenda forward on gender mainstreaming.

Definitions and Concepts

The most widely known and used definition of gender mainstreaming[1] is from the UN Economic and Social Council:

> Mainstreaming a gender perspective is the process of assessing the implications for women and men of any planned action, including legislation, policies or programs, in all areas and at all levels. It is a strategy for making women's as well as men's concerns and experiences an integral dimension of the design, implementation, monitoring and evaluation of policies and programmes in all political, economic and societal spheres so that women and men benefit equally and inequality is not perpetuated. The ultimate aim is to achieve gender equality. *(UNECOSOC, 1997, p. 27)*

In simpler terms, gender mainstreaming is "a process of ensuring all our work, and the way we do it, contributes to gender equality by transforming the balance of power between women and men" (Australian Council for Overseas Aid, 2004, p. 32).

Two dimensions of gender mainstreaming have been emphasized in the literature on this subject:

- 'Operational mainstreaming'—which refers to the integration of equality concerns into the content of policies, programs, and projects, to ensure that these have a positive impact on women and reduce gender inequalities.
- 'Institutional mainstreaming'—which involves addressing the internal dynamics of formal (and informal) institutions, such as their goals, agenda setting, governance structures, and procedures related to day-to-day functioning, so that these support and promote gender equality (UN, 2000).

Both these aspects of gender mainstreaming are closely interrelated. The process of operational mainstreaming depends on the institutional support provided by various structures, starting from formal agencies to family and community units, and, hence, the need for institutional gender mainstreaming.

There are many different perspectives and opinions on what gender mainstreaming is about and whether or not it will achieve the intended end of gender equality in outcome. Jahan (1995) made a distinction between an "integrationist" versus a "transformative" or "agenda-setting" approach to gender mainstreaming (Jahan, 1995, quoted by Porter and Sweetman, 2005). The 'integrationist' approach seeks to integrate gender issues into an already defined and established mainstream agenda. The focus is on technical and managerial aspects of gender mainstreaming. The 'transformative' approach, on the other hand, seeks to reframe the mainstream agenda itself, to better reflect social justice and gender equality concerns. In this approach, gender mainstreaming is not just a technical exercise but a political process that seeks to rearrange power equations.

Gender Mainstreaming in Health (Ravindran, 2000)

Why is gender mainstreaming in health necessary?

Gender inequalities that disadvantage women are observed in every stratum of society, and within every social group, across different castes, races, ethnic or religious groups. Both biological and 'gender' differences between women and men, and the many ways in which the two are intertwined, contribute to differences in health risks, health-seeking behavior, access to and utilization of health services, and health outcomes between the two groups.

Sexual division of labor within the household, and labor market segregation by sex into predominantly male and female jobs, expose men and women to varying health risks. Differences in the way society values men and women, and accepted norms of male and female behavior, influence risk of developing specific health problems as well as health outcomes. Patriarchal norms that deny women the right to make decisions regarding their sexuality and reproduction expose them to avoidable risks of morbidity and mortality, be it through sexually transmitted infection resulting from coercive sex, or death from septic abortion because access to safe abortion has been denied by state legislation. The practice of unsafe sex by large sections of men who are aware of the health risks cannot be explained except in terms of gender norms of acceptable and/or desirable male sexual behavior. Men and women are known to have varying perceptions of health and ill-health and different patterns of health-seeking behavior. Finally, women's access to health services is influenced by factors such as women's unequal access to and control over resources such as money, transport, and time as compared to men, and unequal decision-making power within the family, with men enjoying privileges that women are denied.

Unless research, policy, programs, and services examine, understand, and address these differences and inequalities, they will fall short of their objective of improving the health status of a population.

Accordingly, the World Health Organization's Gender Policy states that the goal of gender mainstreaming in health is to contribute to better health for both men and women, through health research, policies, and programs that give due attention to gender considerations and promote equity and equality between women and men. Gender mainstreaming is expected to increase coverage, effectiveness, and efficiency of all interventions. Further, gender mainstreaming aims to promote equity and equality between women and men throughout the life-course and, at the least, ensure that interventions do not promote or perpetuate inequitable gender roles and relations (WHO, 2002).

According to Gómez-Gómez (2002), gender mainstreaming in health rests on four key concepts: health as a human right; equity in health grounded in principles of social justice and human rights; gender, seen as the social relations of inequality between women and men, intersecting with other sources of inequalities, such as class, race, and ethnicity; and democratic participation; necessary concepts for meeting the "objectives of equity, social justice and health rights defense effectively and sustainably" (Gómez-Gómez, 2002, p. 79). According to this interpretation, gender mainstreaming in health cannot be a top-down agenda, or focus only on gender-based inequities, without attention to other sources of inequities in health.

It may be noted that mainstreaming gender in health calls for a dual focus. One, addressing gender-based differences and inequalities in all health initiatives; and two, implementing initiatives addressing women's specific health needs that are a result either of biological differences between women and men (e.g., maternal health) or of gender-based discrimination in society (e.g., gender-based violence; poor access to health services). Both of these are essential for achieving health equity, which is the ultimate goal of gender mainstreaming.

OPERATIONAL GENDER MAINSTREAMING IN HEALTH

What is Operational Gender Mainstreaming in Health?

Operational gender mainstreaming in health implies the integration of gender concerns in all health information and research, policies, and programs.

Health Research

Gender mainstreaming in health research implies consideration of gender at all stages of the research process, from defining the research questions to developing the study design and data collection tools, the process of data collection and interpretation and dissemination of results.

In many instances, assumptions about gender roles contribute to the invisibility of some health problems suffered by women. For example, gender ideology reinforces the notion that women's work at home is 'not real work.' As a consequence, classical definitions of occupational health do not include the health impact on women of their domestic and childbearing and childrearing roles, although globally women dedicate an important part of their lives to it. Gender mainstreaming health information would require a framework that explicitly takes into consideration women's multifarious roles in production, reproduction, and community activities.

Gender mainstreaming health research also means the adoption of methodologies that have an adequate representation of both sexes, so that sex/gender-specific analysis of data is possible; ensuring that women are adequately represented as respondents in the case of household surveys; eliminating or minimizing bias arising from differential costs and benefits to men and women from participating in the study, and so on.

Health Policies

Health policies are often 'gender blind.' They make references to general categories such as 'communities' or 'the rural poor' without making any distinctions by gender. In effect, they are implicitly male biased. The invisibility of women in occupational health is a good example of why gender-based differences need to be explicitly considered in examining health issues and formulating policies.

Gender mainstreamed health policies would address not only women's special needs but also the health needs they share with men, taking into account gender differences in aspects such as health risks, determinants of health, and health-seeking behavior.

For example, an engendered health policy would recognize spousal violence as a gender-related health problem to which women are disproportionately more exposed because of social norms sanctioning male aggression and their right to control women. It would examine environmental health hazards separately for men and women, and devise programs to prevent and control exposure accordingly. It would provide for active tuberculosis case-finding to minimize underreporting of infection in women, and examine whether or not women's biological differences contribute to their greater vulnerability to the infection or to its consequences. Such a health policy would examine and correct gender disparities in human resources within the health sector and gender biases perpetuated by medical education.

More importantly, in the case of health issues that are specific to women, a gender-mainstreamed health policy would go beyond merely providing a technical service. It would address this 'practical' need of women in a way that challenges existing gender roles and stereotypes transforming women's situation with respect to men. A 'safe motherhood' policy, for instance, would not assume either that women alone are responsible for child care, or that they have access to the resources to ensure their own as well as their child's well-being. It would be designed with awareness that women often do not have a say in whether and when to get pregnant. It would acknowledge that many pregnancies are unwanted or ill-timed from the woman's point of view, and would provide women with the option of safe pregnancy termination. Indeed, the policy would not even be called a safe motherhood policy, but a safer pregnancy policy, allowing for the possibility of safe pregnancy termination.

In other words, a gender-mainstreamed health policy would also seek to transform existing gender relations in a more democratic direction by redistributing more evenly the division of resources, responsibilities, and power between women and men.

A gender-aware health policy would not be blind to other forms of social inequities and treat women or men as homogenous groups. It would be based on the understanding that women and men are divided along class, caste, religious, and ethnic lines, and ensure that the poorer and marginalized sections are not implicitly excluded.

Another issue to bear in mind is that it is not sufficient to design a gender-aware policy in the health sector alone, if policies in other areas that have a bearing on health—all development policies for that matter—are gender blind with an implicit male bias.

Health Programs

While engendering health policies is in itself a complex process, translating these into programs is a far more challenging task. Examples of policies that are progressive on paper but inadequately implemented are numerous everywhere in the world. This appears to be especially true of gender-aware policies that 'evaporate' even by the time that a policy statement begins to spell out concrete program interventions, and almost completely disappear when they get to the stage of implementation. The active involvement of the women's movement and civil society institutions is essential, and not just to ensure that policies are engendered. Without the continued involvement and independent monitoring by these actors, gender-aware policies will never be pursued but be given a quiet burial.

A number of tools have been developed for monitoring how engendered a health program is. A gender-mainstreamed health program would address gender differentials in health risks, health information, and access to health services.

To give one example, a gender-mainstreamed malaria control program would take into account the fact that even though reported prevalence of malaria is higher among men than in women overall, malaria in pregnancy has a much higher case-fatality rate. It would seek to gather and analyze information on malaria incidence and prevalence by sex and disaggregated into various population subgroups so that it becomes clearer whether or not the general pattern of higher prevalence among males is true for all population subgroups. It would engage in active case-finding, i.e., take samples for blood tests within the community, so that women are not underrepresented among those tested.

A gender-mainstreamed health program would not load all responsibilities for improved health on women but rather also involve men. It would be sensitive not to add to women's workload. It would not perpetuate gender biases. For example, strategies for the control of sexually transmitted infections would focus on condom use by men rather than making women responsible for negotiating condom use with their partners.

A health program that has mainstreamed gender would also strive to redress inequities in health by gender across various sections of the population, through, for example, creating women-friendly health facilities or making health care available closer to home, to bridge the gender gap in access to health care. Such a health program would also try to narrow gender gaps in terms of distribution of responsibilities and power among health personnel. A conscious attempt has to be made to ensure that all the workload involved in making health programs address gender concerns does not fall on women workers and that male health workers are also involved in making health prevention and promotion as much men's business as it is women's.

Initiatives in Operational Gender Mainstreaming

In this section, we examine examples of mainstreaming gender in:

- health policies
- health programs/projects
- health research
- health providers' training

Mainstreaming Gender in Health Policies

Sweden is perhaps the only available example of a country with a gender-integrated public health policy. There have, however, been several attempts at gender analysis of national health policies, intended perhaps as first steps towards mainstreaming gender within policies.

Sweden's new public health policy, which came into force in 2003, has integrated gender within the framework of an equity-oriented public health policy. This policy is unique in many ways. Unlike most public health policies, in which objectives are based on diseases or health problems, Sweden's public health policy addresses the broader social determinants of health, including gender (Östlin and Diderichsen, 2003). The policy was developed over a three-year period, which was spent on gathering sound scientific evidence, including gender-based inequalities in health. The policy document specifically highlights its commitment to a gender perspective, and to reducing gender-based inequalities in health (Gunnar, 2003), alongside reductions in inequalities by socioeconomic groups, ethnic groups, and geographic regions. Gender would thus be a crosscutting category within other dimensions of inequalities that the policy seeks to redress.

In Kenya, a Gender and HIV/AIDS Technical Subcommittee, formed in 2002, undertook the task of engendering the National HIV/AIDS Strategic Plan (National AIDS Control Council, 2002). The subcommittee carried out gender analysis of the Strategic Plan to identify areas where gender differences had not been given due consideration. The gender analysis found that:

- In the area of prevention, there was not enough attention on gender-based violence, rape, and incest as pathways to HIV infection; health education materials did not address gender-specific concerns; and female condom had not been prioritized.
- With respect to treatment, the National Strategic Plan had not mentioned setting up rape/incest crisis centers, counseling, and post-rape STI/HIV/contraceptive prophylaxis. The plan was silent on nutritional needs of women and men living with HIV/AIDS, and on the special needs of women who cared for HIV positive persons, but had no information on their own seropositivity.
- Collection of sex-disaggregated data had not been emphasized and no attempt had been made to develop gender-sensitive indicators for monitoring and evaluation of interventions.

Based on this analysis, the Gender and HIV/AIDS Subcommittee outlined, within each of the priority areas of the plan, activities that would pay specific attention to differences between women and men in health needs and access to treatment, care, and support. These were published as a report on which this summary is based.

Systematic efforts to integrate gender considerations into health sector reform efforts were facilitated in the Latin American and Caribbean Region by the Pan-American Health Organisation (PAHO) (Gómez-Gómez, 2002). PAHO's strategy, implemented initially in Chile and Peru, consisted of: helping countries in documenting the implications of health policies for gender inequities in health; disseminating evidence to empower advocates to inform policy makers; and assisting relevant stakeholders and civil society to institutionalize and monitor gender equity priorities into national policies.[2] As part of this project, an observatory of Gender Equity in Health has been set up in Chile to document and disseminate information on gender equity in health (PAHO, 2007).

Mainstreaming gender in health reforms was also attempted in Ghana's Sector-Wide Approach (SWAP). The Ministry of Health carried out gender analysis and held consultations with stakeholders to develop a draft health sector gender policy to readdress gender gaps as part of the SWAP (Theobald et al., 2004).

Timely intervention, through a content analysis study of Ireland's Cardiovascular Health Strategy document carried out by WHO/EURO, helped identify a number of gender gaps. For example, despite considerable data presented on differential gender experiences among men and women in the context of cardiovascular diseases, as well as the health services, there were no references to gender considerations in the recommendations made, wherein the emphasis was on inequalities by geographic regions.

This study has triggered a lot of research in the area of gender and health in Ireland, and drew attention to the importance of including gender in the cardiovascular health policy at the level of the European Union Council of ministers, paving the way for further action to mainstream gender into the Irish cardiovascular health policy (Women's Health Council and WHO/ EURO, n.d.).

Salmon and colleagues (2006) have carried out gender analysis of Canada's Mental Health and Addictions Policy, and outlined directions for integrating sex and gender into the policy. The report demonstrates how the application of sex and gender analyses would be useful in refining the health policy in Canada in terms of treatment protocols, accessibility to care, quality of programs, quality of prevention activity, and help in promotion of good mental health for all Canadians (Salmon et al., 2006).

The preceding policy interventions are among the few attempts at mainstreaming gender in the content of health policies. The impact of Sweden's public health policy on bridging gender gaps in health does not appear to have been assessed as yet. It is not clear if attempts at gender analysis of specific health policies, and of advocacy for integrating gender considerations in health sector reform policies, were translated into policy changes on the ground.

Gender Mainstreaming in Program Interventions

Mainstreaming Gender Within Community-Based NGO Health Interventions

In this section, we examine 27 community-based NGO health interventions that have mainstreamed gender. These include 22 interventions found in the *SO WHAT Report* (IGWG, 2004), and five interventions from the Commonwealth report (Commonwealth Secretariat, 2002). All the interventions are donor funded and community based, and all aim at improving reproductive health, although the entry points for some of the interventions have been through education or economic development.

The interventions have been classified into four main areas: maternal mortality and morbidity, unintended pregnancies, quality of care initiatives, and STIs/HIV/AIDS. The following framework from the *SO WHAT Report* has been used to assess the gender sensitivity of interventions:

- *Gender exploitative interventions*: those that exploit gender inequalities for the purpose of gaining reproductive or family planning targets.
- *Gender accommodative interventions*: those that make it easier for women to perform their gender roles or duties ascribed to them without changing or questioning the inequalities between the roles of men and women in the society.
- *Gender transformative interventions*: changes that challenge gender equalities between men and women.

Table 10.1 summarizes these 27 reproductive health interventions by nature of problem addressed, level of gender sensitivity, and reproductive and gender outcomes achieved according to the assessment. The following are some significant findings:

- The vast majority of the interventions (21 of 27) consist mainly of training and education activities. Interventions mainstreaming gender in clinical or psychosocial interventions are rare, irrespective of the reproductive health issue under consideration.
- Many of the interventions (11 of 27) are 'gender-accommodating': that is, they cater to women's and men's different needs without acknowledging or challenging unequal gender power relations.
- In all 27 interventions, there was more than one positive reproductive health outcome; many of these were tangible changes in behavior, in utilization of services, or in health outcomes.
- Improved gender outcomes were also noted in 20 of 21 interventions that examined this aspect.

These case studies constitute an important source of evidence on the impact of mainstreaming gender within health interventions. However, the quality of this evidence is compromised by methodological limitations. Comparison of baseline data collected before the intervention, with the achievements after the intervention, has been possible in only a small number of interventions. Gender-mainstreamed interventions are not evaluated against a comparison group of interventions that do not integrate gender considerations. There is no documentation of the processes and steps through which mainstreaming gender may have brought about the desired health outcomes. The evidence provided does not clarify whether the positive outcomes were a result of a change towards more equitable gender-power equations or simply the result of better access to services. In terms of gender outcomes, many of the conclusions are based on participants reporting that there has been improvement. Questions remain as to whether these gains would be sustained in the long term, and whether women will be able to address and overcome the gender-based

Table 10.1   An Analysis of Selected 'Gender-Mainstreamed' Reproductive Health Interventions

Characteristics	Number of interventions
Area of reproductive health addressed	
Unintended pregnancies	9
Maternal mortality and morbidity	3
STIs and HIV/AIDS	12
Quality of reproductive health care	3
Target group	
Female	15
Male	2
Female and male	10
Nature of interventions	
Education and training	21
Counseling and social support	2
Clinical services	2
Savings and credit	1
Other	1
Gender sensitivity	
Gender accommodating	11
Gender transformative	16
Reproductive health outcomes[1]	
Improved knowledge of RH issues	13
Changes towards positive attitudes	3
Increase in condom use	5
Increase in use of contraception	7
Better self-care	2
Increase in utilization of RH services	7
Improved quality of RH services	2
Improved health outcomes	6
Gender outcomes	
Improvement in gender relations between partners; improvement in communication and gender equitable behavior	11
Increased empowerment of women	8
Increased awareness of gender issues	1

(continued)

Table 10.1 (continued)

No improvement	1
Gender outcomes not measured	6

Sources: (IGWG, 2004; Commonwealth Secretariat, 2002).
1 Figures do not add to 27 because more than one outcome was reported by some interventions.

barriers they experience in their everyday lives after the short-duration gender interventions.

Mainstreaming Gender Within Government Health Programs

A. THE WOMEN-CENTERED HEALTH PROJECT OF THE MUMBAI MUNICIPAL CORPORATION (WCHP), INDIA

This was a collaborative project between the Bombay Municipal Corporation (BMC), SAHAJ, a nongovernmental organization, and the Royal Tropical Institute, Amsterdam. The Project was implemented in two wards of Mumbai, covering a population of approximately one million (Khanna et al., 2002). The objectives of the project included, among others:

- Implementation of women-centered reproductive health services closer to women, that is, at the health post and dispensary levels, by increasing the range of services on priority reproductive health problems; involving men in ways that will not increase their control over women; improving information, education, and counseling by responding to women's needs and in ways that enhance their control over their bodies.
- Establishment and implementation of quality assurance mechanisms, including better provider–client communication, treatment procedures that respect women and are woman-friendly, and improved referral links.

There were three major categories of project activities: action research, training, and health interventions. The project succeeded in improving both reproductive health and gender outcomes. It put in place 'reproductive health clinics' one day a week in 10 Family Welfare Centers within the project area, and ensured availability of a woman physician, good clinical quality, and availability of relevant drugs. Aspects of quality of care, such as privacy for examining women and respectful and empathetic provider–client communication, were successfully implemented in all health facilities within the project area. In terms of gender outcomes, health providers and senior managers reported that they found gender-sensitization workshops to be informative and thought-provoking, and helped them make changes in their day-to-day work.

The effects of the project spilled beyond the project area. For example, a gender module developed by the WCHP was incorporated successfully in all training provided in BMC. WCHP's training modules on Gender, Men's Involvement, IEC, Provider–Client Communication, and Quality of Care, were incorporated into the final training schedule for Mumbai's Reproductive and Child Health (RCH) Program.

The project faced numerous implementation challenges. The bureaucratic and hierarchical nature of a large public system, such as BMC, did not find it easy to accommodate the participatory, bottom-up approach in planning and execution of gender-mainstreaming activities adopted by WCHP. The officers and health care providers did not have much patience for process-oriented approaches that made heavy demands on their time, and were far more comfortable with top-down orders that could be implemented mechanistically.

Acting on gender mainstreaming priorities identified by the project also proved to be very difficult. For example, changing the timings at health facilities to suit men's work schedules could not be implemented. Starting crèches for BMC employees and increasing the number of toilets for women with sanitary bins on BMC premises were identified as needs, but implementing these was fraught with difficulties. It took enormous time and energy, and much patience and optimism, to achieve any substantive change.

The biggest challenge for this project has been sustaining the initiatives after the project period. Within a year after the project ended, some of the activities initiated were discontinued, including those that did not involve commitment of additional resources (Khanna et al., 2002).

The WCHP appears to be an example of successful 'operational' mainstreaming, which could not be sustained because the institutional structures within which it was functioning—that of the BMC—had not concurrently engaged in gender mainstreaming but continued to be hierarchical and gender blind. The institution treated WCHP as one of its many short-term projects rather than as an attempt to make fundamental changes in the way in which the health services were organized and run. Nevertheless, the contributions of WCHP in terms of gender sensitization of staff at all levels is likely to have brought about at least a few changes in provider attitudes and behavior.

B. HONG KONG GOVERNMENT

Another example of mainstreaming gender within government departments is in Hong Kong. As a result of application of gender analysis to the planning and provision of public toilet facilities in the country, the Food and Environmental Hygiene Department (FEHD) found that females needed to spend a longer time in toilets than males, and it was very common to see queues outside female toilets. Therefore, FEHD increased the WC compartment ratio (female to male) from 1.5 to 1 to 2 to 1 since April 2004, as a general guideline in planning FEHD public toilet facilities. It also included racks, hangers, baby changing counters, and emergency call bells in the toilets (Health, Welfare and Food Bureau, 2006a).

Hong Kong's Electrical and Mechanical Services Department (EMSD) has arranged talks in hospitals, planned for afternoon TV information slots, and posted and distributed materials at public places to make information on the safety of electrical and mechanical gadgets used in households more accessible to women (Health, Welfare and Food Bureau, 2006b).

Both the WCHP and the Hong Kong government's initiatives are examples of gender-accommodative interventions, which cater to the varying needs of women and men without challenging their gender roles: for example, the intervention of EMSD did not challenge the gender division of domestic work.

Mainstreaming Gender in Health Research

In this section we present three examples of gender mainstreaming health research. The first is on the experience of National Institute of Health (NIH) in the US. The second is a summary of a review of experiences in Latin American and Caribbean countries, and the third is an example of a country-level initiative by a school of public health in India.

NIH Gender Policy in Health Research

The NIH in the US set up its Office of Research on Women's Health (ORWH) in 1990. Its mandate included: ensuring that research conducted and supported by the NIH adequately addressed issues regarding women's health; ensuring that women are appropriately represented in biomedical and biobehavioral research studies supported by the NIH; and supporting research on women's health issues and activities related to career advancement of women in biomedical careers (Caron, 2003).

An evaluation of the NIH-funded studies by the Gender Accounting Office (GAO) in 2003 concluded that, although the inclusion of women had been achieved in research processes, the analysis of data did not throw light on whether there were sex or gender differences in the impact of interventions. It was also found that grant applicants were not informed that research studies had to include an analysis of sex-based differences (Caron, 2003).

An independent evaluation of the NIH policy, through an analysis of published material by Harris and Douglas (2000) as quoted in Caron (2003), found that efforts to include women in the clinical trials did moderately increase as a result of ORWH policy. However, closer examination found that the representation of women increased only in large trials that were restricted to women. The underrepresentation of women in areas such as cardiovascular diseases continued unchanged (Caron, 2003).

Integrating Gender in Health Research: The Latin American Experience (LACWHN, 2002)

There exists a substantive body of 'gendered' research in health in the Latin American region, carried out by feminist researchers, either NGO or university based, most of which have been individual work not guided by a cohesive agenda. The broad areas of gendered research have been violence against women; sexual and reproductive health and rights; access to health services and quality of care; and mental health.

According to the review by the Latin American and Caribbean Women's Health Network (LACWHN, 2002), few governments in the region have set an agenda or developed an explicit strategy to integrate gender considerations in health research. Although a number of countries in this region have a commitment to equity in health, this is usually framed in terms of socioeconomic, ethnic, and geographic regions, leaving gender out of the equation. Gendered research does not feature in government-funding policies anywhere in the region. The scenario is one of considerable initiative by feminists and women researchers, not backed by policy commitment.

All the same, gendered research has had some impact on policy-making, especially in the areas of violence against women and sexual and reproductive health. More importantly, such research has contributed to a deepening of understanding of the nature and dimensions of gender inequalities in health by articulating women's experiences.

The Small Grants Programme on Gender and Social Issues in Reproductive Health Research, India[3] (Ravindran, 2005)

This was a modest initiative to build capacity among researchers in sexual and reproductive health to undertake 'gendered' research. A small grant program offered 11 research grants for undertaking research focusing on gender and social dimensions of sexual and reproductive health issues in India.

Each grantee was teamed up with a 'mentor' who reviewed the final proposal, provided critical inputs to the development of data collection instruments, collection, analysis, and interpretation of data, and inputs to the final report. Training workshops for all grantees were conducted at crucial junctures during the research process. The initiative produced 11 research reports on sexual and reproductive health issues, which are good examples of gender-mainstreamed research. Not only the 11 grantees but the 10 mentors also learned firsthand about implementing gender mainstreaming in health research.

There are several such examples of small-scale initiatives. But overall, not enough has been done to change policies that enable the systematic integration of gender considerations in health research in all academic and research settings, and to generate gender- and sex-specific data as part of routine data collection. This is one important bottleneck hampering the identification of priority areas and of monitoring progress towards gender equality.

Mainstreaming Gender in Health Providers' Training

A large number of efforts have focused on in-service training of health professionals on gender issues. Some of the well-known international efforts include: WHO's training on Gender and Rights in Reproductive Health; Pan-American Health Organization's training course on Gender, Health and Development; and WHO-Western Pacific Regional Office's (WPRO) publication of resource guides in gender, poverty, and health, for mainstreaming gender in medical education. Such initiatives are numerous and have yet to be evaluated for their impact.

This section, therefore, focuses on preservice training of health professionals, and is based on a recent review on integrating gender into the curricula for health professionals (Ravindran, 2006).

Much of the work on integrating gender into the curricula of health professionals has been done in relation to the undergraduate medical curriculum, and in the area of women's health specialty, especially in the US. Attempts to integrate gender (rather than women's health) into the medical curriculum are more recent. There are only three known examples of curriculum development and course implementation. Monash University has integrated gender into the curriculum in the five years of its new problem-based and patient-centered curriculum. The Medical School at Chulalungkorn University in Thailand has also made a similar attempt. The Gender and Health Collaborative Curriculum Project in Canada has developed Web-based modules that are resources for faculty who wish to integrate gender into their teaching, and may also be used by interested students. In contrast, many public health programs offer optional courses on gender (Ravindran, 2006).

Other efforts at integrating gender into the curricula have focused on creating an enabling environment, and in capacity building of medical educators. For example, an initiative in India has been training medical educators from six Indian states on the need and strategies for gender mainstreaming the medical curriculum, with a view to creating change agents within the system who would advocate for gender mainstreaming. A similar initiative is being implemented in Southern Africa among schools of public health. Advocacy with senior policy makers is also being undertaken in various settings.

Three factors appear to facilitate the process of mainstreaming gender in medical curricula. The first is the window of opportunity provided by larger curricular changes, such as introduction of problem-based and patient-centered learning, and introduction of new courses. The second is the presence of dynamic leadership committed to mainstreaming gender. The third factor is the extensive preparatory work carried out by such leaders: well-thought-out and sustained advocacy with decision makers; capacity-building and introductory workshops for medical educators and students; and devising ways of integrating gender without overloading the existing curriculum.

Some of the major challenges reported by initiatives include institutional resistance and difficulties of involving key faculty and male colleagues in this process. Another issue is that there are very few faculty members in each institution who have the expertise to teach gender and women's health issues. The limited research on gender issues in health and women's health is another bottleneck hampering the extent to which evidence-based teaching on gender and health is possible (Ravindran, 2006).

INSTITUTIONAL GENDER MAINSTREAMING

Operational gender mainstreaming needs structures, mechanisms, and processes that will catalyze, initiate, and sustain gender mainstreaming efforts. In the first section following, we describe mainstreaming efforts within national health sectors; and in the second section, mainstreaming gender in health within international organizations.

Steps and guidelines for 'institutional' mainstreaming in health

The institutional gender mainstreaming process requires the creation of structures, mechanisms, processes, and resources to initiate it, and once initiated, to sustain the efforts. The Gender Management Systems (GMS) approach proposed by the Commonwealth Secretariat (2002) outlines the following as essential:

- establishment of a lead agency and Gender Management Team
- informed participation of all stakeholders
- availability of statistical data and information to identify priority areas for mainstreaming
- establishment of performance appraisal systems (Commonwealth Secretariat, 2002)

Creating new structures and mechanisms is not adequate to ensure that operational gender mainstreaming happens. The gender mainstreaming structures and mechanisms have to function within and/or in collaboration with existing health system institutions and structures. For gender mainstreaming to happen in policy and program interventions, in health research and training, institutions responsible for these activities have to be gender sensitive and ensure that women are not discriminated against in any way (Government of South Africa, 2002).

The following steps are recommended to help make the transition to a gender-mainstreamed institution:

- Developing a formal gender analysis of the institution in order to identify gender inequalities in rules, resources, gains, activities, and power.
- Developing institutional policy on mainstreaming gender equality. This will specify the goals of the policy, which activities will be

undertaken to address gender interests of staff and constituencies, by when, who is responsible, what resources will be allocated, and how the implementation of the policy will be monitored.

- Establishing a committee and additional mechanisms to manage the entire process comprising all department heads and the chief functionary of the organization.
- Ensuring that female staff does not bear all the institutional responsibility for mainstreaming gender equality but men and women at all levels, including senior management.
- Staff education processes to build staff's understanding that gender inequality can result in violations of women's human rights, and has a negative impact not only on women staff members, but on the organization and its work overall.
- Enforcing existing policies such as policies on sexual harassment in the workplace.
- Changing specific policies that are gender blind or blatantly gender unequal, such as hiring procedures that may discriminate against married or unmarried women (Kabeer, 1994).

Gender Mainstreaming within National Health Sectors

South Africa's gender policy guidelines for the health sector were developed in order to support the Department of Health and Public Health Institutions to systematically identify and address gender considerations in health, and within the organizations responsible for managing and delivering health care services (Government of South Africa, 2002).

The guidelines set a series of objectives for 'institutional' gender mainstreaming, i.e., promoting gender equity and equality within institutions of the health sector. These included: elimination of gender-based discrimination in human resource procedures, such as appointments and promotions; changing institutional rules and culture to create an environment supportive of gender equity and equality; and enhancing the capacity of staff and senior management for mainstreaming gender concerns within health policies, programs, research, and training (Government of South Africa, 2002).

In order to achieve these objectives, structures and mechanisms were created. Full-time gender focal points were appointed at the national and provincial levels to provide technical support for implementing the gender policy. A Health Sector Co-Coordinating Committee (HSCC) was constituted of representatives of health departments at different levels (national, provincial, and local) and civil society actors to help with gender analysis, to develop a gender action plan and a framework for monitoring and evaluation, and to facilitate the development of a Management Information System (Government of South Africa, 2002).

The Gender Equity Strategy of the Ministry of Health and Family Welfare (MOHFW) in Bangladesh was developed through a consultative process and adopted in 2003. The overall objective of the strategy was to enhance the capacity of the MOHFW to address gender inequities in health, which were detrimental to overall health development. Gender considerations were systematically identified, and strategies to address them were outlined within each of five essential components of the Health and Population Sector Program (HPSP). The Gender Equity Strategy included enhancing women's participation in senior management, creating a supportive, safe, and harassment-free work environment for female staff, and promoting skills and sensitivity among managers to identify and address gender issues in the workplace (Government of Bangladesh, 2003).

Institutional Mainstreaming in International Organizations

The World Health Organization

The WHO's Gender Policy was formally adopted in 2002, although work towards formulating the policy had started several years earlier. The policy called for 'integrating gender considerations' into all research, policies, programs, projects, and initiatives, in which WHO is involved (WHO, 2002).

- The lead agency for gender mainstreaming within WHO is the Gender, Women and Health Department at the WHO headquarters in Geneva. This department is responsible for providing technical support to all departments of WHO, for mainstreaming gender in their work through, among other things, the development of appropriate gender analysis tools and building a substantial evidence base.
- A high-level Gender Task Force, consisting of senior managers within the organization, was appointed by the director general to oversee the implementation of the Gender Policy. A WHO Gender Team was constituted, consisting of gender focal points from departments and initiatives at WHO headquarters, and core gender specialists in the Department of Gender, Women and Health.

During the years following the adoption of the Gender Policy, the lead agency, the Department of Gender, Women and Health at the headquarters, has produced an impressive array of publications contributing to building the evidence base on gender and health, and developing and refining tools and guidelines for gender mainstreaming in research. These tools and publications have been the result of successful collaboration with a number of technical departments at the headquarters. The gender units of the WHO Regional Offices have also been engaged in similar activities.

While these achievements are impressive, especially given the relatively understaffed and underresourced character of the lead agency and regional gender units, they are a far cry from 'mainstreaming' or integrating gender into the organization's way of doing business. Gender focal points in different departments carry out their gender-related tasks as an add-on to their regular tasks. Capacity building for integrating gender has not happened systematically and is not anywhere near the scale it ought to be. Gender considerations are not routinely integrated into policies, programs, strategies, or research, or within organizational structures created to implement new initiatives and programs. A quick scan of the organization's Web site will bear testimony to these observations.

The experience of institutional mainstreaming at the WHO is shared by many multilateral and bilateral organizations, as the discussion in the next section will illustrate.

Other International Organizations[4]

A review of gender mainstreaming experiences of 14 international organizations by Moser and Moser (2005) provides comprehensive information on progress made with respect to institutional mainstreaming in international organizations. The review covers bilateral donors, international financial institutions (IFIs), UN agencies, and NGOs. Although these are not institutions within the health sector, their experiences are relevant because the processes involved and the emerging challenges are likely to be similar across sectors. Table 10.2 presents information on the presence of various components of institutional gender mainstreaming across the 14 organizations (Moser and Moser, 2005).

All the reviewed institutions had adopted the terminology of gender equality and gender mainstreaming. Gender analysis, gender training, and development of tools and techniques for monitoring and evaluation were seen as important strategies for mainstreaming by most organizations. In a majority of the organizations, responsibility for gender mainstreaming was shared by a cross-section of staff, supported by gender specialists. However, half or more of the 14 organizations had not allocated financial resources to enable implementation of the gender policy; were not working with men for gender equality; and had not been involved in strengthening the capacity of women's organizations or working with civil society.

Proceedings of an informal consultation of Gender Focal Points from multilateral development organizations confirms these observations, and is much more critical of the limited progress made (MFA, 2002). Many gender focal points reported that gender policies and strategies had been put in place as merely 'cosmetic' changes, without any attempt to allocate the necessary resources or personnel, to guide the processes, or monitor and evaluate what had been achieved.

According to one observer:

> gender has tended to be treated as a passing fad, and especially in between major conferences, been down-played, and resurrected for frantic activity, and dusted over and dry-cleaned like winter clothes in

autumn, just before the institution would be called upon to account for past undertakings. (Chinery-Heisse, 2002)

CHALLENGES TO MAINSTREAMING GENDER IN HEALTH

Major Findings of this Review

The present chapter attempted to review progress made in mainstreaming gender in health policies and programs, research, training, and within health system institutions. We found that many tools and guidelines had been developed on how to implement gender mainstreaming, and that there were many descriptions of gender mainstreaming initiatives. But few publications provided insights on the processes adopted, or on the outcomes of gender mainstreaming initiatives.

Descriptive accounts of gender mainstreaming initiatives indicate that more has been done in 'operational' mainstreaming, as compared to institutional mainstreaming, of gender equity concerns within the health sector. Attempts at institutional mainstreaming seem to be suffering from the apparent tendency to 'appear to do much' rather than making fundamental changes. Institutions seem to have superficially gone through the motions of adopting a gender policy and creating a few structures, without investing any more into making these actually work. Most attempts have been top-down, without scope for democratic participation, both within international organizations and national government institutions. At the government level:

> gender mainstreaming has become a mechanical process to attract funding but does not change practices of discrimination embedded in government institutions. (Sandler, 2002)

These weaknesses in institutional mainstreaming of gender make it difficult, if not impossible, for operational mainstreaming to be large-scale or sustained over a long period of time.

Within operational mainstreaming, service-delivery and training interventions that have been implemented and evaluated are mainly community based and carried out by NGOs with external funding. Many of these tend to focus on women's specific needs without challenging gender roles and norms. Attempts at integrating gender issues in the training of health personnel have also, by and large, remained small-scale attempts initiated in a few settings by committed individuals or advocacy groups.

There are only a small number of examples of planned and system-wide initiatives for mainstreaming gender, guided by policy and implemented by the state. Even when successful in terms of improving health outcomes and promoting gender equity, micro-level, small-scale, or ad hoc interventions are not likely to make the health sector as a whole more gender equitable.

Table 10.2   Components and Associated Activities of Gender Mainstreaming Policies in 14 International Organizations

Components	Activities	DFID	CIDA	Sida	IDB	ADB	WB	UNIFEM	Habitat	UNICEF	UNDP	Action Aid	OXFAM	HIVOS	ACORD	%
Dual strategy of mainstreaming and targeting gender equality	Mainstreaming into policies, projects, and programs (all stages of cycle)	X	X	X	X	X	X	X	X	X	X	X	X	X	X	100
	Actions targeting gender equality	X	X	X	X	X	X	X	X	X	X	X	X	X	X	100
Gender analysis	Sex-disaggregated data and gender info	X	X		X			X	X		X					43
	Analysis of all program cycle stages	X	X	X	X	X	X	X	X			X	X		X	79
	Gender-sensitive budget analysis										X					7
Internal responsibility	Responsibilities shared between all staff and gender specialists/focal points	X	X	X			X		X	X	X	X	X	X	X	79
Gender training	Understanding and implementation of gender policy for staff and counterparts	X		X								X	X	X	X	43
	Staff/counterpart gender sensitization												X			7
	Staff/counterparts gender training skills	X	X		X	X	X	X	X	X	X	X	X	X	X	93
	Manuals/tool kits	X				X	X		X	X	X					43

(continued)

(continued)

Supporting women's decision-making and empowerment	Strengthening women's organizations through capacity building and training			X				X					X	X	X		36
	Support women's participation in decision-making/ empowerment	X	X	X	X			X	X	X	X	X	X	X	X	86
	Working with men for gender equality		X	X						X			X	X	X	43
Monitoring and evaluation	Effective systems and tools for M & E	X	X	X	X	X	X		X	X	X	X	X	X	X	93
	Gender-sensitive indicators							X			X					
Work with other organizations	Strengthening gender capacity at work with government donors, private sectors			X	X	X	X	X		X	X	X	X	X	93
	Capacity building of civil society	X	X	X				X	X		X				14
	Support to national women's machineries		X	X				X							11
Budgets	Allocation of financial resources to staff to carry out gender policy	X			X	X		X			X	X		X		50
Knowledge resources	Publication of knowledge base for best practice and effective strategies			X	X	X		X			X		X		X	50
	Networks		X					X			X				21
	Online databases							X			X				14

Source: Moser and Moser (2005).

Where health policies are concerned, the task of mainstreaming gender in their content has barely begun. More has been done to identify 'gender gaps' within existing policies, rather than address these gender gaps within policies and in their implementation. With the exception of Sweden's public health policy, these have not considered gender as part of human rights and social justice agendas.

This lack of progress is not a phenomenon peculiar to the health sector. A number of reviews of gender mainstreaming undertaken between 2000 and 2005 seem to agree that efforts at gender mainstreaming had not succeeded in putting gender on the agenda in the policy and planning processes and that gender concerns were still in the margins of these processes (Riley, 2004; UNRISD, 2005). The general consensus appears to be that gender mainstreaming has not delivered what was anticipated when the concept was included in the Beijing Platform of Action (Mitchell, 2004); and that the contribution of gender mainstreaming to gender equality "were at best embryonic and at worst, still to become visible" (Watkins, 2004, p. 5).

Factors Constraining Gender Mainstreaming

What are some reasons for the limited progress with respect to gender mainstreaming in health?

The discussion that follows draws on the authors' own experiences, in addition to published literature critiquing gender mainstreaming. Our focus is more on the larger systemic challenges than on issues related to management and organizational structures within institutions. We deal first with the specific challenges in mainstreaming gender in the health sector, and then with factors common to gender mainstreaming efforts across sectors.

Challenges Specific to the Health Sector

Gender mainstreaming is a difficult undertaking in any sector, but mainstreaming gender in health has to contend with some specific challenges:

- Because there are biological differences between women and men in both health needs and experiences, there is a tendency to attribute all male–female differences to biology. The consequence is that maternal health programs are seen as an adequate response to addressing differences in health between sexes. The need for examining gender issues in all health problems, as well as in delivery of health care services, remains unrecognized.
- While the disadvantages experienced by women in sectors like education, employment, or political participation are evident from available data, the case of health is more complex. Women outlive men in most countries of the world, and for many health conditions, male mortality exceeds female mortality. Many policy makers and program managers, therefore, remain unconvinced of any gender-based inequalities

in health, and of the need for gender mainstreaming. Other dimensions of gender inequality in health, such as in morbidity, access to health care, and social and economic consequences of ill-health, are seldom examined.

- Health sectors in many countries are informed by a biomedical approach to health and disease under the leadership of health professionals. Health care providers tend to see themselves as technical persons who solve problems presented to them, and may believe themselves to be free from any gender (or other social) biases. Gender mainstreaming, in their view, may represent a diversion of valuable time and resources away from the far more important task of 'saving lives.'

This makes gender mainstreaming especially difficult because it requires the adoption of a social determinants approach within which gender is one of the determinants. Framing gender as a social determinant of health crosscutting other social stratifiers such as class, race, and ethnicity would also take into consideration inequalities in health among women and men.

It is probably because of these additional challenges that the health sector has been a late starter in gender mainstreaming. The WHO adopted a gender policy only in 2002, seven years after the Beijing Platform of Action.

Challenges Faced Across Sectors

Confusion About Concepts

Lack of clarity about the meaning of the term 'gender mainstreaming' is mentioned by numerous documents commenting on the obstacles to gender mainstreaming. For example, a UN assessment of the system-wide medium-term plan for the advancement of women (1996–2001) mentions "lack of understanding of gender as a concept" among important constraints identified (UN, 2000, as quoted in Mitchell, 2004, p. 9).

In a study of the introduction and implementation of gender mainstreaming in the Republic of Ireland, Carney (2004) finds language to be an obstacle to communicating and understanding the idea of gender mainstreaming among policy makers. She argues that the term *gender mainstreaming* needs to be unpacked to make clear all that it implies:

- Gender equality does not exist at present.
- Gender concerns are in the margins of policy processes, and they therefore need to be brought to the center, i.e., be mainstreamed.
- Policies that are made without explicitly considering gender issues are not 'neutral,' but are likely to be biased against women.

The author concludes that unless these central concepts and ideas are clarified, the implementation of gender mainstreaming will stagnate.

Disappearance of Women-Specific Projects

There has also been the tendency to misinterpret as competing approaches the two complementary components of gender mainstreaming, viz. working on women-specific projects to bridge the gap between women and men, and mainstreaming gender across all areas of work. Consequently only one of the two approaches was chosen and adopted. This has sometimes led to drastically trimming, or even dismantling, Women's Bureaus and Gender Units (Chinery-Heisse, 2002). Some critiques believe that this may be a deliberate attempt to sabotage gender mainstreaming by doing away with a focus on women (Hannan, 2002).

Depoliticization of Gender Mainstreaming

Another reason for gender mainstreaming remaining at a superficial level is the reduction of gender equality work into a set of tools and activities, delinked from the women's movement and from a rights and social justice agenda (Sandler, 2002). Gender mainstreaming is not just about identifying gender gaps through gender analysis and 'including' women where they were previously excluded. It is also about asking why women were excluded in the first place, identifying the forces that perpetuated such exclusion, and challenging these forces. It is about taking on patriarchy, misogyny, and discrimination, and the structures that uphold them.

It is possible that such depoliticization has been the consequence of attempts to 'sell' the idea of gender mainstreaming to powerful and patriarchal organizations by advocates of gender mainstreaming, who then have to frame the project in such a way that gender mainstreaming fits with the dominant frames of the organizations concerned.

Adoption of an 'Integrationist' Agenda

The depoliticization of gender mainstreaming has meant that many gender mainstreaming efforts have been 'integrationist'—politically conservative, merely trying to add women to the existing agendas, without challenging the validity of the agendas themselves (Jahan, 1995, as quoted in Porter and Sweetman, 2005). This is also true of the health sector, where attempts at gender mainstreaming have been made without questioning some of the fundamental problems in the sector, such as health sector reforms promoting commodification of health care services. Some critiques believe that the problem lies in the very term 'gender mainstreaming,' which appears to seek co-option and integration rather than transformation.

> Gender mainstreaming asks feminists not to rock the boat, not to go too far, not to demand anything other than equality of treatment in a badly skewed system, rather than equality of outcomes. (Hawthorne, 2004, p. 88)

The UNECOSOC definition of gender mainstreaming obscures the issues at hand. By not spelling out what counts as gender mainstreaming and what does not, it allows for the appearance of something being done when very little of substance is being achieved (Hawthorne, 2004, p. 88). Bureaucracies in national and regional governments and within international organizations busy themselves with activities they can report on when it is time for the next round of assessments. A plethora of policies, strategies, guidelines, manuals, gender-analysis tools, and frameworks now exist and get counted as "progress made towards gender mainstreaming." When one examines the impact on the ground in terms of gender equality in outcomes, there is practically nothing to show.

The Pervasive Development of Neoliberal Macroeconomic Policies and Paradigm Shifts in Favor of Privatization

A gender mainstreaming agenda is inherently contradictory to a neoliberal frame that believes that there should be no state intervention in the marketplace to influence supply and demand and prices and costs. Gender mainstreaming is about precisely such interventions. In health, for example, the agenda would be to make health services affordable, to change the location and range of services, and so on, which if left to market dynamics would exclude those who do not have purchasing power. We cannot both support privatization on the one hand and gender mainstreaming on the other.

The question to ask is whether gender mainstreaming succeeds while leaving untouched the structures that create and maintain social inequalities and the processes that exacerbate these inequalities. According to Molyneux and Razavi (2005), the answer is a categorical no:

> A world in which the dominant policy models tend to deepen social and economic inequality and reinforce marginalization, in which redistribution has no place, and in which governments compromise the interests of their citizens to accommodate global forces, is unlikely to be a world that secures gender equality. (p. xxi)

Where do We Go from Here?

We believe that rather than doing more of the same, hoping that sustained efforts will bear fruit, it is time to acknowledge that we were probably "working hard on the wrong things" (Sandler, 2002). We need to transform both our agenda and our way of doing business.

- It is time to frame gender mainstreaming explicitly as an issue of equity, rights, and justice, health as a basic human right, and gender and social equity as a basic consideration in health.
- The focus would shift from 'integration' of gender issues into existing agendas to reframing the agenda in a way that promotes gender

and social equity in health. For example, rather than make sure that women's interests do not get excluded from the health sector reform agenda, the attempt would be to transform the agenda to make it equity oriented.

- The approach would emphasize setting agendas that consider gender inequity within the context of inequities by caste, race, class, ethnicity, and so on, as a crosscutting issue; and gender will be a part of the health equity agenda.
- Alliances may be forged with those advocating for attention to and researching the social determinants of health inequity; and with those challenging neoliberal macroeconomic policies and other forces that exacerbate inequalities and compromise well-being.
- Rather than being top-down initiatives, political mobilization to create demand for gender and social equity in health must be seen as necessary groundwork for mainstreaming gender in health.

ACKNOWLEDGMENTS

This chapter is an abridged version of a report submitted to the Gender and Women's Equity Knowledge Network of the WHO Commission on Social Determinants of Health in November 2006. Another version of this chapter was published in the journal *Global Public Health* 3 (S1): 121–142, in the year 2008.

NOTES

1. A wide range of terminologies are found in the literature on gender mainstreaming, such as 'integrating gender considerations,' or 'adopting a gender perspective.' Insofar as they refer to the same processes, described earlier, we have treated these as synonymous to gender mainstreaming.
2. Information on progress of the project is available only in Spanish, and could not be included in this chapter.
3. The initiative was located at the Achutha Menon Centre for Health Science Studies, Sree Chitra Tirunal Institute for Medical Science and Technology, Kerala, India, and funded by the Ford Foundation.
4. These do not work specifically on health.

REFERENCES

Australian Council for Overseas Aid. 2004. Gender mainstreaming: Moving from principles to implementation—the difficulties. An ACFOA discussion paper. *Development Bulletin* 64: 31–33.
Carney, G. 2004. From women's rights to gender mainstreaming: An examination of international gender norms in the Republic of Ireland. *Occasional Paper No*

8. Belfast: Queens University Belfast, Centre for Advancement of Women in Politics, School of Politics and International Studies.

Caron, J. 2003. *Report on Governmental Health Research Policies Promoting Gender or Sex Differences Sensitivity.* Alberta, Canada: Institute of Gender and Health.

Chinery-Heisse, M. 2002. Experiences in promoting gender equality. In *Strategies for the Promotion of Gender Equality—Is Mainstreaming a Dead End? Report from an Informal Consultation of Gender Focal Points in Multilateral Development Organisations*, edited by MFA. Oslo: Norwegian Ministry of Foreign Affairs: page numbers not available.

Commonwealth Secretariat. 2002. Establishment of the gender management systems in the health sector. In *Gender Mainstreaming in the Health Sector: Experiences in Commonwealth Countries.* London: Commonwealth Secretariat: 52–65.

Gómez-Gómez, E. 2002. *Gender Equity and Health Policy Reform in Latin America and the Caribbean.* Washington, DC: Pan-American Health Organization.

Government of Bangladesh. 2003. *Gender Equity Strategy.* Dhaka: Ministry of Health and Family Welfare.

Government of South Africa. 2002. *Gender Policy Guidelines for the Health Sector.* Pretoria: Department of Health.

Gunnar, A. 2003. *Sweden's New Public Health Policy: National Public Health Objectives for Sweden.* Stockholm: Swedish National Institute of Public Health.

Hannan, C. 2002. Promoting gender equality in multilateral development organizations. In *Strategies for the Promotion of Gender Equality—Is Mainstreaming a Dead End? Report from an Informal Consultation of Gender Focal Points in Multilateral Development Organisations*, edited by MFA. Oslo: Norwegian Ministry of Foreign Affairs: page numbers not available.

Hawthorne, S. 2004. The political use of obscurantism: Gender mainstreaming and intersectionality. *Development Bulletin* 64: 87–91.

Women's Commission, Govt. of Hong Kong. In *Gender Mainstreaming, The Hong Kong Experience: Implementing Gender Mainstreaming in the Government of the Hong Kong Special Administrative Region.* Hong Kong: Women's Commission Secretariat: 42–43, 47–48.

IGWG. 2004. *The SO WHAT Report: A Look at Whether Integrating a Gender Focus into Programs Makes a Difference to Outcome.* Washington, DC: Interagency Gender Working Group Task Force Report.

Kabeer, N. 1994. *Reversed Realities: Gender Hierarchies in Development Thought.* London: Verso.

Khanna, R., S. Pongurlekar, U. Ubale, and K. de Koning. 2002. *Gender-Sensitisation of Health Care Providers: Experiences of the Women-Centred Health Project, Mumbai, India.* Mumbai: Women-Centred Health Project.

LACWHN. 2002. *Gendered Health Research for Development: A Vital Contribution to Health Equity.* Santiago: Latin American and Caribbean Women's Health Network.

MFA. 2002. *Strategies for the Promotion of Gender Equality—Is Mainstreaming a Dead End? Report from an Informal Consultation of Gender Focal Points in Multilateral Development Organisations.* Oslo: Norwegian Ministry of Foreign Affairs.

Mitchell, S. 2004. What lies at the heart of the failure of gender mainstreaming: The strategy or the implementation? *Development Bulletin* 64: 8–10.

Molyneux, M., and S. Razavi. 2005. *Gender Equality: Striving for Justice in an Unequal World.* New York: UNRISD.

Moser, C., and A. Moser. 2005. Gender mainstreaming since Beijing: A review of success and limitations in international institutions. *Gender and Development* 13 (2): 12–13.

National AIDS Control Council. 2002. *Mainstreaming Gender into the Kenya National HIV/AIDS Strategic Plan: 2000–2005.* Nairobi, Kenya: Gender and HIV/AIDS Technical Sub-Committee of the National AIDS Control Council.

Östlin, P., and F. Diderichsen. 2003. *Equity-Oriented National Strategy for Public Health in Sweden: A Case Study.* Copenhagen: European Centre for Health Policy. http://www.who.dk/E69911.pdf.

PAHO. 2007. http://www.paho.org/English/AD/GE/Policy.htm (accessed September 16, 2007).

Porter, F., and C. Sweetman. 2005. Mainstreaming: A critical review. *Gender and Development* 13 (2): 2–10.

Ravindran, T.K.S. 2000. Engendering health. *Seminar* 489: 34–38.

———. 2005. Report of the small grants programme on gender and social issues in reproductive health research. *Unpublished Report.* Trivandrum, India: Achutha Menon Centre for Health Science Studies.

———. 2006. Integrating gender into the curricula of health professionals: Experiences and lessons learned. *Paper Presented at the WHO Meeting on Integrating Gender in the Curricula of Health Professionals.* Geneva: World Health Organization.

Riley, J. 2004. IWDA Gender and development dialogue, 3–4 July 2003 summary report. *Development Bulletin* 64: 107–111.

Salmon, A., N. Poole, M. Morrow, L. Greaves, R. Ingram, and A. Pederson. 2006. *Improving Conditions: Integrating Sex and Gender into Federal Mental Health and Addictions Policy.* Vancouver: British Columbia Centre of Excellence for Women's Health.

Sandler, J. 2002. Promoting gender equality in different international organisations (UNIFEM). In *Strategies for the Promotion of Gender Equality—Is Mainstreaming a Dead End? Report from an Informal Consultation of Gender Focal Points in Multilateral Development Organisations, 6–9 November 2002,* edited by MFA. Oslo: Norwegian Ministry of Foreign Affairs: page numbers not available.

Theobald, S., H. Elsey, and R. Tolhurst. 2004. Gender, health and development I: Gender equity in sector-wide approaches. *Progress in Development Studies* 4 (1): 58–63.

UN. 2000. Further actions and initiatives to implement the Beijing declaration and the Platform for action. *Unedited Final Outcome Document as Adopted by the Plenary of the Twenty-Third Special Session of the General Assembly on 10 June 2000.* New York: United Nations. http://wcd.nic.in/bej5plus.htm.

UNECOSOC. 1997. Gender mainstreaming. *Extract from the Report of the Economic and Social Council for 1997 (A/52/3, 18ᵗʰ September 1997).*Vienna: Division for Advancement of Women. UN Department of Economic and Social Affairs. http://www.un.org/documents/ga/docs/52/plenary/a52–3.htm

UNRISD. 2005. Gender equality, striving for justice in an unequal world. Geneva: UN. http://www.unrisd.org/unrisd/website/document.nsf/(httpAuxPages)/E0C CDA6F0D9651CFC1256FB1004AA6E8?OpenDocument&panel=additional.

Watkins, F. 2004. *Evaluation of DFID Development Assistance: Gender Equality and Women's Empowerment. DFID's Experience of Gender Mainstreaming: 1995–2004.* Glasgow: DFID Evaluation Department.

WHO. 2002. *Integrating Gender Perspectives in the Work of WHO: WHO Gender Policy.* Geneva: World Health Organization.

Women's Health Council (WHC) and WHO/EURO. n.d. *Integrating the Gender Perspective in Irish Health Policy: A Case Study.* Dublin: Women's Health Council and Copenhagen, World Health Organization, Regional Office for Europe.

Contributors

Karina Batthyany is Professor of the Social Science Faculty, University of the Republic in Uruguay. She has been the coordinator of the social science research team at the International Secretariat of Social Watch. She has also been consultant to UNIFEM, UNDP, and is nowadays program officer at UNFPA in Uruguay. She is the author of several books and numerous articles.

Sonia Corrêa has a degree in Architecture and a post-grade in Anthropology. Since the late 1970s she has been involved in research and advocacy in the domains of gender equality, health, and sexuality. She is the founder two Brazilian nongovernmental initiatives in this field: SOS Corpo, Gênero e Cidadania based in Recife, and the Commission on Citizenship and Reproduction. From 1992 to 2008 she was the research coordinator for sexual and reproductive health and rights of DAWN— Development Alternatives with Women for a New Era. Since 2002, she is the cochair of the Sexuality Policy Watch. She has published extensively in both Portuguese and English. This list includes, among others, *Population and Reproductive Rights: Feminist Perspectives from the South* (Zed Books, 1994); Sexuality, Health and Human Rights (Routledge, 2008). She has also lectured in various academic institutions as it is in the case of NEPO, the Center for Populations Studies at UNICAMP (Brazil), and the Reproductive Health and Gender Summer Programs of the Colégio de Mexico.

Asha George is currently a health specialist responsible for community-based approaches in the Policy and Evidence Unit of the Health Section in the Program Division at UNICEF, New York. Before this she was a consultant on maternal health and service delivery issues with various organizations in India, including the Indian Institute of Management Bangalore and the Coalition for Maternal-Neonatal Health and Safe Abortion. She started her work in public health in Mexico with UNIFEM and UNFPA providing support for the Cairo and Beijing World Conferences. She is a coeditor with Kabir Sheikh of a forthcoming book *Health Providers in India: Contemporary Perspectives and Practices* (Routledge), and with Gita Sen and Piroska Östlin of the book *Engendering International Health: The Challenge of Equity* (MIT Press, 2002), and is an editorial advisor for the journal *Reproductive Health Matters*. She has a master's in Public Health from Harvard University and a Doctorate of Philosophy in Development Studies from Sussex University.

Veloshnee Govender is currently a lecturer in the Health Economics Unit (University of Cape Town, South Africa). Before this, she was a research consultant at the Indian Institute of Management (Bangalore) and her work primarily focused on maternal health, health systems research, and equity issues in India. She has also worked as a public health specialist for the Global Forum for Health Research (Geneva) and the Initiative for Cardiovascular Health Research in the Developing Countries (New Delhi). Her research interests include health system reform and financing and gender and equity issues in health and development. She holds an MPH in International Health from Boston University and an M.Com in Health Economics from the University of Cape Town.

Aditi Iyer is currently Research Consultant at the Centre for Public Policy, Indian Institute of Management Bangalore, and Fellow, School of Population, Community and Behavioural Sciences, University of Liverpool. Her research interests focus on social inequalities and their intersections in health; social determinants of health; maternal and reproductive health; health systems and policy; and ethical issues in research and field action; and a number of peer-reviewed publications have emerged from her work. She received her PhD in Public Health from the University of Liverpool, and her MA in Social Work from the Tata Institute of Social Sciences, Mumbai. She was awarded the Goran Sterky Fellowship at the Division of International Health (IHCAR), Karolinska Institutet, Stockholm.

Helen Keleher is Professor of Health Science at Monash University, Melbourne, where she leads a research program on health promotion, evidence, and healthy public policy. Her research is focused on change from traditional health practices to integrated, community-based, equity-focused health promotion and comprehensive primary health care, with a focus on the determinants of health, particularly using gendered approaches. She was a member of the Women and Gender Equity Knowledge Network for the WHO Commission on the Social Determinants of Health and convenor of the Australian Women's Health Network from 1998 to 2005. She is a long-standing board member of the Public Health Association of Australia.

A. Kelkar-Khambete has an MPhil in Women's Studies and a PhD in Health Sciences and is working as a Research Associate at the Achuta Menon Centre for Health Science Studies (AMCHSS) of the Sree Chitra Tirunal Institute for Medical Sciences and Technology (SCTIMST), Trivandrum, Kerala State, India. Her research interests mainly focus on poverty, gender, and reproductive health concerns of women and on health systems research that addresses the translation of the gender concerns of the women in their day-to-day lives into culturally sensitive and gender equitable health policies and programs.

Melissa Laurie is a graduate student at Columbia University's Mailman School of Public Health in the Sexuality and Health Track. Her research interests are in sexual commerce and the built environment, sexual humor, and sexual rights. She has worked for the last four years with the NY/NJ AIDS Education and Training Center, first as a training coordinator for the Montefiore Adolescent AIDS Program and now as the Minority AIDS Initiative Coordinator for the Central Office at Columbia.

Ranjani K. Murthy is an independent researcher working on issues of gender, poverty, and health. She is on the Program Advisory Committee of Asia Pacific Resource and Research Center (ARROW), Malaysia. She is on the editorial board of the journal *Gender and Development*. In the past she was part of the Rights and Reforms Initiative, Women's Health Project, South Africa, and coauthored a global paper on community accountability and participation in the context of reforms. She was also part of the team that worked on a training manual to develop capacities of civil society actors to understand the impact of neoliberal health sector reforms on sexual and reproductive health and advocate changes where necessary. She presently builds capacities of civil society actors on this issue.

Piroska Östlin is a public health scientist with a PhD in Medical Science from the University of Uppsala in Sweden. She is Associate Professor in Public Health at the Karolinska Institute and member of the Board of the European Institute of Women's Health. During the last 10 years she has been working extensively for the World Health Organization (WHO) as an adviser on gender mainstreaming and health equity issues. Together with Gita Sen, Östlin was coordinator of the Women and Gender Equity Knowledge Network of the WHO Independent Commission on Social Determinants of Health (CSDH). Her former positions include Secretary of the Swedish Public Health Commission, Expert in International and Global Health at the Swedish National Institute of Public Health, and Member of Board of the Nordic School of Public Health. Her publications include *Gender Inequalities in Health: A Swedish Perspective* (Harvard University Press, 2001; with Danielsson, Diderichsen, et al.)

and *Engendering International Health: The Challenge of Equity* (MIT Press, 2002; with Sen and George).

Loveday Penn-Kekana is a medical anthropologist who is based at the Centre for Health Policy in the School of Public Health at the University of the Witwatersrand. Her research interests include maternal health, health systems, and gender-based violence. She is currently completing her PhD looking at factors that shape provider practice in maternity wards in South Africa.

Rosalind Petchesky is Distinguished Professor of Political Science at Hunter College and the Graduate Center, City University of New York. She is the author of numerous published books and articles in the field of sexual and reproductive health and rights and gender politics, including *Global Prescriptions: Gendering Health and Human Rights* (Zed, 2003) and *Sexuality, Health and Human Rights* (with Sonia Corrêa and Richard Parker; Routledge, 2008). In the 1990s she developed and directed the International Reproductive Rights Research Action Group, whose seven-country field research was reported in the volume *Negotiating Reproductive Rights: Women's Perspectives across Countries and Cultures*. More recently she has worked with a number of transnational organizations, including the Women's Environment and Development Organization, the journal *Reproductive Health Matters*, Sexuality Policy Watch, and the Coalition for Sexual and Bodily Rights in Muslim Societies. Petchesky is the recipient of a prestigious MacArthur Fellowship.

T.K.S. Ravindran, Honorary Professor at the Achutha Menon Centre for Health Science Studies, has a PhD in Applied Economics from the Centre for Development Studies, Trivandrum, India. Sundari was a coeditor of *Reproductive Health Matters* from 1993 to 1998. She is a founding member and secretary of a grassroots women's organization—Rural Women's Social Education Centre (RUWSEC), India, founded in 1981; a member of the Steering team, which launched in 2006 the Coalition for Maternal-Neonatal Health and Safe Abortion (India). She has worked as a consultant with the World Health Organization, Geneva, since 1984, and was a Gender Specialist in its Department of Gender and Women's Health from 2001 to 2003. She is editor of *The Right Reforms? Health Sector Reform and Sexual and Reproductive Health*; and of WHO's training manual *Transforming Health Systems: Gender and Rights in Reproductive Health*; and has authored a number of WHO publications including *Women in South-East Asia: A Health Profile*, and WHO's gender and poverty training resource for medical educators on domestic violence, ageing, and gender-sensitive and pro-poor health policies.

Gita Sen is Professor of Public Policy at the Indian Institute of Management in Bangalore, India, and Adjunct Professor of Global Health and Population at the Harvard School of Public Health. Together with Piroska Östlin, she was coordinator of the Women and Gender Equity Knowledge Network of the WHO Independent Commission on Social Determinants of Health (CSDH). Her books include *Engendering International Health: The Challenge of Equity* (with Asha George and Piroska Östlin; MIT Press, 2002), *Women's Empowerment and Demographic Processes—Moving Beyond Cairo* (with Harriet Presser; Oxford University Press/IUSSP, 2000); and *Population Policies Reconsidered: Health, Empowerment and Rights* (with Adrienne Germain and Lincoln Chen; Harvard Center for Population and Development Studies, 1994). She is a member of the Governing Council of the United Nations University, and cochair of PAHO's Technical Advisory Group on Gender. She has been vice-chair of the International Women's Health Coalition (US), a member of WHO's Global Advisory Committee on Health Research. She received the Volvo Environment Prize in 1994, an honorary doctorate from the University of East Anglia in the UK in 1998, and an honorary doctorate in medicine from the Karolinska Institute in Sweden in 2003.

Rachel Snow has been on the faculty at the University of Michigan (US) since 2003, where she is Associate Director of the International Institute, Associate Professor in Health Behavior and Health Education, and Associate Professor at the Population Studies Center. An international specialist in reproductive health, Rachel Snow has conducted clinical, epidemiologic, and social research on the successful implementation of reproductive health technologies and services in resource-poor countries, with sustained work in Burkina Faso, Ghana, Nigeria, South Africa, Nepal, India, Bangladesh, and China. Snow has worked extensively at the intersection of sex, gender, and vulnerability, and is currently focused on sex differences in the use of HIV care in Africa and strengthening human resources for health in Ghana. Snow has served on numerous expert committees at the World Health Organization and the Women and Gender Equity Network for the WHO Commission on Social Determinants of Health. She is coauthor of the WHO curriculum *Transforming Health System*, and a founding editor of the *African Journal of Reproductive Health*, now published from Nigeria. Snow received her doctorate in Population Sciences from Harvard in 1988.

Index